PRAISE FOR HEATHER

WHAT FRESH HELL IS THIS?

"We rely on Heather Corinna for clear, funny, inclusive, and zero-nonsense writing about sex and sexuality, and it's no surprise they've delivered again—brilliantly. *What Fresh Hell Is This?* contextualizes and investigates what we think we know about menopause before blowing our minds with a compendium of facts and observations that people facing menopause urgently need. A truly comprehensive, anti-shame, pro-embodiment resource for our time."

—*S. Bear Bergman, author, publisher of Flamingo Rampant, advice columnist, and general-duty trans pride activist*

S.E.X.

"Not only would my own adolescence have been vastly less painful and confusing if I'd had access to the accurate, comprehensive, and above all nonjudgmental information that Heather Corinna so carefully provides, but *S.E.X.* is, literally, a lifesaving book: Corinna's vast commonsense wisdom—especially on topics relating to gender roles, queer sexuality, and gender identities—has the potential to improve the physical and emotional health of anyone who reads it, and to help heal our culture's unhealthy, conflicted approaches to sex, sexuality, and gender."

—*Lisa Jervis, cofounder,* Bitch: Feminist Response to Pop Culture

"The best book about sex and sexuality: It covers everything from puberty to sex to social and emotional health. It also addresses more complicated issues such as relationship dynamics as well as topics around sexual abuse. *S.E.X.* is also an excellent text for LGBTQ+ teens, as it covers sexual and gender identity and outlines different ways of being physically intimate, from kissing to anal and vaginal intercourse."

—New York *magazine*

"*S.E.X.* is a positive and informative all-embracing guide to sexuality by a dedicated author. Heather Corinna challenges adolescents and young adults alike to be proactive in owning their sexuality by being true to themselves, all the while laying the foundation of knowledge and acceptance key factors for the development of a healthy sexuality."

—*Dr. Lynn Ponton, author of* The Sex Lives of Teenagers

"Much like the authors of *Our Bodies, Ourselves* and its spinoffs, Corinna answers every possible question teens and young adults could have. . . . [They] also address topics that are often overlooked, e.g., transgender and inter[sex] identities, realistic teen relationship management skills, and pornography."

—*Deborah Bigelow*, Library Journal

WAIT, WHAT?

"*Wait, What?* is straightforward and clear, exactly what's needed to help kids develop authentic awareness and conversation about bodies, relationships, feelings and sexuality."

—*Peggy Orenstein, author of* Girls & Sex: Navigating the Complicated New Landscape

"Inclusive, respectful, accurate, and informative. . . . Expert sex educators Corinna and Rotman are funny but never flippant when answering typical tween questions. . . . [T]he authors are never confrontational, making room for all points of view."

—*Paula Willey, Baltimore County Public Library, Maryland*,
School Library Journal, *starred review*

"This book consistently puts the needs of its readers first, meticulously working to emphasize gender diversity, individuality, and the messiness of adolescence. . . . Body parts are intentionally ungendered, sexual orientations are shown as fluid and joyful, and there is a constant emphasis on the importance of friendships and mutual support. While brief, this guide manages to cover crucial topics thoroughly and humorously, reassuring readers that while all of this is a big deal, it's something they can handle."

—Kirkus Reviews, *starred review*

"It brings a loving, essential lens to matters of heart and soul, offering a road map not only to physical changes, but the complex social and emotional terrain of consent, crushes, and identity."

—*Rabbi Danya Ruttenberg, author of* Nurture the Wow

WHAT
FRESH
HELL
IS THIS?

Also by Heather Corinna:

S.E.X.: The All-You-Need-to-Know Sexuality Guide to Get You Through Your Teens and Twenties

Wait, What? A Comic Book Guide to Relationships, Bodies, and Growing Up—with Isabella Rotman and Luke Howard

WHAT FRESH HELL IS THIS?

PERIMENOPAUSE, MENOPAUSE, OTHER INDIGNITIES, AND YOU

written by a deeply perimenopausal **HEATHER CORINNA**

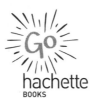

Go

hachette
BOOKS

New York

Copyright © 2021 by Heather Corinna

Interior and author illustrations by Archie Bongiovanni
Cover design by Amanda Kain
Cover illustration © CSA Images/Getty Images
Cover copyright © 2021 by Hachette Book Group, Inc.

Hachette Go, an imprint of Hachette Books
Hachette Book Group
1290 Avenue of the Americas
New York, NY 10104
HachetteGo.com
Facebook.com/HachetteGo
Instagram.com/HachetteGo

First Edition: June 2021

Hachette Books is a division of Hachette Book Group, Inc.

The Hachette Go and Hachette Books name and logos are trademarks of Hachette Book Group, Inc.

The publisher is not responsible for websites (or their content) that are not owned by the publisher.

Print book interior design by Amy Quinn.

Library of Congress Cataloging-in-Publication Data
Names: Corinna, Heather, author.
Title: What fresh hell is this?: perimenopause, menopause, other
indignities, and you / Heather Corinna.
Description: First edition. | New York: Hachette Go, 2021. | Includes
bibliographical references and index.
Identifiers: LCCN 2020058525 | ISBN 9780306874765 (paperback) | ISBN
9780306874758 (ebook)
Subjects: LCSH: Menopause—Popular works. | Perimenopause—Popular works.
Classification: LCC RG186 .C67 2021 | DDC 618.1/75—dc23
LC record available at https://lccn.loc.gov/2020058525

ISBNs: 978-0-306-87476-5 (trade paperback), 978-0-306-87475-8 (ebook)

Printed in the United States of America

CW

10 9 8 7 6 5 4 3 2

This one's for you, Mom.

CONTENTS

CONTENTS

PART 1

AND IN THE BEGINNING WAS THE WORD, AND THE WORD WAS "DAMMIT"

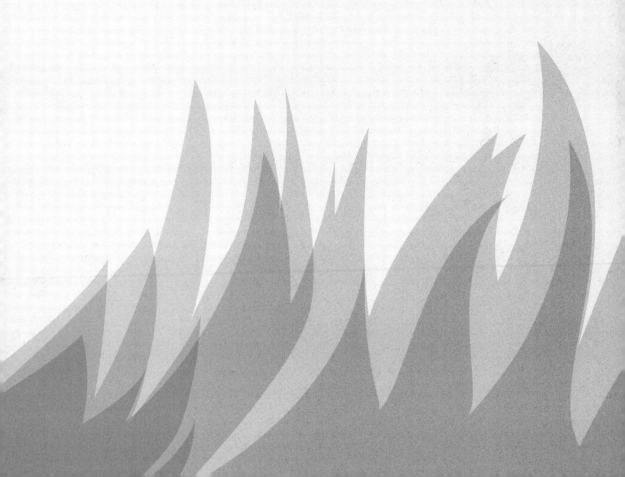

CHAPTER ONE

ARE YOU KIDDING ME? A PERIMENOPAUSE STORY

"This wasn't just plain terrible, this was fancy terrible.
This was terrible with raisins in it."
—*Dorothy Parker*

Did you see the title and flame-filled cover of this book, and did your weary, sweaty, confused, and exasperated soul scream, *That one! That is the book for me!!*?

If so, I'd first like to extend my deepest sympathies, an ice pack, and some of these very helpful edibles. If it's three in the morning as you're reading this, as it may well be, you likely want those more than a book. But since I can't really give you the other stuff, I can at least offer you this book until the sun comes up and you can go get your own coping necessities, whatever they may be.

In the event that is not your situation and you have this book in your hands (1) before your perimenopause has started, (2) after it's started but before it's bothered you, or, you lucky freaking duckie,

(3) only because someone you know is going through menopause, as it is a thing you will never yourself experience, you should pony up and buy the ice and the edibles for the rest of us.

I HAVEN'T EXACTLY BEEN HAVING A great time with perimenopause.

In fact, much of the time it's been not great in the way that, say, the 2016 US presidential election was not great. It's been a losing-my-ability-to-walk-or-to-even-lie-down-without-agonizing-pain kind of not great. It's been not great in a relationship-I'd-invested-all-of-myself-in-blowing-up-in-my-face—one I'd tried at three times over thirty years no less, with my heart, spirit, and life broken exponentially more each time—kind of way. It's been the kind of not great where

I lost my ability to stay living in my home and on land I loved, which it had taken me decades to find and be able to move to. It's been not great in a pandemic, climate-change-catastrophe-every-five-minutes, eldercare-nightmare sort of way. Those are some of the delightful things that have happened during my perimenopause so far.

Of course they have: If they hadn't, would it really be *my* menopause, or yours, for that matter? Doubtful.

Oh! And I've been in it for freaking ever, and it still isn't over for me yet. Of course it isn't.

AT THE END OF 2013, I WAS FINALLY able to get health insurance for the first time since my late teens. I remember that very clearly because I also remember the hospital bill I got for over *$10,000* from a terrible, fruitless clinic-to-emergency-room one-night stand that year, just a few freaking weeks before I had access to that insurance, which would have covered most of that bill.

I also remember when that was because, looking back with the irritating clarity of hindsight, a grueling amount of research, and no small measure of bitterness, it's something that should have made clear to everyone involved—but did not, including to me—that I was probably in perimenopause.

I was living on a rural Washington island with no hospital. It did have a small,

surprisingly affordable community clinic. The doctor I saw there was a very nice man but a very not-excellent doctor, not for me, anyway.

Like anyone who's lived decades without healthcare coverage, I was skilled at avoiding care unless it was absolutely necessary or I could work out some way to swing it and still pay all my other bills. I first started seeing him because of one of the ten million terrible, horrible, no-good, very bad urinary tract infections of my life. I was impressed at first because he was so open to my ideas and suggestions. I also was able to get an Ativan prescription from him, so I may have been momentarily blinded by the heady lust of deep, pharmaceutical gratitude. Looking back, it seems clear that unless I could mostly be my *own* doctor and tell him what was wrong with me and what to do about it, he was not going to have any idea and would make a couple big bad calls once I wasn't the one with the ideas.

One afternoon in that first week of November, at the increasingly tender age of forty-three, I suddenly felt dizzy. I lost a little time, I think. I was having a hard time breathing: my solar plexus and the area around it felt tight. I tried to slow down, take deep breaths: it didn't work. My neck and face felt weird, like I had a really bad sunburn. My head was rolling. I started to freak out. I tried to level myself out and calm the hell down.

I went through reasons I could be feeling that way:

- The mysterious chronic pain I'd been living with for a few years
- A migraine
- The fact that I ran an always-barely-afloat grassroots nonprofit and so had valid reasons to panic every minute of every day
- My on-again, off-again seizure disorder
- Smoking too many cigarettes (something I thought of while smoking after this happened to try and calm myself down)
- Too much coffee (see above)

Or

- Was this the Big One? The nervous breakdown that would finally break me, which I had always figured was a when in my life rather than an if?
- Did I forget to eat?
- Was I just looking for an excuse for a day off?

I didn't have any way to get myself to the doctor and didn't want to call an ambulance because they're expensive as hell. I tried to wait it out so as not to bother my then-partner-now-ex. I got too scared, so about an hour later, I gave up and called. We went to the clinic and waited a million years, as you do. When I got to see the doctor, I told him what I had experienced and explained that I was still feeling out of sorts and panicky. He and his staff took my pulse and my blood pressure, which were low as always. They did an EKG: it was also normal.

You've got to wonder why, then, he chose to send me to a hospital across the water in Seattle, by ambulance, to have possible heart issues evaluated. You've got to wonder why that hospital ran somewhere in the vicinity of six grand worth of tests on my poor, uninsured heart. They were making sure I wasn't having a heart attack, obviously, but god knows why, because that bill sure gave me one.

I saw about ten different healthcare providers that night. I heard a lot about how this was so *confusing*, how they couldn't figure out what was going on, what a *mystery* it all was. Despite my age, my assigned sex, and what I was presenting with, **no one mentioned perimenopause**. No one considered the possibility that I might have been experiencing a hot flash paired with a panic attack, a notoriously common experience in perimenopause.

I didn't know that then. It appears no one else did either.

It clearly did not occur to my doctor or any of the clinical staff that the episode might have something to do with menopause.

It did not occur to the EMTs in the ambulance, who were making a great game of trying to play detective about my symptoms but didn't ask *any* questions about anything pertaining to menopause.

(While we're here, if you haven't had to piss into a bedpan in front of three people while squatting in an ambulance on a moving ferry, you truly haven't lived.)

It did not occur to anyone at the hospital, who *also* did not ask any questions that might lead them down that road: I know now, having since had thousands of them, that I'd obviously had a hot flash, but no one asked me about that. Had someone asked and described one to me, the night—and probably years after—would have taken a very different turn.

How didn't I know about this? I was in my forties when this happened. I still have ovaries and a uterus. I'm nonbinary, but there's an *F* on my medical charts and my ID, a thing that generally leads people to certain anatomical assumptions. I've spent about half my life working in and around sexual, reproductive, and feminist health. I basically grew up in a hospital and have always been a compulsive reader, so doctor's office pamphlets, medical journal blurbs, parts of nursing books (and the ingredients of many cereals and shampoos) have taken up residence in my head since I was wee. I talk to a lot of people who have or have had a uterus in a lot of different life stages on the regular. Not only have I worshipped at the altar of *Our Bodies, Ourselves* for as long as I can remember, but I was on the editorial team for the last edition, for crying out loud.

I'd both seen and read *Fried Green Tomatoes* so many times.

So many.

TOWANDA!

I KNEW MENOPAUSE EXISTED, BUT NOT much else. Before the last decade, my expectations of menopause for myself were that it would end my periods and, I'd hoped, the pain they cause and probably make me less interested in sex.

I didn't have any idea how long the transition could last. I didn't even think of it as a transition at all so much as something that happened all at once when periods stopped. I didn't know all it could involve, how I could feel in it, the array of options I had for managing it, or what I could ask of others and insist on for myself. I didn't know how past and current health and life issues of mine would impact it and vice versa. I didn't even know the basics of what happened: I just thought it was about having less estrogen (it's so not).

I didn't know anything about *peri*-menopause, including that I was in it, until I had already been in it for years, despite having an array of hallmark impacts: painful cystic acne, hot flashes, night sweats, anxiety, depression including a resurgence of my suicidality, menstrual changes, digestive issues, body-composition shifts, an increase in headaches and other kinds of pain, exhaustion, and some serious cognitive challenges. There could have been other reasons for some of those things, sure, and some of them may have even had more than one cause, but once you know *anything* about perimenopause and you look at that list, it seems ridiculous not to see clearly that's what was going on.

Approximately two million people go into perimenopause each year in the United States alone. Only a fraction of that number (around 15 percent) are diagnosed with breast cancer in the United States every year. Fewer people have heart attacks and strokes here annually than go into perimenopause. How do all of us—you, me, our mothers, healthcare providers, the ladies on *The View*—usually know so much *less* about something so much *more* common, something that will **absolutely** happen to everyone born with a uterus and ovaries in some way at some point, most often as an unavoidable part of the life cycle, than we do about things less common that are only, and frequently even avoidable, maybes?

How did we get to this place of cluelessness about our own bodies and lives? It's not that complicated.

Any of us reading (or writing) this book, no matter where we live or where our families are from, are experiencing menopause under patriarchy because that's the whole damn world.

If we're experiencing this in the colonized West or anywhere else steeped in male dominance and capitalism, we're experiencing it in an overarching culture that barely values any of us, and even then only conditionally, *before* menopause. Once that's on the horizon, and with it the farewell tour of our known or assumed reproductive capacity and its companions, the story history so far tells is one of, at *best*, neglect, glib mockery and dismissiveness, and, just as frequently, mistreatment, commercial exploitation, denial and gaslighting, further marginalization and oppression, abuse, torture, and death.

While everyone who experiences it doesn't identify as a woman, from the standpoint of the men who snatched women's healthcare out of the hands of midwives and indigenous providers, menopause has always been a women's health issue: one that does not directly impact them or their bodies and so has been treated the way most things that don't impact them directly have. Regardless of my appreciation for its existence, the history of Western medicine on the whole is gruesome. Untold numbers of people have been harmed, and not just women: men have absolutely been harmed too, particularly men who were Black, indigenous, and otherwise of color (BIPOC), poor, immigrant, prisoners, and disabled. It's been extra gruesome, of course, to those who aren't, or who haven't been considered, men at all.

One of the biggest things that got us here is, put plainly, a profound lack of empathy and care on the part of folks with all the power for something that only happens to those of us without power. As author of *Care Work: Dreaming Disability Justice* and *Dirty River: A Queer Femme of Color Dreaming Her Way Home* and coeditor of *Beyond Survival: Stories and Strategies from the Transformative Justice Movement* Leah Lakshmi Piepzna-Samarasinha, also themself in perimenopause, put it so well when we talked, "I think that for a lot of people, menopause is kind of a collision course with parts of the patriarchy and sexism and oppression."

THAT'S NOT ALL, OF COURSE. THE related legacy of silencing shame that runs through all things reproductive and assigned women's or female—or not-male, no matter how you slice it—sex or roles, the intentional mystification of our bodies, and how much how many of us, especially in generations before ours, have been denied not just information about our own bodies but the ability and the freedom to share that information with each other: these have all been and are still players too.

Medical and cultural gatekeeping have been at play here as well. For most of history, and until very recently, when doctors and scientists have bothered to research menopause, they often haven't shared their findings freely with menopausal people or allowed us to be stewards of that information. Gatekeeping is why we didn't know almost anything about what really goes on with perimenopause until the last few *decades*, information we have women—in medicine and other science, in the feminist health movement and other communities—to thank for.

We're now going on two generations of broad, diverse studies and more accessible information. We have representative organizations like the North American Menopause Society. A standalone *Our Bodies, Ourselves* volume devoted to menopause was released in 2006. Many people who have been writing or distributing menopause information and doing studies over the last thirty or so years have also themselves experienced menopause, like Canadian feminist health trailblazer Centre for Menstrual Cycle and Ovulation Research founder Jerilynn Prior, women's health researcher Dr. JoAnn Manson, women's health writer and advocate Barbara Seaman, *Menopause: A Positive Approach* (1977) author Rosetta Reitz, and *The Silent Passage* (1998) author Gail Sheehy. Over the last decade, more theoretical or historical books on menopause, like Louise Foxcroft's *Hot Flushes, Cold Science* (2009) and Susan Mattern's *The Slow Moon Climbs* (2019), and menopause memoirs, like Sandra Tsing Loh's *The Madwoman in the Volvo* (2014), Darcey

Steinke's *Flash Count Diary* (2019), and the comic anthology *Menopause: A Comic Treatment* (2020), have shown up on the scene. Websites, podcasts, and apps are emerging, as are menopause clinics, telehealth services, and menopause-specific product lines.

Even in media, where menopause has been, on the whole, so woefully absent and, when it's barely appeared, so horribly represented, we're starting to see big changes in both visibility and representation, especially over the last couple years. I wouldn't be surprised if soon enough we see the rollouts of *Bridget Jones's Menopause*, *My Big Fat Greek Menopause*, *Sex and the City Is Too Damn Loud for Menopausal People to Get Any Sleep Why Even Bother Trying*, and whatever menopause series Reese Witherspoon and Shonda Rimes inevitably produce.

Even with all this information having been on the horizon for a while now, so many of us **still** don't know jack. Some of that is because, of course, all information isn't good information. As is the case with everything, a lot of misinformation about menopause abounds, especially in popular media.

We have to know *to* look for this information in the first place. Someone would ideally direct us to it before we need it, or at least once perimenopause is probably starting for us. The information also has to be useful and accessible for *all* of us, not just those for whom it has almost exclusively been tailored so far: white, straight, married, able, economically privileged, cisgender women. When you already feel shitty, the last thing you want is information that's supposed to help you but only makes you feel worse. Things are chang*ing*, but they are still far from changed, and no doubt all this change won't be positive either.

So, here we are: historically without what many of us and those before us have needed for so long but after enough change that you now have this book, of all things, in your hot little hands. That, whatever its flaws—and I assure you it has them, for I am not only human but also deeply menopausal and have been sweating into this keyboard while writing, locked in a small room during a pandemic—is, I believe, a good thing for you.

If my own experience, and maybe yours, is any indication, perimenopause without realistic expectations or preparation can bear an embarrassing resemblance to the epically terrible movie *Castaway*.

There you are, just going about your life, and then there's a rumble, a couple weird bumps, and then—HOLY SHIT THE PLANE IS CRASHING. You wake up in unfamiliar terrain, your hair a mess, drenched in sweat, in a panic, and probably also mysteriously without your top, because isn't that always how it goes. You're freaked out, but you see a coconut or two and expect a quick rescue, so you think you've got this, sweet, naive you.

Soon, you discover you do *not* have this. You don't know what is going on, what you are doing, or what will help, and there are also no more coconuts. You may flood your porch or lobby with shamefully wasteful boxes full of mostly useless, not to mention money-costing, crap that might work for someone else but sure doesn't work for you. If you find one or two things that *do* work for you, you may hold on to them with a questionable attachment and a paranoid ferocity, ready to slice the fingers off anyone who comes near them. This very much includes the thermostat.

This can be *that* kind of adventure, and it pains me to say so, including because I *really* hate that movie.

It might not be: for some people, it really isn't. For some people, it's only a bad vacation, if that. For some, it's totally mellow . . . until it isn't. And if that's how it goes for you, you're sure going to kick yourself if you weren't gathering what you needed to make a raft while everything was so lovely and delightful.

FROM EVERYTHING I'VE READ AND OTH-erwise taken in, from everyone I've listened to and my otherwise now massively expanded sense of things, I have absolutely had a harder time with this than most. I would not say that my experience

of perimenopause has been a good approximation of average. Thus far, mine has been *A Very Castaway Perimenopause.* I have known love for more than one proverbial bloody volleyball. I didn't have to learn how to make fire, because I was, as I often still am, *on* fire. I existed in a solitary and desperate survival mode for a long time there, but I have survived. So far, anyway.

Those of us who have the *most* difficult of times, though, appear to be the minority. What we know from research so far is that more people will have an easier time or have it last a shorter period of time, and some of you will even have little to no trouble at all.

On top of some of the other things I already mentioned earlier, I was a life-long smoker with preexisting disabilities, including severe spinal degeneration and injury, chronic pain, chronic fatigue, and mystery reproductive issues, and I also have a brain and neurological system that've never been all that keen on the rules. I am sensitive to hormonal shifts and have a history of depression, suicidality, and sexual, physical, and emotional trauma. I spent my first five years or so of perimenopause very unsupported emotionally and gaslighted on the daily. I've had nonstop crises throughout, unexpectedly semi-acquired two adolescents in my personal life and very small apartment . . . you get the picture. I was also highly uninformed and completely unprepared.

CHOOSE YOUR OWN MISADVENTURE: MANAGING YOUR MENOPAUSE

Luckily for us both, I now know some of why I have been having such a hard time. I know that those things I mentioned are parts of what's made it tougher for me. I know some of what I could have done about it, which I didn't know before, too. I now know a lot more, period, which, all by itself, makes a surprising amount of difference. I also know a lot more about what we all still don't know, which, despite being awfully annoying, is sometimes oddly helpful too.

You can't change history, including your own life history. You can't change your genetics. You can't change how your life has gone up until now, and, if you're like a lot of us, you probably can't change a great deal of your current circumstances either. That means there's some of perimenopause and postmenopause you can't change. But you *can* change some of it, including just by accepting it and yourself in it, and you can manage a lot of it.

A great deal of research makes clear that when we come into this phase even just basically educated about it and realistically prepared and supported, we will have better experiences. If it hasn't even started for you, just reading this book is very likely to make it all go better when it does, and I don't say that just to flatter myself. Even if it's already started for you, even if it already stinks, you can probably improve the experience you're having just by *finding out* more about it.

THIS IS NOT ONE OF THOSE BOOKS WHERE I, the Great and Powerful Corinna, have solved the mystery of menopause— *tada!*—for myself and now can solve it for you so that we all have a wonderful time and experience and revere this phase of life as nothing but a glorious passage of sparkly wisdom and wonder.

I did not solve that mystery. The idea of my being the master of menopause is also HILARIOUS, because, let me tell you, I am menopause's *dog*. You're going to have to look elsewhere for mastery.

This isn't the everything-you-need guide. Everything you need isn't going to be in *any* book, let alone this one, and even if it were, we both know that you wouldn't have half the patience you'd need to read its eight thousand pages, let alone the energy to drag it up three flights of stairs from the lobby.

Understanding, acceptance, and management (or not!) of your choosing really are the names of the game here: they are what's actually doable and also won't make you feel even shittier about yourself than perimenopause can make you feel already. As disability activist, writer, and my genius friend s.e. smith pointed out when we talked about this, just like with disability and disabled people, so much historical—and current— messaging about menopause and those of us in perimenopause or postmenopause treats it and us as something capital-B broken in need of repair. There's this idea that to be "right" or "balanced," we need to try and keep or make ourselves, our hormones, and our bodies as premenopausal as possible, rather than accepting that we, our bodies, and our hormones are *always* right, even if we don't always feel comfortable or love (or are valued by our culture in) every phase of them. This book isn't about fixing you, your hormones, or any other part of your body. I think you're just right, even if you, probably like me right now, happen to be fucking miserable in this particular moment. I'm not here to fix you. I'm just here to try and help you get through this hot mess.

Whether it's about helping you avoid getting stranded in your menopause in the first place or, if that's already happened, getting you through it and helping you learn to groom your beard, I think I can help. The good news is that even if I can't do either, you probably spent less on this book than you spent on those ten bottles of herbs or creams that didn't do shit either, and this burns real pretty and doesn't reek if you throw it on a fire.

THERE'S A LOT OF NARROWLY PRESCRIPtive advice in Menopauslandia. If someone found what worked for them, they will often believe and say that will solve all the things for you. If someone had something that did *not* work for them or

that they just couldn't do, they will frequently make that the big, bad thing *no one* should do and maybe even scare you out of using it despite its working very well for you and your having every assurance it's safe for you. And if someone wants to *sell* you something, well, god help you.

Our lives, our bodies, and the whole of our experiences are simply far, *far* too diverse for everything or anything to work for all of us (or not work for all of us) or to feel the same way for all of us. If anywhere in all this I—or anyone else, for that matter—say something that simply doesn't square with your experience of your own body and how things have (or haven't) worked or felt for you, I want you to trust yourself, your body, and your own expert knowledge of both.

I worked with nutritional therapy consultant and community organizer kiran nigam of Fortify Community Health in Oakland, California, for help with the nutritional portions of the book. She adds, "Our bodies are complex, with lots of things going on inside them. And they are wise. Most people are socialized in such a way that their ability to listen to that wisdom has been compromised. So much of my work with my nutrition clients is in healing that connection and ability to listen. If something doesn't feel good or right for you, don't do it."

About halfway through my soul-sucking research for this book, I came across this passage of perfection at the end of Sandra Tsing Loh's *The Madwoman in the Volvo*:

> Have no shame. The middle-aged women I know, clawing their way one day at a time through this passage, have no rules—they glue themselves together with absolutely anything they can get their hands on. They do estrogen cream, progesterone biocompounds, vaginal salves, coffee in the morning, big sandwiches at lunch. They drink water all day, they work out twice a week, hard, with personal trainers. They take Xanax to get over the dread of seeing their personal trainers, they take Valium to settle themselves before the first Chardonnay of happy hour. They may do with just a half a line of coke before a very small martini, while knitting and doing some crosswords. If there are cigarettes and skin dryness, there are also collagen and Botox, and the exhilaration of flaming an ex on Facebook. And finally, as another woman friend of mine counseled with perfect sincerity and cheer: "Just gain the 25 pounds. I really think I would not have survived menopause—AND the death of my mother—without having gained these 25 pounds."

Setting aside that we're not all women and that some of the things on that list maybe aren't so smart to do for one's health, ability to remain out of jail, or both, this is some of the best advice I came across in writing on menopause spanning five centuries.

I want you to do whatever it is you need to do to get yourself through this in ways that you can access, that are effective for you, and that dovetail as much as possible with who *you* are, what you want, and what you feel comfortable with. There is no one thing everyone can get or use that fixes all the things for everyone. No such sorcery exists. If there were one thing, it would be puppies, *obviously*.

In other words, I want **you to do you**.

The same goes for however you *feel* about your menopause experience. I'm not going to tell you how to feel about or view perimenopause, menopause, and life after. That's yours to feel. If we're entitled to anything, having reached this stage of life or otherwise found ourselves here, it should be the right to own and contextualize our own experience of this.

There remains—as has always existed in the colonized West and under patriarchy at large—social, cultural, and even medical pressure to have a "good" menopause. A lot of covert and overt sentiment out there over the last hundred years or so suggests that good, low-maintenance women have a good, low-maintenance menopause, and bad, difficult women (and certainly those with the audacity to have a uterus and not be women at all) have a bad, difficult one. Similarly, I've often felt an invisible finger wag for having what is apparently an unacceptably unsunny view of my experience so far or for not seeing this as the purportedly magnificent journey and wonderful experience it would be for me if I would just stop being such a negative Nancy already.

There is no right or wrong way to experience menopause; there's only however we do.

If you're presently having or at some point have a hard time with menopause—whether that's about physical, mental, emotional, social, or practical impacts, or all of the above—it's not likely because you are a bad or difficult person, don't have the right attitude, or are otherwise doing or have done something else wrong. It's mostly going to be about your genetics and your life and health history and circumstances to date, all of which you can do little about now and mostly couldn't do much about before. You aren't likely only having a bad time of it because you have a bad attitude—a deeply dismissive, patronizing, and presumptuous idea brought to you by the exact same kind of bullshit that suggests all anyone depressed needs to do is exercise.

If you're having an easy time with it, chances are that isn't just because of your winning attitude, what you weigh, or your exercise regimen. Of course, an easy time now can always change in the future. But so can a difficult one.

No matter how it's going or how it goes, here's what I think this book can do for you:

♦ I can tell you about the current understanding of how perimenopause and menopause happen; what can happen to your body, mind, and life as a result; and why that stuff does or might happen.

♦ I can fill you in on some history that will make you feel stabby but is important to know and, I think, fascinating, especially if you can't sleep right now and need some dead people to direct your anger at. A lot of those dead people are why so many of us are so ignorant and have such horrible ideas about menopause and people in and beyond it. It's helpful to know how this particular sausage got made and which sausage makers to curse until the end of time.

♦ I can regale you with tales of my many menopausal fascinations and irritations, which you will either love or skim while you get to what you actually need, and that, my friend, is your call. I promise not to take it personally.

♦ I can give you a lot of optional things to consider for understanding, processing, and managing your experience. This is a buffet, not a fixed menu: you get to try what you want, leave what you don't, mix it all up, and use it however works for you.

Most of what's here is aimed at people born with ovaries, a uterus, or both, who are in or around midlife, and who will arrive at menopause by way of perimenopause. Plenty of it may be useful for those who came to this by way of sudden menopause instead (like as a result of a reproductive surgery or cancer treatment) or early menopause, and some of it may even be useful for trans women, who can find themselves in a similar spot by choosing or having to stop using estrogen therapies. But for those of you in the latter groups, you just won't likely feel as seen here as you will with other resources targeted specifically to you, which also will likely have more of what you need.

Reproductive aging is obviously something that happens to everyone, including people born with a testicular system, though it isn't analogous to menopause. You can read about that in the appendix (Menopause for the Rest of Us, page 285) from someone who's lived in that kind of body herself.

"All I needed for the mind was to be led to new stations. All I needed for the heart was to visit a place of greater storms."
—Patti Smith

POSTMENOPAUSAL PUNK

Our experience of a menopausal transition is just one of those things that most often lives somewhere on the spectrum between not being a big deal to being downright catastrophic. I'll say it once, I'll say it a thousand times (and I really will, just you wait), but this is of course all influenced by what we know about it (usually very little), what we know to do about it (see previous), and also how we feel about it, very much including what we think it is a transition *to*.

If we have the idea that menopause is the beginning of the end of our body, our chutzpah, our sexuality, our value, our beauty or desirability, our place in the world, the end of us, period, well, of course we're going to dread it.

I've got more to say about all this later, but since reading about some of my personal experiences probably won't help much with dread, I want to make sure you know that it really is going to be okay. Eh, let's try that again. To poorly paraphrase Pema Chödrön, even if it isn't all okay, and it may not always be, you're still going to get through this and to the other side. But that's cold comfort if you feel just as full of dread, terror, or despair about what's on the other side. And that often seems to be the real kicker.

And of course it is. The Atwoodian reality we live in that makes the value of anyone born with a uterus or vagina primarily or solely reproductive tells us that when it ends, or if we never had that ability or desire in the first place, we and our lives are effectively over.

Institutionalized and internalized ableism also teaches us that we are not supposed to accept, enjoy, or love our bodies and ourselves if we have lost *any* of our expected utility in some way—like by losing the ability to provide labor or to move or think in certain ways—and if we also no longer meet beauty standards imposed upon us.

We get clear messages that menopause means that we will not continue to want or be wanted for—let alone have!—a sensual or sexual life, alone or with partners, especially if we no longer meet sexual standards made for us primarily by cisgender men.

Menopause can be a great and dignity-defying feat, especially in the world we experience it in. We are not supposed to like, love, or accept ourselves more or better after menopause. We're not supposed to be happy or relieved that menopause may free, or make us freer, from some things. Our emotionally intimate

relationships aren't supposed to become *more* intimate. We're expected to continue to tamp down our biggest, scariest, and rawest feelings, as we've been expected to do our whole lives, even in this phase, when they can grow like wildfire. We are not supposed to feel, let alone express or share, our anger, grief, frustration, resentment, or even many kinds of joy unless they support the status quo.

We're not supposed to get better at taking care of ourselves and better at asking for help and centering our own needs thanks to menopause. We are **by no means** supposed to stop taking so much care of everyone else so we can focus on ourselves. We're also not supposed to decide that now would be an excellent time to radically change our lives or relationships so that they better suit us.

Messages we get about menopause more often tell us we must keep ourselves from much of what we want and need in this time. It's easy to get the idea that life in and after menopause is going to be little, dreary rituals of desperate maintenance and exacting control over food, exercise, the shape and size of our bodies, our skin, our intimate relationships, our sexuality, our leisure, our moods, robbing us of what pleasure we might have found in these things before.

We are not supposed to be, nor do we expect to be, curious or otherwise anticipatory about what menopause might change and bring for us.

We are not *supposed* to find freedom, liberation, or a whole new world of badassery through and on the other side of this. What many of us so often don't know is that even despite so many barriers and blockades, **a great many people do**.

As Black southern feminist mother, leader, and organizer Omisade Burney-Scott, also host of *The Black Girl's Guide to Surviving Menopause* and author of the zine *Messages from the Menopausal Universe* (and my birthday twin), said, "I'm not saying you won't be transformed, but you will come out whole."

We may have it in our heads that Sid Vicious, Exene Cervenka, Henry Rollins, Poly Styrene, Kathleen Hanna, and maybe our younger selves are the ultimate punk representations. And yet, postmenopausal people *everywhere* are being punker than anyone decades younger (including Exene and Kathleen) all the time, and we often don't even see it. If you thought coming through adolescence whole took great acts of nonconformity, wait until you meet menopause and life beyond. Postmenopausal people are *punk as fuck*.

My mother worked at a women-only eldercare facility in my early teens. I spent a lot of time there by my own choosing. I remember feeling like some of those elderly women saw and understood me, even through all my eyeliner, hairspray, and rage, more than almost anyone else

back then. In hindsight, and particularly now that I've seen and known many more postmenopausal people since, it seems so obvious. They'd been where I'd been, and they'd all come through it—at least twice, no less!—the fascinating, awesome, unique people whom I can never get enough of.

We're not less of ourselves on the other side of this. We're *more*. In part that's because this is another sometimes massive, and often longer than expected, life experience, phase, and process we had to get ourselves through to get there. It's also because we had a whole, much more complicated, much more experienced, much more done-with-everyone-else's-bullshit self to get ourselves through it with than we had to get ourselves through puberty. And if we get ourselves through this not by white-knuckling it, but by making ourselves, our own care, and our own well-being a real priority?

Well, as Aretha Franklin said of her own many crucibles, "I paid my dues, I certainly did." Aretha was already a badass of epic proportions at twenty-five when she literally taught women and girls everywhere how to *spell* self-respect. But the postmenopausal Aretha who was that fur-shrugging, swaggering queen? She showed us how to fully **inhabit** it. That's the kind of *more* I'm talking about.

Writer, storyteller, and author of *Fat, Pretty and Soon to Be Old: A Makeover for Self and Society* Kimberly Dark told me,

"Menopause gives us an opportunity to really see that the way society is organized was messed up to begin with. I would love to see more menopausal people trying to change the world because they've realized, I've got to opt out of this game. The game kicked me out anyway right now, but I've still got to opt out. We are ripe to be leaders in social change around this hierarchy business." **Exactly.** Menopause is being kicked out of the proverbial house, saying, "Good riddance!" and turning what would otherwise be a painful kick into a powerful catapult.

I NEVER PROMISED YOU A ROSE GARDEN: MENOPAUSE AND PUBERTY

While we're on teenage rites of passage, now's as good a time as any to mention that menopause and perimenopause are frequently referred to as "puberty in reverse." That's not entirely accurate, and also really fucking terrifying for those of us who had a horrible time of puberty and adolescence.

Puberty, too, is a long, often chaotic life phase that involves an array of changes primarily because of steroid hormones and reproductive systems. Our bodies in childhood start with very low levels of estrogen, progesterone, and testosterone. Levels of those hormones usually show up and increase with puberty and are erratic until the process starts winding down, those hormones settle into more consistent patterns and predictable levels,

and our bodies and brains settle with them. On the other side of it, our bodies and often we, as people, are changed. A menopausal transition—which I'll soon explain in gory detail—*is* a sort of flip of all that. But there are a bunch of differences, and that analogy misses a lot of diversity in biology, physiology, and life experience. Too, even though the levels of estrogen and progesterone are similar in postmenopause to those in prepuberty, we don't go back to how or who we were before puberty. Menopause isn't *Cocoon.* Sorry.

That said, and as much as my surly inner teen hates to admit it, the comparison does hold some water. Some similar things are happening not just physiologically but emotionally and socially. Perhaps even more importantly, it'd be great if we could at least know to expect that some of the exact same shit we found frustrating, upsetting, literally awful, or insufferable during puberty we may also find frustrating, upsetting, literally awful, or insufferable in menopause.

◗ It can be disorienting and disembodying and even sometimes—or entirely—feel like a violation.
◗ It's not often consensual, and it can be traumatic or retraumatizing.
◗ You wanted people to STFU, stop being gross, and leave you alone then, and you want people to STFU, stop being gross, and leave you alone now.

- Like puberty, it can be highly gendering.
- Body and other kinds of shame are often in the mix.
- It can be stressful, isolating, demoralizing, and disheartening.
- You're going to act like a total freak sometimes, even by your standards.
- There will be tears. And anger. And tragically unfortunate haircuts.

But even more importantly, it'd be *extra* great if someone told us that many of the things that helped us get through puberty—things we already know how to do because we did get through it or have learned since—will also help us get through and manage all the parts of menopause.

I'm talking about things like these:
- Access to comprehensive, accurate information about what is happening to us
- Agency and control over our own lives so we can manage this in the ways *we* can and want to, centering **our own needs and abilities**
- Environments that are normalizing, shame-free, and accepting of the process our bodies and the rest of us are experiencing
- Access to what we need to care for ourselves, starting with at least our most basic needs (shelter, clothing, food, water, rest, safety)
- Emotional and social support and healthy, mutually beneficial, and equitable intimate and peer relationships (This is no time for the jerk from college you had the great misfortune of hitching your proverbial wagon to or the adult version of your junior high nemesis.)
- Respect, sympathy and empathy, compassion, and kindness from others for what we are going through, however our experience may be at the time
- Our own goddamn room where anyone who wants to come in needs to knock first
- Realistic expectations and comforts that are in alignment with our own unique genetics, abilities, disabilities, and other unique life circumstances
- Best of all, even just the simple and constant reminder that, like puberty, a menopausal transition is temporary and will end (I say, still not entirely convinced), and the person on the other side of it and their body, life, and all the rest of them will not be half or less than a person at the end of all the good stuff.

SOME MENOPAUSE LINGO

Menopause language is confusing, and not just to me because I'm exhausted. I'll explain a lot more about what each of these things means and how they all work in a bit, but I want to do a quick lingo rundown before I say anything else to spare you (or me) any further confusion.

Menopause is a term with two meanings, a maddening linguistic situation. Neither of those is pausing men, but if you want to and you can, by all means, go for it.

Menopause is shorthand for the whole experience of a menopausal transition or change, whether that happens for someone by way of perimenopause, surgery, or another route and whether it happens as part of the aging process or not.

Menopause also, much more precisely, means the single moment in time when it has been 365 days since a person has had a menstrual period *expressly* because of the ovaries going into retirement, be that on their own or by way of surgery or medical treatments.

Perimenopause (or when we're being pally about it, "peri") means "around menopause." In most current frameworks, it describes an often long phase of life and the reproductive system that starts as premenopause is coming to its end and exists as the great in-between before you and your reproductive system reach menopause.

Menopausal transition: The (often long) road through perimenopause, or another route to menopause, to postmenopause and all the phases that includes.

Postmenopause: The other side. The golden fleece. The Promised Land. Where we just need to make it to without killing anyone or dropping every single thing we're juggling while we go through this. Where we land and start settling into when our body's done with the wild ride of transition, and where we'll remain until we shed this mortal coil.

There are some things I *won't* be saying here:

"Natural" menopause: This is often used to differentiate between gradual menopause, which happens because of aging, and other ways menopause happens, like via total hysterectomy or oophorectomy,

> Language for body parts is tricky. I don't assign gender to body parts (including my own) or people with certain body parts. As much as possible, I also use gender-neutral terms for certain parts. But I often need to get specific about parts and places and don't have a lot of options, so when that happens, I use clinical terms (like vagina, vulva, or breasts). The "utero-ovarian system" is the shorthand I use to describe a system that includes or once included the uterus and cervix, fallopian tubes, ovaries, vagina, and vulva.

radiation, or testosterone use. Intended or not, "natural" implies that every other way of experiencing menopause is unnatural, a framework that is not only false but stigmatizing.

"Surgical" or "induced" menopause: While these terms work for some people, many people who experience menopause because of surgeries or treatments didn't have those surgeries expressly to make menopause happen, and some have hard feelings about menopause as an outcome, which that terminology can feel unsupportive of.

It's grown on me to think about menopause as being either **sudden**, without a longer process of perimenopause, as happens after total hysterectomy or oophorectomy, some medical treatments, or otherwise, or **gradual**, as it goes for people who come to it by way of some kind of perimenopause process.

As you may have picked up on already, I talk about perimenopause and menopause as things that can happen to *people*. The majority of those people have been and still most often are women, but menopause and perimenopause also can and do happen to intersex people, to trans men and otherwise transmasculine people, and to nonbinary, genderqueer, agender, and other gender-diverse folks like myself.

That said, there's a lot to talk about when it comes to women and femmes, sexism and misogyny, menopause and aging. For some people, too, this is an experience that's about femininity, gender, or both, and women are the ones talked about in almost literally all the history of this and all the existing literature to date. I talk about women, misogyny, sexism, and gender in this book a lot, because they come up with menopause a lot, even if and when they might not otherwise come up for a person were they experiencing menopause in a different world than the one we live in. I don't myself feel an internal sense of gender, but since I was assigned female sex at birth and was and still often am assigned the roles and social status of a woman, as it so often is for trans and nonbinary folks, this is complex for me. Alas, no matter who we are or how we identify ourselves, the cultural sexism and misogyny that menopause has long been and is still often steeped in tend to impact pretty much everyone and anyone who experiences menopause or who is presumed to, as you're about to find out in lurid detail.

CHAPTER TWO
WHAT WERE THEY THINKING?

"I like a view but I like to sit with my back turned to it."
—Gertrude Stein

BIENVENUE À LA FUCKERIE! A BRIEF HISTORY OF WESTERN MEDICINE AND LA MÉNÉPAUSIE

You may hear that your attitudes and feelings *about* menopause greatly inform and influence your *experience* of menopause. If anyone gives you the idea that your attitudes and feelings about menopause are the *only* or even the primary drivers in your experience of menopause, please know that's a bunch of baloney, and it's high time for some stink eye.

How we experience menopause is about a *lot* of things: genetics, our health and whole life histories, and our current physical, emotional, social, and other conditions. But it's also irritatingly clear, including from a great deal of empirical evidence, that our attitudes *do* also play a part.

The sources of our feelings, ideas, and attitudes vary and aren't limited just to menopause itself. We gather and construct them from all the places we gather all of our ideas and feelings about anything like this: our larger culture, our smaller communities and relationships, you know the drill. Yet, while a lot of that context can be very diverse, how menopause has been conceptualized, considered, treated, and presented in and by Western culture—particularly by two of its most influential pillars, medicine and media—is often a primary source of our ideas and attitudes and, not at all coincidentally, much of our ignorance, misinformation, and misunderstanding. We've only acquired comprehensive, diverse, and accurate information about menopause, perimenopause, and the people in them over the last twenty-five or so years. That information has only been shared widely for maybe half that time, an estimate that is far more generous than the sharing has been.

THOSE OF US IN ANY PART OF PERIMENO-pause right now have had at least half a lifetime to acquire and internalize ideas and attitudes about menopause and menopausal people that were seriously incomplete or inaccurate physiologically, emotionally, and socially and whose messaging was rarely supportive, normalizing, or empathetic. I say only half a lifetime because even though more correct, complete, less horrifyingly sexist, and otherwise just objectively better information has existed for this last quarter century or so, that doesn't mean we, or the menopausal before us, were able to access that information or even know it was there to access. Especially if you or your circles weren't medical professionals or fans of some specific wings of feminist geekery, it may be you've only started to access decent information and attitudes about menopause over the last decade or maybe even only in the last handful of years. This book could easily even be your very first gateway to that.

Knowing this, it should come as no real surprise that how we understand menopause and the menopausal transition is often wrong, and how we feel about it and ourselves in it is often demoralizing. If our ideas, attitudes, and feelings are primarily fearful or otherwise negative, if they mostly make us feel bad or doomed, the hate-on the globe as a whole has long had for the people who experience menopause has likely played a starring role.

THE HEART OF MANY OF OUR MOST NEG- ative attitudes about and expectations of menopause and ourselves as menopausal people was effectively grown in a lab by some of the worst dudes (and the very occasional nondude) who had anything to do with menopause in the last three hundred years, most of whose ideas or practices were anything from laughably boneheaded to deeply abusive and harmful.

As *Menstruation and Menopause* author Paula Weideger said in the 1970s, "The majority of doctors have an elevated opinion of their worth and an underdeveloped ability to respect their patients." This couldn't be more true of many doctors who've had anything to do with menopause for the bulk of colonial Western history.

The history is as you'd expect: It's sexist and misogynist, and those two things alone guarantee it's also often just been really boneheaded and wrong. It's essentialist. It's ableist and often eugenicist. It's racist, xenophobic, and classist. It's capitalist. It's often so, *so* patronizing and really could not be any more presumptuous if it tried, and boy, did it ever. It's mostly been written and codified by people it's personally enriched who couldn't even themselves experience menopause in the first place. It's been exploitive, abusive, violent, and sometimes even fatal.

UP UNTIL AROUND THE SIXTEENTH CEN- tury, there's little to speak of about menopause in the recorded canon of Western medicine.

I won't be doing an "It's a Small World"–style anthropology micro-review here. Taking up this much space with the colonial West over the last few hundred years and then cramming literally *everything* else that is about a thousand times bigger and longer into a few punchy tidbits is insulting as hell and not a thing I think we need yet one more white person doing. Also, while I'm here, if you couldn't give less of a shit about history if you tried and just want to know what's happening to you and your body in the present day, feel free to skip ahead to page 37.

In the mid-sixteenth century, Giovanni Marinello and Jean Liébault chronicled a number of things that often occurred for those whose bodies had stopped menstruating: hot flashes (Liébault called them "little reds"), night sweats, joint pain, fatigue and lethargy, headache, and changes in sexual desire (in this case, increases). Around the same time English physician Thomas Sydenham added "hysterick fits" and heavy menstrual flow ("Like a Candle burnt to the Socket, which gives the greatest light just as it is about to go out") to that list. His preferred treatment was eight ounces of blood taken from the arm for several nights in a row, with the ludicrous idea that taking blood from any part of the body reduces menstrual flow. He did pair that with a narcotic syrup made from poppies, so one at least got a cocktail first.

In 1710, the first known Western dissertation on menopause—*On the End of Menstruation as the Time for the Beginning of Various Diseases*—was published by Simon David Titius of Prussia. In 1774,

John Fothergill published another, *Of the Management Proper at the Cessation of the Menses*. Fothergill opens by talking about menopause in a relaxed way and discusses how expectations of and attitudes about menopause had an impact on how people experienced it. He lists impacts we'll recognize today: "Some are afflicted with the well-known symptoms of plethora, heat, flushings, restless nights, troublesome dreams and unequal spirits; others are attacked with inflammations of the bowels, or other internal parts, spasmodic affections of various parts, stiffness in the limbs, swelled ankles, with pain or inflammation, the piles and other effects of plentitude."

He suggests some healthy approaches—increasing nutrition, for example—but any optimism about Fothergill should end there. He was a bloodletting evangelist who felt any patient with what he perceived as foolish objections to it—like that it was not only painful but useless—should be talked into it.

He was a fan of purgatives, too, because of course he was.

In 1816, Charles Pierre Louis de Gardanne coined the term "menopause" in his article *De la ménépausie, ou de l'âge critique des femmes*. He dedicated about one hundred pages to the subject and apparently—my French is *trés terrible*, so I have to take others' word for it—set a fire under the butt of the new norm of treating menopause as disease. And unfortunately, as was true of so much medicine of the time, his contemporaries and many who came after them treated women with that "disease" horribly.

AUTHOR OF *EVIL ROOTS: KILLER TALES OF the Botanical Gothic* Daisy Butcher describes the treatment of women in menopause during this century as parallel to how female mummies were treated in horror literature of the same era: as objects of revulsion, fear, and disdain, of great danger to men, ultimately disposable, and routinely subjected to barbaric experimentation.

In the early 1800s, Scottish surgeon John Lizars's answer to menopause was to debut the newly invented ovariotomy, a very rudimentary, dangerous, and often deadly form of what we now call the oophorectomy. Mortality rates were as high as 86 percent with some surgeons who performed the practice. Thousands of women suffered and died from these kinds of surgical "discoveries," and likely far more were killed or otherwise harmed than we'll ever know, given the convention of surgeons of the era—like James Marion Sims in the United States, "the father of modern gynecology"—to experiment on Black slaves and poor immigrants, whose lives were so devalued that even their deaths most often went unrecorded.

In 1840, C. F. Menville de Ponsan, a charmer who called menopause "the death of the womb," wrote *The Critical Age of Women, the Maladies They Can Undergo at This Stage of Their Life, and the Means to Combat or Prevent Them*. Working in Britain, Scottish gynecologist Lawson Tait saw what he called menopausal "dementia" as something to try and prevent with a combination of purgatives and asylum commitment.

Isaac Baker Brown was Lawson Tait's rival and one of James Marion Sims's fave colleagues. His idea of prevention for problems with menopause was surgical removal of the clitoris. "The operation," as he politely called his practice of brutal genital mutilation, would keep menopausal and other women from developing hysteria and everything associated with it, like sexual desire. In 1866, he published *Curability of Certain Forms of Insanity, Epilepsy, Catalepsy and Hysteria in Females*—clitoridectomy was the proposed "cure" for all of these. This, apparently, was a bridge too far and, paired with the fact that he hadn't had consent from his patients, was apparently his professional undoing. Chalk one up to the not-really-good-guys-but-at-least-a-little-better-than-this-guy. When Baker Brown died, his rival Lawson Tait volunteered to do his autopsy. What a pair.

EVERY NOW AND THEN, AN OUTLIER showed up in this mix, like Samuel Ashwell, who, in his 1844 *Practical Treatise on the Diseases Peculiar to Women*, said, "It has become too general an opinion that the decline of this function must be attended by illness; but this is surely an error, for there are healthy women who pass over this time without any inconvenience and many whose indisposition is both transient and slight." Nice try, Sam. Unfortunately, Samuel and others like him were vastly outnumbered.

IN 1857, EDWARD TILT PUBLISHED ONE of the first Western medical books about menopause, *The Change of Life in Health and Disease*. The term "climacteric" apparently belongs to him. So does a whole lot of crap.

Tilt's treatments for menopause included rectal douches with Dover's Powder (a combination of opium and ipecac), morphine, laudanum, carbonated soda, belladonna plasters on the abdomen, and lead acetate injections into the vagina. He thought women being sexual in menopause was especially terrifying, gross, and literally insane. As far as Tilt was concerned, any excitement in women was to be avoided at all costs, which perhaps explains why he

was so into drugging them into a stupor as a regular practice. Tilt considered the uterus "the keystone of mental pathology." And yet, he didn't have one, and look how pathological he turned out to be.

You can find him describing those in peri- or postmenopause as having a "dull, stupid astonishment," a "sacrifice of feminine grace," and a "failure of ovarian energy"; he issued warnings for them to avoid becoming "peevish, harsh, dismal . . . viewing everything through a jaundiced veil," a state of being that seems impossible to avoid were this winner your doctor. Tilt described postmenopause—if you could survive him to reach it—as a return to health, with even "a very great improvement of personal appearance, when bones become covered by a fair amount of fat." But, of course, even in that glimpse of patronizing positivity, we're warned that this can't be the case for all of us (especially the poor), who "do not recover health without some sacrifice of feminine grace, their appearance becoming somewhat masculine, the bones projecting more than usual, the skin is less unctuous, and tweezers may be required to remove stray hairs from the face."

W. W. Bliss held the ovaries responsible for everything and anything to do with a woman's body, appearance, and the rest of herself. For Bliss, good ovaries resulted in "good" things—like beauty, fidelity, tenderness, intelligence, and nobility. Bad ovaries resulted in "bad" things

In the mid-1800s women's voices began to emerge on the subject. While not always (but often) more correct, their ideas were often at least considerably more humane, less misogynist, and less vile.

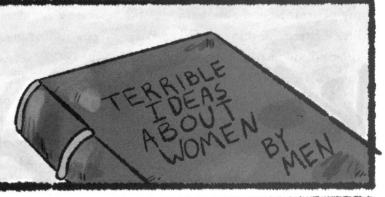

TERRIBLE IDEAS ABOUT WOMEN BY MEN

Feminist, and prison and asylum abolitionist Eliza Wood Burhans Farnham, in 1864:

"This misinterpretation of the annulling of a set of bodily functions has cost the sex countless ages of dread of the inevitable, such humiliation, and nameless martyrdoms. It is actually a transmutation of power, a transfer of capacity to enter into a more exalted department of life; the winding up of a physical series, and the opening of wider channels for the outflow of the affectional and spiritual nature; the closing of one set of avenues, and the broader opening of another, lying above them."

Inventor Lydia E. Pinkham rolled out her Vegetable Compound in 1873, a tonic that claimed to help a myriad of "female complaints," including menopause.

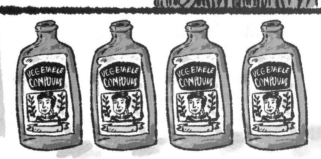

It included black cohosh, pleurisy and unicorn root and fenugreek—and was 20 proof.

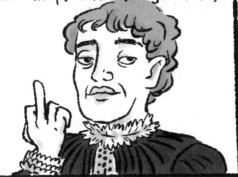

Pinkham's image was on the bottle. She was trolled horribly for having the audacity to use her own plain middle-aged face.

Anna M. Longshore-Potts was one of the first to describe a link between hot flashes and the vasomotor system.

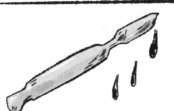

In Discourses to Women on Medical Subjects in 1896, rather than surgeries, enemas or bloodletting, she suggests nutrition, exercise in open air, and rest.

In 1913, educator, feminist and minister Anna Garlin Spencer talked of how, when the "childbearing age is passed, there may be, and now increasingly is, a fresh start given to the mental and emotional life. It cannot be too soon realized that in the lives of women, there is a capacity for a second youth."

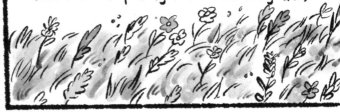

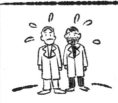 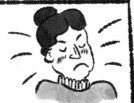

In 1923's What A Woman Of Forty-five Ought To ' Know, Emma F. Angell Drake called out male doctors for making women fearful, shameful and anxious.
She said menopause is just a matter of one of your organs going into retirement, and that this time of life and beyond holds some of your best work and best years.

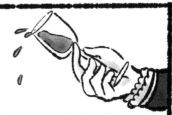

Thanks to institutionalized sexism and misogyny, the ideas and gentler approaches to menopause and those in it of these and other women were not highly influential in their era. They were before their time. Let's raise a glass of boozy patent medicine to them.

like masturbation or sexual desire, periods, the desire to eat, menstrual cramps, a bad menopause, and—as Louise Foxcroft aptly, but more gracefully, added—a persecution complex. If you were bad, your ovaries were bad and, thus, should be removed so you could be good again. In a slut-shaming variation on the theme, 1883's favorite eugenicist read of the summer, *Ladies Guide in Health and Disease: Girlhood, Maidenhood, Wifehood, Motherhood* by John Kellogg (yes, *that* John Kellogg), says women who had "transgressed nature's laws" would find menopause "a veritable Pandora's box of ills, and may look forward to it with apprehension and foreboding."

You will be in no way shocked to learn that the emerging field of psychotherapy didn't help. In 1901, Charles Reed, president of the American Medical Association, deemed menopause "a mental condition," and according to George Savage in *The Lancet* in 1903, even women who were not mentally ill were likely to offer "insane interpretations" of their menopausal symptoms. A decade later, in his volume on "obsessional neurosis," Sigmund Freud spoke of those in menopause as "quarrelsome, vexatious, and overbearing, petty and stingy; they exhibit typically sadistic and anal-erotic traits which they did not possess earlier." Personally, my hat's off to any woman of that era whose vagina was probably giving her grief and thought she might try exploring

her anus instead. Good for her. As for the sadism, well, consider the source.

ALONG CAME HORMONES

Despite the fact that Chinese medicine included what we call hormones—chemical messengers produced by the endocrine system that help regulate all the body's processes—by at least 200 BC, conventional medicine didn't really identify or understand the endocrine system until the mid-1800s. That understanding and study didn't extend itself to utero-ovarian systems until 1929, when Adolf Butenandt and Edward Adelbert Doisy "discovered" estrone and, soon after, the other estrogens. Butenandt shared the 1939 Nobel Prize in Chemistry with Leopold Ružička, recognized for their work synthesizing testosterone.

Estrogen produced from human placenta was already being used to treat menstrual cramps. In 1938, synthetic estrogen, diethylstilbestrol, was developed. This dropped the cost of estrogen significantly: it was now available to a much greater number of people than it had been before. In the early 1940s, synthetic production began, and in 1943 James Goodall developed what would become Premarin—a conjugated estrogen made from the urine of pregnant mares—which the Food and Drug Administration approved for the treatment of hot flashes.

In *How to Treat a Menopausal Woman: A History, 1900 to 2000*, Judith Houck

WHAT FRESH HELL IS THIS?

explains, "There was a divide in this era between those who had the idea that problems with menopause were problems with attitudes about it—fix your attitude, fix your menopause, in other words—and those who thought it a problem that needed a medical solution. Sedatives, much like opiates of past eras, were one of the common front-line responses, and secondarily, hormone therapies."

Ads—some of which masqueraded as journalism—for menopause treatments are what brought menopause to mass media. Images of concerned, scared, sad, tired, or harried looking women in menopause—or their magically transformed cheerful, energetic counterparts—promoted the medical menopause treatments of the time: schizophrenia medications like Thorazine, Benzedrine and other uppers, Butisol and other downers, antidepressants of the time, Premarin and other conjugated estrogen brands, and even new-era advertising for Lydia Pinkham's tonic. Articles in *Good Housekeeping, Ladies' Home Journal, Vogue,* and other popular magazines were usually written by men and mostly hormone-therapy propaganda pieces that held up the notion of menopause as a disease rather than a normal body and life transition.

In 1963, author Maxine Davis—an unsung rebel who founded her own women-focused news service in 1923, *Capital News*—took a positive approach to menopause. She talked about menopause in ways that both sound modern and echoed some of the women of the generation before her: she talked about the ability to be freed of ways menstrual and fertility cycles can limit us, feeling more stable when it comes to moods by way of not being influenced by cycling, and even how cool and exciting maturity can be. "The menopause is a normal event in the life of every woman—normal as morning and evening, normal as summer after spring."

Unfortunately for Maxine and a whole lot of people who could have benefitted from her approach becoming the popular view, it was the views of the guy who said this about her that became the norm instead: "How could such a serious deficiency disease as menopause seem 'normal' to her? Very likely, like millions of other women, she has not yet had the opportunity to learn the facts. It is my own responsibility, however, not to let statements of hers go unchallenged."

I am afraid it is time to talk about Robert A. Wilson.

Lydia Pinkham's tonic would be just the thing right about now. If you do and can still drink, make it a double. If you don't or can't, inhale, grab, or otherwise have at the ready whatever your equivalent is, like maybe a switchblade. You're going to need it.

In 1954, "The Use of Estrogen After the Menopause" by Dr. Kost Shelton was published in the *Journal of the American Geriatrics Society*, an article gynecologist Wilson spoke of as "one of the first beacons of enlightenment in the engulfing sea of ignorance." Shelton had gone on at length about the essential need for women's egos to "not just capture, but to hold a husband," that estrogen is what makes women desirable, and more of the usual tiresome fare. In 1963, Wilson and his wife, Thelma, published a paper in the *Journal of the American Geriatrics Society*, "The Fate of the Nontreated Menopausal Woman: A Plea for the Maintenance of Adequate Estrogen from Puberty to the Grave." Yes, that was really the title. This debuted the premise that systemic estrogen should be used from "puberty to grave," which was expanded in Wilson's 1966 book *Feminine Forever: The Amazing New Breakthrough in the Sex Life of Women*, which is about five hundred times more awful than the title suggests.

Wilson calls menopause a "staggering catastrophe" and claims it is a disease of estrogen deficiency, not a normal phase of life and change of body. He claims lifelong estrogen therapy can keep women "feminine forever" and fix things like empty-nest syndrome, the burden a depressed woman is on her male partner, the difficulty of finding or keeping jobs one is qualified for, and other common manifestations of ageism and sexism, which, if estrogen had fixed them, would have also spared us more from Robert A. Wilson.

Here are but a few more charming lines from *Feminine Forever* that will have you reconsidering your stance on book burning:

- "This transformation, within a few years, of a formerly pleasant, energetic woman into a dull-minded but sharp-tongued caricature of her former self is one of the saddest of human spectacles. The suffering is not hers alone—it involves her entire family, her business associates, her neighborhood storekeepers, and all others with whom she comes into contact. Multiplied by millions, she is a focus of bitterness and discontent in the whole fabric of our civilization."
- "The unpalatable truth must be faced that all postmenopausal women are castrates," and "the Woman becomes the equivalent of a eunuch."
- "In a family situation, estrogen makes women adaptable, even-tempered, and generally easy to live with."
- "No woman can be sure of escaping the horror of this living decay."

In perhaps the most hideous passage of the book, Wilson recounts what he calls an "amusing incident." A man who was "a prominent member of the Brooklyn underworld" brought his wife into his office and said, "Doc, they tell me you can fix women when they get old and crabby. She's driving me nuts. She won't fix meals." This man also says his wife has asked him to leave their house but tells Wilson that if anyone is going to leave, it's her. "It's *my* home," he says.

In *The Future Is Menopausal*, Ann Neumann writes,

It sounds like the set-up to a joke—of the Rodney Dangerfield "my wife's a lousy cook" vintage. Here's the punch line: the aggrieved husband pulls out a .32 automatic and tells the doctor, "If you don't cure her, I'll kill her." Cue the laugh track. This story . . . is worth repeating for a few reasons. One is Wilson's strange self-reported reaction: "I have often been haunted by the thought that except for the tiny stream of estrogen, this woman might have died a violent death at the hands of her own husband." And his conclusion— in my menopausal paraphrase, *drug the bitch*—is breathtakingly irresponsible. He hears a threat of domestic violence and immediately pathologizes the victim.

Wilson finishes that passage by saying, "Outright murder may be a relatively rare consequence of the menopause—though not as rare as most of us might suppose."

Lucky for you, I've spared you his talk about sexuality, how not being in love with a man told him everything he needed to know about why his women patients were ill, what the body of a "fully sexed" woman looks like, his odes to the value of breasts and legs, how screwed you are if someone in menopause is your boss, his descriptions of "the lower-class woman," frigidity, how women should dress, that part where he likens himself and others promoting estrogen therapies to Moses (*let my ovaries goooooo*), how all of what he says apparently comes from a place of *empathy* for women, and other topics where he's exactly as terrible as you'd imagine.

Wilson's methodologies have long been considered weak. He was wrong in some very big ways. He claimed that estrogen therapy keeps menopause from ever happening, that a pap smear can take a "femininity index" that shows the amount of estrogen in the body, that systemic estrogen should be taken at high dosages until death, and that synthetic estrogen couldn't possibly pose any dangers to women because they've had estrogen in their bodies their whole lives.

He massively popularized estrogen therapy, and his particular regimens with it, for menopause. He also popularized his noxious attitudes and ideas about women, femininity, and menopause: hundreds of articles, including in popular women's magazines, promoting his ideas and estrogen regimen were published over the following decade. He wasn't the first to suggest lifelong estrogen regimens or to be wrong in some of the ways he was. There were others suggesting similar things before him, but none so loudly, staunchly—he and his wife claimed estrogen "cured" menopause—and influentially as he. Wilson obviously did not invent the sexism, misogyny, gender essentialism, and ableism he promoted, but he certainly helped to cement this flavor of it and made it awfully profitable, including for himself. The bestselling *Feminine Forever* and its widespread influence had women (and their husbands) running to their doctors begging for estrogen to save them from everything Wilson threatened would happen otherwise.

Wilson's wife, Thelma, used his estrogen therapy regimen too. According to their son, Ron Wilson, she died of breast cancer in 1988 after several battles with it and kept her cancer secret to protect her husband's reputation. Ron Wilson has also exposed unsurprising information that Wyeth-Ayerst Laboratories had funded all of Wilson's work (they claim to have no record of this), including *Feminine Forever*. Ron is still working today to expose animal abuses involved in the manufacture of Premarin.

IN 1969, IN HIS BOOK *EVERYTHING YOU Always Wanted to Know About Sex but Were Afraid to Ask*, psychiatrist David Reuben doubled down on the creepy, super-patronizing, and misogynistic gender essentialism by writing, "Once the ovaries stop, the very essence of being a woman stops," adding that the postmenopausal woman comes "as close as

she can to being a man." Or rather, "not really a man but no longer a functional woman. . . . Having outlived their ovaries, they have outlived their usefulness as human beings." And, yes, if that title sounds familiar to you, it is because Woody Allen made a movie inspired by that book, because of course he did.

The strong messages Shelton, Wilson, Reuben, and others like them sent that femininity was all about ovarian function and estrogen and that womanhood literally ended with menopause—unless you forever medicated to the contrary—stuck. You probably have some of them stuck in your own head, even: it'd be hard not to.

THANKFULLY, BOTH THE BROADER emerging feminist movement of the time and, more specifically, the women's health movement started shouting out and ushering in some radically different attitudes and approaches and some much-needed backlash and oversight.

In 1972 *Ms.* magazine published a pro-menopause article. In 1973, in *Feminist Studies*, Carroll Smith-Rosenberg dissected the essentialism inherent in the prevailing view of menopause and femininity: how womanhood was thought to be constructed by and to arrive with menarche and thus, presumably, to be lost at menopause. She noted that womanhood was deeply defined by ideas about the utero-ovarian reproductive system and presumed experiences of it: as sexual, beautiful, and romantically "blossoming" but also as weak, dependent, fragile, and even infantile, an extreme contrast to how men were described in relationship to their burgeoning reproductive systems, as "vigorous" or "noble." She talked about menarche and menopause as sources of ongoing and chronic shame, insecurity, isolation, and punishment.

That same year, *Our Bodies, Ourselves* included a chapter on menopause. It opens by sharing quotes that the writers—all far too young at the time to be anywhere near menopause—gathered when "a few of our older friends sat down and told some of us what their experiences with menopause had been like." The chapter is normalizing, just like the book is with everything else; the scientific and health information given is highly accurate (given what was known at the time), and issues that impact quality of life with menopause—the quality of life *for* the person themselves *in* menopause, for a change—like depression, sex, and self-esteem, were discussed.

In 1977, Rosetta Reitz published *Menopause: A Positive Approach*, which was exactly that. It includes an array of information gathered from consciousness-raising groups, respect and support for a range of feelings, encouragement to talk about it, strong feminist critique of the estrogen pushers without withholding support for those who want to use it, and

a section on sex and masturbation that even features a mid-forties Betty Dodson talking masturbation at the dawn of her life's work with it, no less. Reitz was very aware of the legacy of menopause to date and wanted to do something to try and repair it and give menopausal people something empowering. (Reitz also wrote a mushroom cookbook and a piece for the *Village Voice* titled "The Liberation of the Yiddishe Mama" and founded Rosetta Records, a label exclusively for woman jazz and blues musicians of the early twentieth century, including Bessie Smith, Ida Cox, and Ma Rainey. She died in 2008, was obviously amazing, and I am in love with her.)

Around the same time, popular general media, including the *New York Times*, and medical journals started voicing cancer concerns. Also in 1977, women's health writer Barbara Seaman published *Women and the Crisis in Sex Hormones* and lit a fire under a growing critique of estrogen therapy. Paired with growing might from the rest of the women's health and feminist movement and more mentions in mass media, all of this work helped get large-scale studies of people in menopause going and helped us reach our current ways of thinking about and understanding menopause.

But even though *Ms.*, Smith-Rosenberg, *Our Bodies, Ourselves*, Reitz, Weideger, Seaman, and some of their other contemporaries were seemingly the first in the Western canon of menopause to point out the discrepancies between how men, medicine, and the culture as a whole represented the menopausal experience and how the people who themselves were actually experiencing it felt about it, crummy attitudes and frameworks still held up. Through the 1970s, the *Merck Manual* still called menopause an "ovarian dysfunction," and in 1980, *Drugs of Choice* and other medical references classified it as a disease of the endocrine system.

Now seems as good a time as any to put history behind us for a minute and get to the present day. We finally know a lot more about what happens with menopause and why it's happening, even if our culture still has a lot of work to do on—*and is there a more menopausal thing to say?*—its attitude.

CHAPTER THREE

THE MENOPAUSAL TRANSITION

WHEN, WHY, HOW, WHERE, AND WHAT THE LITERAL HELL

"You never know what is happening to yourself when it is happening."
—*Elaine Stritch*

PRELUDE TO A PERIMENOPAUSE: PERIODS AND MORE

To grok what happens when utero-ovarian systems start to wind down and eventually retire, it helps to know how they typically operate *before* that happens.

Before anyone pulls a *"Shouldn't we all already know this?"*: yes, everyone with or who's had a uterus, ovaries, or both should, ideally, know how that system basically works. But because most of us were raised and stayed living in *this* world, not

What follows describes the endocrine system, central nervous system, an intact utero-ovarian reproductive system, and other systems of the body when they exist and are operating in the most typical ways and without anything added to the mix—like hormonal contraceptive methods, cancers, or nervous system disorders—that does or can alter how those systems behave. It's currently estimated that by 2025, there will be somewhere in the neighborhood of one billion people experiencing a menopausal transition worldwide: that's way too many people with way too much diversity for any one description like this to fit. More people's bodies with utero-ovarian systems operate as I'm about to describe than not, but many don't or won't: "average" can only do a passable job of describing billions of bodies. The following is how this can go with some intersex conditions but not others. It doesn't describe what's going on for folks with testicular systems at all: if you want to find out a little about that, the appendix has you covered.

Themyscira where Wonder Woman grew up, a lot of folks don't. And yes, that *is* bullshit, which is why I'm explaining it here.

IF WE'RE BORN WITH A PRETTY TYPICAL utero-ovarian system and a body that influences and responds to it in pretty typical ways, within a few years after puberty begins, menstruation and ovulation will start.

Both ultimately begin with the hypothalamus, a part of the brain that, like my patience these days, may be small but still is mighty. Its big jobs are to link the nervous system and the endocrine system and to maintain homeostasis of the whole body and all its systems. It's constantly working to try and keep a balance between our bodies and our external environment, including body temperature, blood pressure, and stress. It's a switchboard between the rest of the body and the pituitary gland. The hypothalamus signals and helps regulate hormones produced by the pituitary and other organs and also secretes hormones of its own, including oxytocin, prolactin-releasing and -inhibiting hormone, growth-hormone-releasing and -inhibiting hormone, and gonadotropin-releasing hormone (GnRH).

Before puberty, progesterone is nonexistent. Estrogen, testosterone, and GnRH levels are very low. As puberty begins, the hypothalamus increases the frequency with which it releases GnRH, and those levels start to rise. Eventually, it gets to a level that signals the pituitary gland to start releasing follicle-stimulating hormone (FSH). The organs of the utero-ovarian system then continue to develop more fully with other parts of the body. These are puberty Tanner stages 2 and 3, for you human development dorks in the audience, where things like breast budding, the start of pubic and underarm hair, and height growth usually happen. The menstrual cycle usually begins a couple to a few years after puberty starts, in Tanner stage 3 or 4.

FIRST BLOOD

A menstrual period marks—leave it to periods to be so literal—day one of each menstrual cycle. At the start of each cycle, both estrogen and progesterone are very low. (In fact, they're about where they'll always be postmenopause.) FSH is what gets the ovaries and the follicles within them going, and with the hypothalamus, they make and release a specific estrogen, estradiol. Estradiol is the estrogen that most of us have probably thought of as *Estrogen, The*, even though it's not the only one.

The first few to several years of menstrual periods and the whole of that cycle, including all the hormones that go with them, are usually spaced further apart than they will be later. Those hormone levels and patterns are usually erratic and irregular for the first three to five years, as are menstrual periods and the timing and experience of menstrual cycles.

There are four kinds of estrogen that can be produced by the body:

Estradiol: the estrogen predominant during the time of life someone is having menstrual/fertility cycles, produced by the ovaries

Estriol: a kind of estrogen most predominant during pregnancy, produced by the placenta

Estetrol: a kind of estrogen *only* produced with and during pregnancy, produced by the fetal liver

Estrone: the primary form of estrogen in the body after menopause, produced by the ovaries, fat, and adrenal glands

THE INCREDIBLE INEDIBLE EGG

At birth, the ovaries usually contain anywhere from one to three million oocytes—undeveloped ova (egg cells). By the time menstrual cycles begin, there are only about a half million to a million left.

As a menstrual cycle begins with a period, FSH starts to stimulate and develop ten to thirty of the follicles that encase those cells. Those developing follicles raise estrogen levels, which sends a signal to the uterus to start building up the endometrium (uterine lining). About the same time the period is winding down, the pituitary gland starts to release some luteinizing hormone (LH) too. The hypothalamus releases GnRH again, and LH levels increase as the cycle continues. LH and FSH work on those follicles for a few days. As they develop, one of them usually takes over, and estrogen keeps rising from the developing big boss follicle, while FSH and LH levels decline. The rest of the follicles start to degenerate and will be reabsorbed by the body like other kinds of cells are all the time.

Nearing mid-cycle, rising estrogen changes the consistency of the cervical fluid and the position of the cervix and its opening. Ovulation usually happens around now (the most average of averages for that is around day thirteen). There's a big surge of LH, followed by a less impressive rise of FSH and a rise in testosterone. That big boss follicle ruptures and flings the ovum out into the uterine cavity, where it gets swept up by the fimbria of the fallopian tubes and slowly and smoothly dunked into the uterus. Swoosh, swoosh. The area that follicle came from—the *corpus luteum*, made up of leftover ovarian cells—creates and releases progesterone, which grows more of the endometrium.

Were sperm cells deposited in the vagina at or right around ovulation, should one of them (with a few hundred other sperm cells helping, credit where credit is due) fertilize that ovum, *and* if that fertilized egg implanted into the endometrium of the uterine wall—usually around a week later—you'd have yourself a pregnancy.

Or not. When an ovum *isn't* fertilized (or was but didn't implant), it disintegrates like the rest of the cells and follicles from that cycle. The progesterone and estrogen, clearly as prone to flights of futility as the rest of us, keep working on and sustaining the endometrium for about another week. FSH and LH levels drop and, with GnRH, will stay very low for the rest of the cycle. Once that happens, the corpus luteum starts to disintegrate. There's little estrogen and progesterone left: they're at the same very low levels as when the cycle started. The lack of progesterone signals the body to discard that endometrium it built up for a pregnancy, and voilà, it's the shedding of that lining and its by-products that makes up a menstrual period, and we're back where we started in a new cycle. And so on and so on.

Not accounting for pregnancies and postpartum, methods of contraception or other medications or devices that change or disrupt cycles, or other times this cycle is on hold or works differently, this is basically how things will typically go for many folks for somewhere between three and four decades.

PERIMENOPAUSE: RIDE THE ESTROGENIC RICOCHET!

Perimenopause is a normal part of aging, is outside our control, and occurs all by itself, not because of something we did. It can suck, but hey, at least it's not *our* fault.

It took long enough, but after such a long history of mostly dudes who had no clue about what was really going on, in the mid-1990s, thanks primarily to the (separate) work of genius researchers Dr. Nanette Santoro and Dr. Jerilynn Prior, we *finally* got a real understanding of what goes on in the menopausal transition. Dr. Prior recently described perimenopause for the Canadian Broadcasting Company as "misunderstood, confusing and long," if you want a quick take on just how very much she gets it.

A lot of folks had and still have the idea that what's happening from perimenopause into menopause is about a steady, gradual downward slide of estrogen, a growing estrogen "deficiency," and estrogen withdrawal as a result. That's not what happens. **If only.** Most of us wouldn't even notice it if it were, because it'd be a *much* smoother ride.

Perimenopause—and what's happening hormonally during perimenopause—is more like a roller coaster than a slide.

It's got ups; it's got downs. It's got twists and loop-de-loops, and if your perimenopause experience is anything like mine, it also has someone's barfing

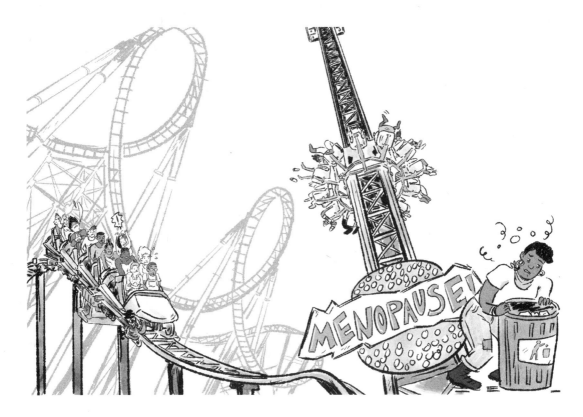

kid, a jerk behind you who won't stop kicking your seat, and some sexist asshole berating his girlfriend you're wishing a seatbelt malfunction on.

For some people, the roller coaster is the short, gentle kind for little kids—some people even manage to sleep through that ride without even knowing they were on it. For others, it's one of those where you feel sick and terrified just *looking* at it. Most people will have something in between.

By the time most of us start to transition into menopause, our stockpile of oocytes is down to around ten or twenty thousand. That might sound like a lot, but the ones left are disinterested slackers: they just aren't the ova most likely to do . . . well, *anything*. That combo—the relatively few ova left and the fact that the ones left are not into it—is what's generally agreed kicks off perimenopause.

Those remaining egg cells now send weaker, more chaotic signals—the signals that previously kept cycles running pretty predictably and smoothly—to the hypothalamus. As a result, levels of estrogen and progesterone start to become erratic, unpredictable, and disoriented, much, perhaps, like your aunt Goldie when she's had more than her fair share of Chardonnay.

This Aunt-Goldie-on-a-bender endocrine situation can result in numerous impacts across all systems of the body throughout perimenopause. These are the things people often talk about or think of as "symptoms" of perimenopause or menopause: hot flashes and night sweats, body shape or size changes, constipation, fatigue, joint pain, and mood swings. Author, menopause researcher, and Women Living Better cofounder Nina Coslov always wants to be sure people know that the notion that perimenopausal impacts like those can only start once periods start getting weird is incorrect. Menstrual changes aren't always the first changes people experience in perimenopause.

THE IDEA THAT PERIMENOPAUSE HAS started only once people start having *longer* cycles or *missing* periods is also outdated: that's not usually what periods are like in early peri. As perimenopause gets started, those who have had fairly regular menstrual cycles *will* often start to see some changes. Most commonly, that first looks like cycles that are shorter, though, where you're having *more* periods, not fewer. Some people also experience very heavy or long periods during this time. That's because it's typical to have *high* estrogen during this time, not low estrogen. Dr. Prior says, "When all of the studies are put together, and the average perimenopausal estrogen levels are compared with average levels in young women, it is clear that the levels are higher, and significantly so."

When we move into later perimenopause, that's when those remaining oocytes start to produce less and less estrogen, so FSH goes high and starts staying elevated in a way it normally wouldn't. That FSH elevation is effectively screaming to the entire neighborhood for estrogen to come home for dinner, and it's not uncommon for our bodies to respond with things like headaches and hot flashes.

It's common to have periods of time when you're doing all right, with what feels like relatively little impact from perimenopause, and then to find yourself in a phase of some big impacts or new impacts you didn't have before. It's just often so unpredictable, which is why any of you who are talking about how easy this has been but are not all the way through it should not be so confident it's going to stay that way for you. (Of course, you should not ever say how easy it's been for you to those of us who are struggling because even though being an asshole sometimes does go hand in hand with the menopausal transition, it's just good manners to save that shit for the people who *aren't* going through this.)

In studies, a pattern appears that shows impacts like hot flashes and perimenopause-sparked depression are at their most intense in the one to three years before and the one to three years after the final menstrual period. In other words, they show that some of the worst of perimenopause may be closest to the end of it, a fact that is often oddly presented like it should be comforting.

This all might not have been such a surprise if, from early on, we'd had a more realistic sense of the usual timeline of our reproductive systems and their impacts on us. It's hard to be prepared for changes when not only is your sense of what they are skewed but your idea of when they'll start coming isn't right, either.

Many of us got the idea that these stages are effectively divided into life before periods, during periods, and after periods. Or that it's about when we're first unable to make babies, then able to make babies, then making babies (or trying very hard to make babies or very hard not to make babies, sometimes periods of both), not making babies, then unable to make babies again. Or periods, pregnancy, menopause, death. You gotta love a life cycle framework that makes death sound like the best part.

The Stages of Reproductive Aging Workshop (STRAW) classification system was developed in 2001 in a meeting sponsored by several health organizations and bodies: the National Institute on Aging and the Office of Research on Women's Health of the National Institutes of Health, the North American Menopause Society (NAMS), the American Society for Reproductive Medicine, the International Menopause Society, and the Endocrine Society. It's based in broad, objective data and has been updated since. It's a widely accepted standard for defining the stages of menopause and the basic life cycle of a utero-ovarian system. It's not perfect and absolutely does not fit all, but it's helpful as a broad overview. (It should be noted that it's a specifically bad fit for those with polycystic ovary syndrome and others without reliable or any menstrual patterns.)

It divides the whole of a reproductive life cycle into seven main stages under three umbrellas and notes the most principal, observable, or measurable differences between them. The high points go like so:

Reproductive (the duration of each of these first three stages varies):
Early Reproductive—Menstrual periods start variable and become regular (or as regular as they will get, anyway).
Peak Reproductive—Menstrual periods are regular (see above).
Late Reproductive—Some subtle changes in menstrual flow or cycle length may begin at the tail end of this stage, FSH levels start to be more variable, and ovarian reserve (how many egg follicles are left) will start to become low.

Menopausal Transition:
Early Menopausal Transition—This is where perimenopause starts. Menstrual periods and length of cycles will more consistently vary. FSH levels are variable. The duration of this stage varies.

Late Menopausal Transition—This is when periods start to be skipped or missed for sixty days or more and when vasomotor symptoms become likely. FSH is both variable and rising to an eventual higher ground over the next two stages. The duration of this stage is listed as one to three years. Here's sure hoping. This stage ends, and postmenopause begins, with the final menstrual period (FMP).

Postmenopause:

Early Postmenopause—There now aren't any more menstrual periods, vasomotor symptoms are *most* likely, and ovarian follicles are very low. Early postmenopause is divided into three smaller substages, and the duration of them combined is anywhere from five to eight years. That first substage, however—and with it perimenopause—ends exactly one year after the FMP.

Late Postmenopause—Vasomotor symptoms have resolved for most by now, and FSH has also stabilized. There may be increasing genitourinary symptoms of menopause, and the duration of this phase is from when it starts until the end of life.

I once went to a haunted house as a kid where I completely lost my shit. It was just one horrifying thing after another after another. I was screaming and barf-sobbing so much that they made some unfortunate teenager who worked there walk with us to get me through the end of it, while I continued to scream nonstop in her face. I remember her telling me the MOST TERRIFYING THING OF ALL was about to happen but *after that, it was over*, like that should make me feel better instead of even more terrified. This "comfort" feels like that to me, since I'm still in this, and I'd really hoped I'd already seen the scariest things. Apparently not.

MENOPAUSE

By the time you have a final menstrual period or, if you weren't having periods, your ovaries go into retirement silently, estrogen and progesterone are settling into the low, stable levels they'll be at for the rest of life. An estrogen switch has also started to happen in the body: moving from getting most of its estrogen from the ovaries (estradiol) to getting most of it (as estrone, via a conversion process by the steroid hormone androstenedione, which also helps create testosterone) primarily from body fat instead.

Then 365 days after that last endometrial hurrah, you'll have arrived at menopause.

Don't yell at me: We're probably going to feel the same that day, and for a lot of days after it, as we did for a while before. Menopause happening doesn't mean that everything we've been experiencing will magically and suddenly stop. It still usually takes a few years or so for us and our bodies to get adjusted to how different the biochemical landscape, and everything that impacts, is.

The good news is that once we do get to menopause, we're basically on a plane that's coming in for a landing: the landing might be bumpy, but we *are* landing, and our perimenopausal flight will be over. All of the big hormonal chaos is done; levels of estrogen and progesterone are lower, FSH higher, and are all now slowly and much more gradually settling into a stabler place, which is how they'll be (unless you are using hormone therapies) for the rest of life.

But hold up a minute—*why*, you might reasonably ask, does reproductive hormonal business during menopausal transition impact the whole body, including systems that seem completely unrelated to the reproductive system?

WHY ARE ESTROGEN AND PROGESTERONE CAUSING SUCH A RUCKUS, ANYWAY?

It's mostly all about what estrogen and progesterone can do or be part of and which systems of the body they impact.

Some people call testosterone, estrogen, and progesterone sex hormones and think some of these belong to only one sex, while others belong to another. There are more than two sexes to begin with, but, regardless, all these hormones can and usually do exist in the bodies of people of any assigned sex and of any gender. Hormones don't have sex or gender: there aren't "female" or "male" hormones, only fluctuating and different ratios of these hormones coexisting within each of us.

They do a lot, and they impact **all** of our systems, god help us. Hormonal changes that we might have thought were just reproductive are *not*, and have never been, just reproductive.

Most hormones come into contact with all the cells of our body as they go through our bloodstream, but only cells with hormone receptors—proteins on the surface of or within a cell that bind to specific hormones—for a given hormone respond and bind to that hormone. If you've ever watched someone work a whole bar until they find someone who wants to go home with them, you know how this works. Cells also often have receptor cells for more than one kind of hormone: almost everyone is pansexual at the hormone bar. Score!

We have three basic types of hormones: amino acid–derived, or *amine*, hormones (like melatonin, thyroxine, epinephrine, and norepinephrine), *peptide* hormones (like insulin, prostaglandins, vasopressin, and oxytocin, as well as GnRH, FSH, and LH), and lipid-derived, or *steroid*, hormones (like cortisol, testosterone, estrogen, and progesterone).

WHAT ARE SOME OF THE THINGS ESTROGENS AND PROGESTERONE DO OR ARE PART OF?

Estrogens

- are a key player in the development of secondary sex characteristics, like breast tissue, body hair, and the menstrual cycle;
- are part of vulvovaginal development during puberty, keep vaginal walls thicker, and play a part in vaginal acidity and vulvovaginal lubrication;
- are messengers for numerous circuits throughout the central nervous system and boost the synthesis and function of neurotransmitters that affect sleep, mood, memory, sexual desire and response, pain, and cognitive factors such as learning and attention span;
- have a relationship with dopamine and endorphins—the often slut-shamed

neurochemicals you may know as the "feel-good" hormones—and other neurochemicals and, relatedly, help decrease the perception of pain;

◊ help balance cortisol, the "stress hormone";

◊ increase serotonin and serotonin receptors;

◊ play a role in mental health, with decreased or fluctuating estrogen levels understood to play a role in postpartum, (peri)menopausal, and menstrual depression or psychosis and also in obsessive compulsive disorder;

◊ help maintain the lining of the uterus and provide the fertilizer, as it were, for the ovum and the green light for ovulation during fertility cycles;

◊ stimulate the muscles of the uterus to develop and contract, including with menstruation, orgasm, and infant delivery, and play a part in the muscular growth and the contractions of the fallopian tubes;

◊ stimulate the body to produce cervical mucus;

◊ influence body hair and how voices sound;

◊ help maintain and regulate body temperature and also are involved in blood flow to our skin and sweating;

◊ have a lot to do with breasts, particularly the mammary glands;

◊ help regulate cholesterol and balance water and salt;

◊ often influence bloating, irritable bowel syndrome (IBS), and inflammation;

◊ influence body shape, particularly when it comes to breasts/chests, hips, and thighs, and also increase fat storage;

◊ increase insulin;

◊ regulate oil glands of the skin, maintain moisture and hyaluronic acid levels and collagen production, help protect the skin from sun damage, and help heal wounds;

◊ support lung function;

◊ protect the heart and bones.

Progesterone

◊ grows and regulates the endometrium;

◊ brings about menstruation when its levels dramatically drop;

◊ is essential for maintaining pregnancy, usually keeps any more ova from being released by the ovaries throughout pregnancy (in other words, is why you can't usually get pregnant when you're already pregnant), and stimulates the development of the glands of the breasts for milk production and lactation;

◊ relaxes smooth muscles (like those of the uterus and gut);

◊ helps with sleep, including by increasing production of GABA, a sleep-helping neurotransmitter;

◊ helps prevent seizures;

◊ helps regulate moods;

◊ helps build new bone;

- is required for brain function, protects the brain from damage, and promotes repair after brain injury;
- helps facilitate memory and ease anxiety;
- can be the why of constipation and can influence bloating;
- is a player in body-temperature regulation;
- with estrogen, is a common player in IBS;
- impacts metabolism;
- may help you quit smoking and other sticky habits;
- protects against breast and endometrial cancer as well as cardiovascular disease.

Very high levels of progesterone are often found with adrenal or ovarian cancers, ovarian cysts (which is why cysts often resolve with menopause), and congenital adrenal hyperplasia. Very low levels are associated with infertility, ectopic pregnancy, preeclampsia, miscarriage, missed or skipped periods, and unusual or unexplained uterine bleeding.

Estrogen and progesterone also work best in a specific balance to each other. So, when they aren't in that balance, we generally won't feel good.

Here's where we find our inner Ethel Merman and bring it all home.

Those two hormones can or do play a part in all of those things across all those systems of the body because of the staggering number of places we have estrogen and progesterone receptors in the cells of our bodies.

Where do we typically have estrogen and progesterone receptors?
- In the brain and central nervous system
- In the cardiovascular system
- In muscles and bones
- In the reproductive system and breasts
- In the gastrointestinal system
- In the immune system
- In the lungs
- In the eyes, skin, and hair
- In mucous membranes

In other words, we have them freaking *everywhere.*

This is why perimenopause and menopause can wreak such havoc for us and our whole bodies and why so many seemingly disparate things can go on because of and during either or both. If it feels like this is not sparing a single part of our bodies, minds, or lives, that's because it isn't.

WHEN DOES PERIMENOPAUSE START AND END?

Most typically, perimenopause starts somewhere in our forties; but it can also start in the thirties or, though more rarely, in the fifties.

The average age of official menopause—that anniversary of menstrual retirement, the day the perimenopause dies—varies a little by region and ethnicity, but fifty-one is the mean age

Perimenopause or menopause may happen earlier due to

- smoking, especially heavily or over a long time, including secondhand smoke;
- epilepsy;
- not having any pregnancies or births;
- malnutrition, being low weight, or having low body fat;
- thyroid conditions;
- autoimmune conditions like some types of diabetes, rheumatoid arthritis, or fibromyalgia;
- fragile X syndrome or Turner syndrome;
- partial hysterectomy;
- surgical removal of the ovaries or ovatestes;
- chemotherapy, radiation, or other medical treatments; or
- genetics.

Either may happen later due to

- later-life pregnancies or births;
- thyroid conditions;
- having higher body fat; or
- genetics.

people are when they get there, and it's been that age for a long time.

People who reach menopause before forty-five are usually said to have experienced "early" menopause. Those who don't start to transition into menopause until age fifty-five or later are sometimes said to be experiencing "late-onset" menopause. These time windows seem awfully arbitrary and not particularly useful to me, but in the event they're useful to you, there they are.

HOW DO YOU KNOW IF YOU'RE IN PERIMENOPAUSE?

You can't reliably test for perimenopause most of the time.

Figuring this out is more like following the rules of the *Final Destination* franchise. It's about looking for the signs, whether the person looking is you, a healthcare provider, or both. And if you hear John Denver playing, run.

If you've had fairly regular menstrual cycles up until recently, have they been changing, like getting closer and closer together or spreading further and further apart?

Are you skipping cycles or having any superheavy flow?

Are you having hot flashes or night sweats?

Do you feel otherwise inexplicably (I said *in*explicably) more irritable, more depressed, or more anxious? Do you just feel like something's different?

If you know the history of any relatives who went through perimenopause, did it happen around your same age?

Are you in or around your forties?

Did you cry once already over something in this book? Are you crying right now? Are you crying right now alone, on the cold (oh thank goodness) kitchen floor?

Did you buy this book?

You're probably in perimenopause.

BECAUSE HORMONES AND THEIR LEVELS are all over the place in perimenopause, but levels are also very fluid *pre*menopause, there's usually just no point in running a test because those levels can be so different from day to day either way. Until you're either *post*menopause or getting very close to it, you're not going to have the sustained low estrogen and high FSH levels that make clear you're either already past or near the end of perimenopause.

Dr. Judith Hersh, an OB/GYN, NAMS-certified menopause practitioner, and International Society for the Study of Women's Sexual Health fellow, says that even if and when she *could* run a blood test, "I don't treat a blood test or a number, I treat a person. So we'll talk about what's going on, and if it's interfering with quality of life, then we'll treat that." She calls perimenopause "Never-Never Land: because you just don't know. What I generally do with patients who aren't on medications that would affect their menstrual cycle, is say, 'When you've gone six months with-out a period, check in with me.' At *that* point, **then** I'll test hormone levels."

Healthcare providers like Dr. Hersh can and may also run *other* tests to rule out that it's not something else that can act like peri—like thyroid disorders or reproduc-tive cancers—and can help you go through the signs that you might be in this, but you can often do the latter all by yourself.

But by and large, Dr. Hersh and other menopause-literate providers figure that if you've got a uterus and ovaries and you're in your forties, just by those to-kens alone, you probably are going into or have already begun perimenopause. In the United Kingdom, the National Insti-tute for Health and Care Excellence offers a series of guidelines healthcare providers are supposed to follow when working with people who are currently or potentially peri- or postmenopausal. The guidelines make clear that no one over forty-five having vasomotor symptoms or irreg-ular periods, who hasn't had a period in twelve months and isn't using a hormonal method of birth control, or who doesn't have a uterus anymore should be given FSH tests to determine if they are in peri-menopause or postmenopause. That's not because it isn't safe but because it's usually just unnecessary. It's fine to presume that people showing a certain common profile are probably in perimenopause.

If you're one of those people who wants to know things absolutely, positively, for sure, I'm sorry to tell you that you have to be all the way on the other side of this to get that kind of certainty. There's also no test you can take or other way to know when it will be over once it's started. But you don't need a test to manage impacts of perimenopause like mood or mental health issues, sleep issues, hot flashes, or constipation. All the things we—or a care provider—can do to help with those things are things we can do merely be-cause they're happening.

HOW LONG DOES THIS WHOLE THING LAST?

Who the hell knows. No seriously: **Who knows?** Can they call me? Unfortunately, this is something where *everybody* says something different. That's probably be-cause it's both so diverse and so hard to quantify that a super-specific answer is impossible, but it's still really annoying.

Anecdotally, some people report that it didn't happen to them at all, that they just stopped having periods (it seems more likely their perimenopause was instead both uneventful and short and/*or* they had something else going on that had their attention, but who knows: bodies are weird, unpredictable, and diverse), so that's a theoretical albeit unlikely length of zero years. Some people report they have been or were in this for twenty-five years. It's not common, but some people who have been postmenopausal for de-cades will say they feel like some parts of this—like hot flashes—just never ended for them. That gets us to its ending in anywhere from zero years to never, which feels extraordinarily unhelpful and also saps my will to live.

Equally unhelpful is the fact that when sources give estimates, they're often unclear about how they're defining perimenopause or menopause. Some only consider perimenopause to begin when menstrual irregularities begin (and also don't account for those who don't have periods, period, or who already had irregularity for other reasons). Others have a more modern take that looks at an array of possible changes and impacts. For all these reasons and more, even reliable sources have a wide array of answers.

Our Bodies, Ourselves: Menopause and Toni Weschler in *Taking Charge of Your Fertility* both say perimenopause lasts around a decade. The Centre for Menstrual Cycle and Ovulation Research says, "On average the perimenopause lasts several years and commonly lasts six or seven." NAMS says four to eight years. *The Menopause Myth* by Dr. Ariana Sholes-Douglas says one to eight. On its website, Harvard Medical School says, "The average duration is three to four years, although it can last just a few months or extend as long as a decade." And the scientists in a mid-1990s study, "The Influence of Age on Symptoms of Perimenopause," who clearly have a death wish, say, "According to some experts, it can span a 25-year period from approximately age 35 to 60 years."

Based on all that and my greater confidence in some sources, and taking the STRAW staging and data from other studies into account, I'm inclined to say we're looking at somewhere between half a decade and a decade and a half.

I know that's not the best news you've ever heard. Maybe figure that if you prepare yourself for twenty years of this and it only lasts five, you're going to be in for a wonderful surprise. I don't think anyone should figure they'll only have just a few months of this, because it seems guaranteed to really, really piss you off when it's years instead. I also feel like Menopause's Law is that if you assume it's going to be over fast, it will take ninety million years to be over. I think it's most sound to think about this like an informed person might think about divorce: it's probably going to last longer than you want it to and longer than your lawyer gave you an estimate for, so it's probably best to prepare for the worst just in case.

OTHER ROUTES TO MENOPAUSE

For many who experience it, menopause occurs both spontaneously because of aging and with some kind of gradual transition, and that's the kind this book focuses on. But there are other ways of experiencing menopause too. This isn't an exhaustive list and only very briefly summarizes each of these.

"PREMATURE" MENOPAUSE OR PRIMARY OVARIAN INSUFFICIENCY (POI)

You may also hear this called "premature ovarian failure" or "decreased ovarian reserve."

POI is menopause that happens when people reach menopause considerably earlier than expected. If you are or were in perimenopause in your twenties or thirties—it can even happen to some in their teens—or found yourself on the other side of menopause before forty and haven't had any kind of surgery or medical treatment that can cause menopause, you're probably someone experiencing or who has experienced POI.

It's understood to happen because of medical conditions like chromosomal disorders or certain intersex conditions (such as Turner syndrome or Fragile X syndrome), thyroid conditions, diabetes, autoimmune disorders, surgeries, or medications that have affected the blood supply to the ovaries. It's sometimes used to describe menopause due to radiation or chemotherapy treatment when that happens for younger people. Very early menopause can also be genetic.

POI is said to occur for anywhere from 1 to 5 percent of people with utero-ovarian systems, but since diagnosis is rare, that number might be higher. Blood tests can verify it the same way they can show menopause has happened: with high FSH and low estradiol levels.

SUDDEN MENOPAUSE

I'm talking about menopause that can occur due to radical hysterectomy (removal

There are some increased risks for people who experience early menopause. Many of these increased risks can be prevented, forestalled, minimized, or treated with recognition and care:

* Depression
* Heart disease and stroke
* Lower bone density and osteoporosis
* Feelings of social isolation (this can particularly happen around pregnancy and childbearing as well as exclusion from other age-normative lifestyles or events)
* Autoimmune disorders (or additional autoimmune disorders for those who already have one or more)
* Cognitive function issues

of both the uterus and ovaries) or bilateral oophorectomy (removal of both ovaries), as a result of some treatments for illness, or anything else that damages the ovaries. These can lead to what is sometimes called "surgically induced" or "treatment-induced" menopause, respectively. Either permanent or temporary menopause can result from some medical treatments, such as chemotherapy (aka "chemopause"), pelvic radiation, or medications like tamoxifen, leuprolide, or Zoladex.

Whereas gradual menopause is often like riding a roller coaster, sudden menopause is like that ride where you shoot all the way up and are then quickly dropped all the way down: it's faster and usually also way more intense.

How sudden it is depends on how someone got there. Menopause due to chemotherapy or other medical treatment often occurs over months; menopause that happens due to surgical removal of both ovaries happens instantly. But just as the case can be with some who come to menopause gradually, a minority of those who come to it suddenly can experience some menopause impacts, like hot flashes or fatigue, for a long time.

Those who experience sudden menopause, especially those who aren't already in or very near perimenopause, can have a harder time with it—particularly if they lack proper medical support—than those who experience menopause with a gradual transition. Most people who experience sudden menopause will need ongoing medical care and treatment, often including hormone therapy. Sinéad O'Connor recently talked about how lack of proper medical support after a total hysterectomy to treat her endometriosis brought on extreme mental illness, including suicidality, for her. "I was told to leave the hospital two days after the surgery with Tylenol and no hormone replacements and no guidance as to what might happen to me," she said. There's long been a clear consensus about hormone therapy after hysterectomy, oophorectomy, or both: for those who are able to use it safely, either estrogen, progesterone, or both are typically advised to help with both short- and long-term impacts.

OOPHORECTOMY AND HYSTERECTOMY

Oophorectomy is the removal of one or both ovaries and sometimes the fallopian tubes too. Hysterectomy is the removal of the uterus, sometimes with the cervix, sometimes not. Sometimes hysterectomy has been, and still is, wanted; sometimes it hasn't been and is not. Sometimes it hasn't even been consensual.

Hysterectomy has a long and sordid history (and oophorectomy doesn't have a great one either). It's a procedure that at times is and has been necessary or sound and has also often been hastily pursued when less invasive options were available. Additionally, it has a deeply awful and traumatic origin as a part of the systematic oppression of Black women and those with developmental disabilities. As you may recall, modern American gynecology originates from the "work" of James Marion Sims who operated on enslaved Black women without consent or anesthesia. This kind of abuse continues today in disproportionate use of hysterectomy in these communities and others. Mass hysterectomies of immigrant women without their full, informed consent in an Immigration and Customs Enforcement detention center in Georgia were just recently exposed.

America has the highest rate of hysterectomy in the world, with around six hundred thousand hysterectomies performed annually. Approximately twenty million American people have had a hysterectomy. By the age of sixty, more than one-third of all women in the United States have.

About 90 percent of hysterectomies now are done electively, rather than as an emergency or lifesaving procedure. There is an array of reasons for either or both of these surgeries, including fibroids, endometriosis, pelvic inflammatory disease, prolapse, reproductive cancers, hyperplasia, and ovarian cysts; they can also be a means to manage certain cancers or prophylactically to prevent them, to control

severe childbirth complications or severe, uncontrollable uterine bleeding, and as a method of gender affirmation.

People who have only a hysterectomy, without removal of or damage to the ovaries, will typically still come to menopause via perimenopause, as they would have had they retained their uterus. Because of the lack of hormonal feedback from the uterus to the ovaries, however, it may occur earlier.

If, as it does about half the time, hysterectomy includes bilateral oophorectomy ("radical" or "total" hysterectomy) of both ovaries or ovotestes, sudden menopause will occur as a result. If only one ovary has been removed and another remains, it's a hybrid gradual/sudden menopause experience, and menopause often occurs earlier. Unless hormone therapy is used afterward (or has already been used leading up to the surgery, as with those using testosterone), estrogen levels will quickly drop to around half as much as the ovaries or ovotestes were jointly producing before. Whenever it happens after that, the menopausal transition may be a little easier because the body has already adjusted to less estrogen, and you've already got a head start on managing the whole thing.

TEMPORARY MENOPAUSE

This is an impermanent pause of the reproductive system, sometimes called medical menopause. It can happen sometimes with radiation or chemo, use of selective estrogen receptor modulators, or ovarian-suppression therapy used for conditions like endometriosis, fibroids, or breast cancer. With treatments that can bring about either temporary or permanent menopause, menopause is more likely to be permanent the closer a person is to the time of life they'd start to experience menopause due to aging and more likely to be temporary the further away from that time someone is. This term is also sometimes applied to people who stop ovulating and menstruating for other reasons, including long-term use of hormonal birth-control methods or because of eating disorders or very high levels of exercise.

People who experience temporary menopause will still go through menopause as a result of aging. You can also experience temporary menopause more than once and then menopause due to aging. I have no words to adequately describe the grave injustice of these situations, so I'm not even going to try. Let's just say I think sainthood and a pension should be on the table.

TESTOSTERONE USE

If you've been using testosterone at levels typical for gender transition or affirmation for at least six months, your body has already started a gradual menopause transition. If you've been on it for a couple years or more, even without radical hysterectomy, you're probably already all the way done.

The menopause that can happen with testosterone therapy will usually be similar to later perimenopause and pretty quick comparatively. Setting aside the range of effects testosterone brings to the table itself, the erratic estrogen and progesterone fluctuations common in early perimenopause probably won't happen, because of increasingly higher levels of testosterone from the HT. Some of the emotional volatility a lot of people feel when they start T is because of T, but some of it is also because of the change in hormone balance that results in dropping, and then eventually minimal, estrogen levels. So, in some ways, it may feel like sudden menopause. A menopause transition without testosterone in which all the biggest hormonal shifts happen in just one year would be considered fast.

SYSTEMIC ESTROGEN WITHDRAWAL

Suddenly or gradually withdrawing from estrogen hormone therapy, either by choice, because of surgeries or health conditions, or due to lack of access, can be similar to suddenly or gradually going through menopause, regardless of one's gonads or assigned sex at birth. Similar physical impacts can occur—like hot flashes and night sweats, sleep disturbances, and genital dryness—as can similar possible psychological impacts, like anxiety, depression, or dysphoria, particularly for transgender women (for more, see the appendix).

Some people who started hormone therapy during and for their menopausal transition will also sometimes describe coming off of it as feeling like they've picked up where they left off in terms of menopause. Some people who withdraw from estrogen therapy cold turkey seem to do okay, but others experience this way of "finishing" menopause as more difficult than they found menopause before using estrogen. Coming off estrogen can be especially difficult for those who have been using it for ten years or more.

CHAPTER FOUR

YA BASICS

"Always start out with a larger pot than what you think you need."
—*Julia Child*

Until the last couple years, I did almost nothing to take care of myself with menopause. I did plenty for other people, even when it came to *my* menopause, but little for myself.

My root concept of both menopause and myself in menopause positioned us both as burdens. When I *did* think about how I was going to manage it, my thoughts were focused on how I would keep our burden on others as minimal as possible. Sound familiar?

I feel a need to defend myself to you and my inner feminist overlord. There were some less pathetic, less eldest-daughter syndrome reasons too. I had no freaking **idea** how long this could last and when things *started* happening I thought that meant I was at the end. How quaint. I had massive healthcare and economic fatigue and strain because of my spine and chronic pain, and my healthcare coverage was limited. I couldn't get around.

I felt like shit from enough other things, and I figured I'd still feel shitty anyway, so why bother. Also, go figure, once you are in menopause and having a Very Bad Time, you may find yourself too exhausted to find care, too irritable to ask people in your life to make more room for you as you go through this, and too damn hot and dry to do just about anything.

I didn't know what my options were or that the options were far more than just estrogen therapy or no estrogen therapy. I didn't know the ways the healthcare providers I'd tried to talk to had wrong, outdated, or incomplete information, and I didn't know the right things to ask for. I didn't know that this wasn't all about doctors in the first place, that a lot of things I could start on my own were probably going to be the most impactful and accessible, and that they were things I needed to be doing, working on, or privileging more for myself and my long-term health anyway.

I think the biggest thing, and the only universally best thing, you can do for yourself in this is to immediately start **taking more care of yourself**. Only you can sort out how much more "more" needs to be and what that care looks like for you. You may or may not need or want physical or mental healthcare in this, or any specific kind of it. You may not be into taking any kind of medicines, buying anything, or even talking that much about it. But unless you have the shortest, most uneventful menopausal transition of all time (up yours, by the way, if so), I think it's safe to say you are going to need to take some more care of yourself.

YA BASICS

There's a handful of (seemingly) super-duper basic advice that care providers and others, solicited or no, commonly offer to people in menopause, especially those of us who are expressing, in the parlance of our times, that we are not fucking okay. Receiving this advice is often accompanied by a strong desire to slug its author, a wholly understandable response.

That advice is usually some or all of the following:
- "Reduce and manage stress."
- "Improve your sleep."
- "Hydrate."
- "Get active."
- "Get emotional support."
- "Quit smoking."

- "Get on hormones," or, its alter ego, something like, "Don't touch hormones with a ten-foot pole; are you crazy, they'll kill you!"
- "Lose weight."

I'll get to hormone therapy in a bit (but if you don't want to wait, it starts on page 95). Polarized and forceful universals are never useful, those about hormone therapy very much included. I'll also deal with the weight loss advice later. I'm in no mood. I never am, but we need to talk about it, so I will. Later. And resentfully.

To the great annoyance of many, myself included, the remaining suggestions all appear to be objectively excellent advice for everyone during and *after* menopause. Based on what we know to date, and supported by science, these things can often help with many, if not most, menopausal impacts, the whole of our menopausal experience and its outcomes, and life postmenopause. It's so irritating when everyone is right.

These suggestions aren't magic. They won't likely make a wholly dismal menopause experience dreamy, but they will usually at least improve things. Most of them are also low-cost or free, but they do demand some investments of time, attention, and energy. But since they're all associated with better health outcomes during menopause *and* on the other side, they're solid investments.

They also aren't all easy for everyone. Some of these things, sometimes all of these things, are seriously challenging for some of us and can even require pretty heavy lifting. Sometimes they're just not a lift we can manage at all at a given time or in a given period. Each to their ability.

But. Once we get into the impacts and what can help, you're going to see these coming up again and again. I figured you might want an explanation. I did. I thought you might need some help with some of these too. I ~~did~~ do. (Who do I think I'm kidding?)

Here's the scoop.

"REDUCE AND MANAGE STRESS"

When things create stress for us—whether those things are external, like money, kids, or traffic, or internal, like chronic illness, trauma, or major physical or psychological change, even the positive kind—that stress creates chemical changes throughout our bodies, namely, an increase in cortisol and other stress-related hormones.

For the uninitiated, cortisol is a steroid hormone like estrogen and testosterone. It's produced and regulated by the hypothalamus and the adrenal and pituitary glands. Just as the body has estrogen and progesterone receptors, it has cortisol receptors. Just as all those estrogen and progesterone receptors mean those hormones can be felt across the body and impact nearly all its systems, the same is true of cortisol. When we get stressed, the brain sounds an alarm across the sympathetic nervous system that triggers the release of adrenaline. Once that adrenaline increases, our heart rate goes up, taking our blood pressure with it, and a bunch of other systematic changes occur. If that stress and our heightened response keeps up long enough, cortisol and a couple other supporting hormone players are released.

Cortisol isn't a problem in and of itself. It's good we have cortisol and that our body increases it sometimes. If our body is stressed because we have low blood sugar, cortisol helps pick it up. If blood pressure rises, cortisol helps to lower it. It helps with memory. In the right balance, it manages and stabilizes inflammation. It and adrenaline are how we can react fast, like when, say, we're about to get run over by a car because we walked into a busy street while only paying attention to that cute person crossing on the other side, a thing I don't know anything about.

The problems arise when stress becomes chronic and our cortisol levels stay sustained, fly up often, or both.

Having increased cortisol during any phase of menopause can amplify some of the common impacts: hot flashes, mood issues or disorders, cognitive function issues, and also some of the long-term health risks that increase once we're postmenopausal, like bone loss, insulin resistance, and cardiovascular risks. When cortisol elevates, progesterone also decreases, so the benefits of progesterone, which we're already getting less of during and after perimenopause, decrease even more.

Increased cortisol can make it tougher for us to do other things that usually make menopause go better. It makes it harder to sleep. It increases inflammation. It makes it easier to get upset—and then even more stressed—and harder to get our shit back together.

MANAGING STRESS IS TWOFOLD. I explain this because if I know anything in this world, it's that people experiencing menopause are stressed beyond stressed, and few of us have been raised in a world or environments where people taught us how to manage stress and reminded us often, and with care, that we should.

Managing stress is about doing what we can to avoid, limit, reduce, or dump things that create stress for us in the first place and doing what we can to respond to stress when it does occur so it has less of an impact.

You may already know the drill with all this, and you probably also already have a good idea of what your stressors are. Just in case you don't, or it's helpful to have someone back you up in what you already know, here's a top ten:

1. **Take on fewer things.** Chances are good that some of your stress comes from biting off more than anyone should chew. Inventory your life and the things in it that cause you stress, and start doing what you can to delegate, share, change, or eliminate them. Fewer stressors = less stress.

2. **Deal with your tough stuff, especially any trauma and its impacts.**

3. **Give less of a fuck.** There's a lot of talk from well-adjusted people on the other side of menopause about how they care a lot less about a lot more things than they did before. I believe this is often a survival skill picked up in perimenopause, one that likely kept them from yelling at other people and helped them carve out the time, space, and energy to care for themselves, often after a process of figuring out they gave way too many fucks to adequately deal with any of this.

4. **Insist other people manage themselves.** See Chapter 13 plus also #1, #3, and #5. My mother told me her friend Maggie's dream job is to be the person who pushes people out of the plane during skydiving lessons. We could all stand to think more like Maggie.

5. **Take out the trash.** If it's garbage, get rid of it, get the hell away from it, or at least protect yourself as best you can in the meantime and do what you can to get ready to dump it as soon as it's safe or otherwise feasible

for you to do so. Maybe the garbage is your job, a friend, a partner or spouse, a belief, an interpersonal dynamic, pants, or a way you beat up on yourself. Whatever it is, try and find a way to get it out of your life, head, or heart.

6. **Move, rest, and pursue positive social interactions, even if they're tiny.**

7. **Do things you like that help you relax your body and your mind.** Maybe that's coloring, a shower, masturbation or sex with a partner, or making or listening to music. Maybe it's stretching; maybe it's benzodiazepines; maybe it's taking a walk. Whatever it is, so long as it feels like a physical and emotional exhale, that's the stuff.

8. **Breathe.** I literally forget to do it all the time. I mean I forget plain old breathing, not even deep breathing, which is even better to do to manage stress.

9. **Whatever it is, take a break from it.**

10. **Close the stress cycle.** When it comes to how to manage stress when or as it's happening, there are about a million things you can do, but they generally boil down to three basic groups: chilling your body and mind out, getting some kind of social support, or revving your body up (so you can then chill out). Here's how you do the last one.

Nutritional support for stress aligns with some things recommended for people in menopausal transition. Go figure. B vitamins (B1, B2, B6, and B12) can help reduce stress. Vitamin C can help regulate cortisol and clear it from the body. Magnesium is a mineral that can get depleted by stress and helps us and our muscles to de-stress, and zinc helps keep our digestion from adding stress to our bodies. You can also check out some of the herbal chiller-outers in the mini-herbal on page 279.

Any time I talk about nutrients, know that it's always best to get them straight from the source via food as much as possible. But if and when you can't, supplements can work too. Just be sure that (1) you don't take more than is recommended and try only to supplement what you're actually missing in your diet, and (2) that you're using quality supplements. As kiran nigam advises, "You want to get supplements in their bioavailable, rather than synthetic, forms so that you can integrate and absorb them, rather than burdening your liver with more toxins to clear. This can often come with a big price difference. My recommendation to my clients is if the bioavailable, high-quality supplement is twice as expensive, get it, and just take it every other day."

CLOSING THE STRESS CYCLE

Emily Nagoski, PhD, and Amelia Nagoski, DMA's *Burnout* is a wildly helpful book I strongly encourage you to read in its entirety.

Here's one longer story from it made short: all that chemical stuff our bodies do under stress and all the systematic impacts are all about preparing us—and our muscles—for fight, flight, or freeze responses to danger. Once all of that happens, if we don't use that whipped-up energy—even if the thing that was causing us stress is itself gone or no longer has an immediate effect on us—our bodies can get stuck in the middle of that stress response. It sticks around, and with it, chemicals and their impacts, which don't do us any favors.

The more stress we experience or hold, the more this all just keeps piling up. This is not good, especially when we are in at least one something (menopause) that, in and of itself, often causes stress.

One efficient way to resolve this cycle and put accumulated stress away is by doing the things our bodies would have done intuitively way back when, as Emily and Amelia say, we were running from lions instead of from Zoom meetings. Ideally, we want to do something physical that gets us breathing more deeply and gets our hearts pumping in a good way—anything safe for us that we can do for twenty to sixty minutes a day. We can also do it right after something stressful for quick relief. What we do to take care of this will obviously depend on our abilities, opportunities, immediate needs, or limitations. Some people may jog; others may dance, box, or ride. Someone else may run into a bathroom stall at work and jump up and down or scream into a pillow, and others still may do an upper-body chair or bed workout. I have found that aerobically flailing Kermit arms can be very effective.

PHYSICAL ACTIVITY ISN'T THE ONLY WAY to do this. Another way to get your body and mind to a relaxed, stress-resolved place might be intentional breathing: I'm talking about breathing techniques like those in yoga traditions, box breathing (breathing through your nose to a count of four in, holding gently for four, exhaling through your mouth for four, then pausing for another four before you start again), or a shorter inhale (count of four) and longer exhale (count of eight), or just slowing yourself down with a couple big, deep breaths instead of yelling.

More ways are things like meditation, or prayer—I typed "medication" there first, for at least the second time in writing this book, which tells you something about me, but it should be noted that medication does certainly belong in this list, if things like anxiety medications, selective serotonin reuptake inhibitors (SSRIs) or serotonin-norepinephrine reuptake inhibitors (SNRIs), cannabis, or other kinds of medications work for you. Being in nature; soothing movement like stretching, massage, or other bodywork; t'ai chi, yoga, or progressive muscle relaxation/body scanning; reading a comforting book; taking a bath; having sex; or napping can do it too. A long kiss may even do the job. So can a primal scream. I don't advise trying both at the same time.

Social support and other positive social interactions are other ways. That's talk and other kinds of therapy, affection, hanging out with people who make you feel happy, playing with your pets, even just saying "good morning" on the street to someone who says it back (and definitely does not say, "Up yours, lady").

Emily and Amelia also add creative expression and both crying and laughing to this list. Those of us already rapidly cycling through both on a regular basis may appreciate this call for our special talents.

The other bit of good news here is that all of these things help us to be more resilient to stress, so we've less accumulated stress to manage in the first place. All the more reason to prioritize and do these things that we and our bodies often really want to do anyway.

"IMPROVE YOUR SLEEP"

Since one of the things that is often highly disruptive to sleep during perimenopause *is* perimenopause, this advice may seem deeply dense. It's not, I swear, but you can feel as irritated with me as you want.

Trouble with sleep is one of the most common issues for people in every phase of menopause. Studies of menopausal sleep show it often becomes progressively more difficult to sleep through each phase, from premenopause to postmenopause. *Fantastic.*

If we're in our forties and fifties as most perimenopausal folks are, we likely *already* have too much on our plates and, as a result, too much stress, which impacts our sleep. Also, we're women, trans, and other gender-diverse people who have been living under patriarchy for decades already and are now experiencing menopause, and usually aging too, in its context. This hasn't, and doesn't, exactly make it easy to sleep soundly.

Never one to arrive to the party without a horribly chosen gift, menopause often brings its *own* sleep challenges.

If you didn't already have them, menopausal sleep disruptions can include
- hot flashes, night sweats, and chills;
- anxiety and panic attacks;
- heartburn, acid reflux, and other gastrointestinal issues;
- deeply unreasonable urinary system demands and reactions, like urgency or urinary tract infections;
- sleep apnea;
- restless leg syndrome;
- dry, itchy skin;
- genital discomfort or pain;
- heavy periods;
- a persistent low-grade level of rage and dread;

- if you drink, the way booze interacts with your body, especially at night, and the same for things like many yummy snacks, including oily, sweet, or spicy foods; and

- exhaustion, which really *should* help with sleep, and yet here we are, with me writing this and you reading it at this hour.

Erratic hormone levels like those in early peri mess with sleep, given all the systems that respond to those changes and that inconsistency.

Progesterone plays a big part in sleep, all by itself. When progesterone is low, we tend to feel more anxious and restless. During perimenopause, progesterone often gets and starts to stay lower earlier on. Low progesterone messes with sleep because it messes with our ability to chill out enough *to* sleep.

Sleep deprivation or crummy sleep makes a mess of us in the best of conditions. kiran nigam summed it up: the amount and the quality of our sleep have an impact on almost every system of our body, some of which you'll recognize as particular issues during menopause—our endocrine and immune systems, metabolism, cognition, neurological issues, cell regulation, and stress levels. Sleep loss and sleep disruption are themselves major stressors. And in and around menopause, a lack of or low-quality sleep can do even more damage.

Sleep trouble can elicit or worsen menopausal impacts, including cognitive issues, hot flashes, irritability, impatience, depression, anxiety, and sexual desire and function. A lot of people diet to address weight concerns, but improved sleep is more likely to help maintain our own, unique healthy size range and, unlike dieting, does us no harm. Sleep also helps protect us from some long-term menopause health concerns like increased risks of diabetes and cardiovascular issues; if those are already present, it is a help in managing them.

HOW THE BLEEP DO YOU IMPROVE YOUR SLEEP?

I, perhaps like you, consider sleep to have gone very well when I can get to bed around the time I should, fall asleep within a half hour or so of trying, stay asleep most of the night, when weeping is not part of the process, and get more than five or six hours of it.

I've got a long history of big sleep trouble that includes chronic pain, anxiety, trauma and post-traumatic stress disorder, bladders and other organs, housemates, work, a stalker, midwestern summers, periods and pregnancies, an array of animal life, including bedbugs, construction, quote-unquote creativity, tequila, heartbreak, poverty, patriarchy, sex (the having of it, the lack of it, the waiting for someone to show up at 2 a.m. for it), the bus, the drunk outside the window (including the times I *was* the drunk outside the window), other people's children, gunshots, mufflers, this eerie random thump we hear from our upstairs neighbor's place at night and only during winter, three household fires, two late-night floods, and a mad squirrel in a pear tree.

Oh, and lest we forget, which we might, as we do so much else, perimenopause.

Recently, I've started to figure out how to play the games it seems my sleep appreciates. Even with some suboptimal changes in sleeping conditions (when apartment hunting, always count how many kinds of dumpsters are under the bedroom window), my efforts have been paying off. I am now semi-reliably having nights of excellent sleep. This is great timing, because after three to four decades of sleep deprivation and horrible sleep, I am exhausted. I'd even say, though I'm afraid to jinx it, that my sleep has improved enough that it's probably played a big role in making some parts of peri less miserable for me. If figuring out how to get more and better sleep doesn't make a big dent in *your* level (or lack!) of menopausal misery, you *will* at least be sleeping through more of it. I'd give just about anything to Rip Van Winkle my way to the other side of this if that were an option.

So, how do you make sleep, and better sleep, happen? It's mostly basic stuff you may already know, but maybe you need an extra nudge of permission to review and then do some of these things for yourself. There are also some things that are more specific to what is often called "menopausal sleep." As if. Some of those things may not make that oxymoron an alternate reality, but they might at least help.

Before, around, or at bedtime:

- Within your abilities, increase how much movement you get in a day. Cardio and other high-key stuff are best earlier in the day from a sleep standpoint, but something mellow, like gentle stretching, restorative yoga, a chill evening walk, or a very light swim, closer to bed shouldn't interfere and might even make it *easier* to sleep. More movement usually = more sleepiness and sounder sleep.

- If it's okay for you, consider a buffer of three to four hours between eating and bedtime, or avoid or limit things that ask a lot of ye olde gastrointestinal system or make you wired before and while sleeping. Eating when you wake up in the middle of the night can be emotionally comforting but makes getting back to sleep tougher.

- Try to stick to the same bedtime and waking time each day. If you can't manage it with bedtime, a consistent waking time is apparently the most important of the two when it comes to sleep.

- Bedtime rituals or routines help tell the body and brain it's time for sleep.

Brushing your teeth, turning your ringer off, reading, telling your kids you weren't kidding and they need to go to bed too, having a wank, meditating, praying for insomnia absolution, whatever it is you do to get ready for bed each night—doing them all as regular, repeated habits helps.

🍃 Screens and bright lights before bed are generally not friends of sleep because they tell the brain to **STAY AWAKE**!!! Besides ditching or limiting phone and computer lights before bed, you can gradually turn down all the lights as you're making your way to bedtime, just like they do on the airplane. It feels fancy and can become part of a sleep routine.

🍃 Rolling over and falling asleep after masturbation or sex with a partner can be nature's Ambien. Just saying.

🍃 Pharmaceutical sleep medications and other kinds of medicines are also options. That can be anything from teas, tinctures, supplements, or other forms of herbal or nutritional medicine *to* pharmaceuticals like Ambien, depending on what is okay for you and you have access to. It can even be a placebo. Cannabis and sexuality educator and *The CBD Solution: Sex* author Ashley Manta told me that tetrahydrocannabinol (THC) (one of the primary compounds of cannabis) can have thermoregulating effects: "Cannabinoids like THC work with our bodies'

endocannabinoid systems to create homeostasis. Folks having night sweats, hot flashes or insomnia might find consuming a THC product right before bed helps with sleep." Ashley suggested a quicker-acting consumption method like inhalation before you go to bed if falling asleep is a problem and pairing it with a cannabis edible if staying asleep is a problem, since it'll hit later. Whatever you may use, taking it as part of a bedtime routine will usually bump up its efficacy. Just be sure to look out for interactions and be safe.

The "sleep environment" (aka that soft place under the laundry and the dog):

🍃 Try and keep where you sleep sleep-only or sleep- and sex-only. The fewer things that happen there during waking hours, the more our impressionable minds will associate it with sleep and rest and will feel readier to snooze just by being there.

🍃 Don't wear a ton of clothes to bed if you can help it: better to keep extra layers next to the bed that you can grab while half-asleep. That may work better when they're blankets rather than clothes. Whereas kicking off or pulling up a blanket probably won't wake you up, trying to get pajama bottoms on over your head in your sleep probably will. I learn these things so you don't have to.

🍃 Better ventilation = better sleep. Open windows, doors, a fan, or all of the above: anything that keeps air moving around should help with sleep. Especially if you're sweating your ass off. Truly, *whatever* you think could make your sleep space more conducive to your sleep, you're probably right that it'd help, and you should try it.

◊ Sleeping with another human may make sleep more difficult for you. Sleeping with *you* may make sleep more challenging for them too. Kimberly Dark lived with a partner who was in perimenopause. Peri wasn't that big a deal for her partner. They had a flexible life in which they could make a lot of adaptations, including work and sleep hours. They said perimenopause wasn't a problem unless they said it was a problem. Kimberly told me, "That was a pretty funny thing to say to me, especially with hot flashes where she'd fill the bed with sweat and rip off all the blankets or turn on all the lights to change the bedding in the middle of the night. I'd be like, well, as the person sleeping next to you, don't I *also* get to say what's a problem?" If sleeping alone makes sleeping easier for you, those who would otherwise be your co-sleepers, or both, go for it.

SOME POTENTIAL PURCHASES

If you don't have one already, get yourself a fan for where you sleep. You're probably going to want it to have some different levels and some flexibility with where it can be (versus, say, a fixed window fan). Wheeled fans are the bomb.

The bed itself and bedding tend to make a difference. When I got to the point in my spinal degeneration that I was in bed full-time, I did myself and my body the service of getting an actually good mattress. I was still at thinking any mattress was better than a cheap American futon. I needed to graduate.

If you're dealing with vasomotor stuff (hot flashes and night sweats), you probably want what stays coolest or feels coolest in both a mattress and bedding. If you've got the budget for linen sheets, everyone I know who does never shuts up about them. Not even when I beg. Cotton, eucalyptus, and bamboo fibers and natural or poly blends that specifically advertise themselves as wicking can do the job, and the more menopausal we get, the more of these seem to crop up. (Though we may wind up resenting menopausal marketing less in this area than others.)

I have a cooling pillow that I carry with me, very like I did my teddy bear when I was a kid. I had him with me *always*, and I would have cut you if you came for him. Just so we're clear, stay the eff away from my pillow.

There's a bunch of options with these, including just making your existing pillow cooler. You can put a big, rectangular ice pack—the soft mushy kind—inside

Ode on a Cooling Pillow

Thou divine frigid cradle of promised
    sleep,
Thou frosty bear of squishy, quiet time,
Oh coldest mistress, oh counter of sheep,
Whose snow-bitten cheeks touch mine:
What mem'ry foamed legend creates
    thy shape
Of cubes or fluff, or of both,
In what remains of melting
    Greenland?
What polyester gods are these?
    What chilly oath?
And I, now more hirsute, with such
    sweet fire escape?
What soothing icicles? What cool
    command?

Ah, happy, happy cold! that doth put out
The overheated head, the igneous
    brow;
And, downy crown, who be no layabout,
The fevered sear you disallow;
Beloved bleakness! Dream of penguins!

Forever freezed and thus to be enjoy'd,
Forever wintry, and forever unsung;
All shivering passion far above,
That refuses to leave me annoy'd,
By burning forehead, and a parching
    tongue.

O arctic heritage! Glacial hammock!
    with brede
Of man-made materials so lovingly
    overwrought,
With silken floof that doth intercede
The blistering fevers my wicked
    biochemistry hath brought
As doth eternity: Cold Pastoral!
When overuse shall this cushion waste,
Thou shalt remain, in midst of
    other woe
Than ours, a friend to menopause, to
    whom thou say'st,
"Your raison d'etre is my midlife
    cliché—that is all
Ye know on earth, and all ye need to
    know."

your pillowcase before you go to sleep or under the pillow, if you're more of a flipping-to-the-cold-side person. Because night sweats often start on or around your head and upper body, as hot flashes do, a cool pillow can make a big difference at keeping you from overheating in the first place.

Never underestimate the power of pillow / wedge / bolster / rolled blanket / body pillow architecture, especially if you're having joint pain, headaches, apnea, or gastrointestinal bleck. Being most comfortable going to sleep and while sleeping—like via a rolled blanket under your knees to better support your back, a wedge to raise your head to help prevent or manage acid reflux—obviously helps. Guides to restorative yoga often include a lot of suggestions about props and body positioning for rest.

You might want to experiment with sleeping positions besides your Old Faithful too. Our bodies are changing: sometimes we need to change how we physically support them.

THE BATTLE OF MOUNT THERMOSTAT

In my humble opinion, if there's only one person in menopause in your home, that person trumps everyone else when it comes to the temperature of the domicile, or, at the very least, the room they sleep in. Extra blankets for everyone (except us)! If you feel more magnanimous than I, you can perhaps find some kind of mutual compromise. I'd just reserve veto power for The Worst Nights Ever.

If you aren't the only one in menopause and your temperature needs don't always match, you might make an agreement about whoever's got it worse that night getting their way, see if you can't get a bigger bed, or sleep in different rooms where you can each make your own temperature adjustments.

If not, you duel at dawn.

If you can't get to or stay sleep ("If." "Or." Ha.):

❥ If you can't fall asleep within a half hourish, get out of bed and go somewhere else where you can do something that makes you feel sleepy, then try again. UK-based meditation and mindfulness resource Headspace says, "The goal of this technique, called stimulus control, is to break the association of bed as a place of frustration and worry."

❥ Try faking yourself out by trying to stay awake instead of trying to go to sleep. Sometimes sleep can work like orgasm: if you focus too much on trying to make it happen, it's less likely to happen. Good night, and good luck.

P.S.

❥ If you have chronic pain, chances are good you already have sleep issues because you have chronic pain. If they're getting worse with peri- or postmenopause, don't forget to say something to your care providers.

I NEED TO PREPARE YOU FOR SOMETHING

All this work on sleep may not work right away. It may not work for weeks or even months. It may not work period.

It may be in a process of desperate sleep-improving experimentation that you find yourself in what I consider the five stages of menopausal sleep. I feel compelled to mention that Elizabeth Kübler-Ross introduced the original five-stages-of-grief model in her book *On Death and Dying* while likely in her perimenopausal era.

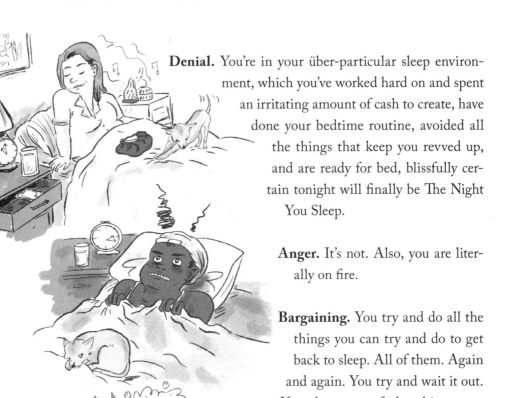

Denial. You're in your über-particular sleep environment, which you've worked hard on and spent an irritating amount of cash to create, have done your bedtime routine, avoided all the things that keep you revved up, and are ready for bed, blissfully certain tonight will finally be The Night You Sleep.

Anger. It's not. Also, you are literally on fire.

Bargaining. You try and do all the things you can try and do to get back to sleep. All of them. Again and again. You try and wait it out. You do some of the things you know won't help. You do all the things again. Nothing else is working, so you put your soul on the market.

Depression. Even *that* doesn't work.

Acceptance. In an hour, everyone else is going to start waking up, and there's no chance in hell you're going to get to sleep then. Good morning, I guess.

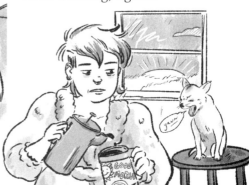

"GET ACTIVE"

Movement is often presented as one of the easiest things we can do for ourselves to help with any part of menopause. Yet there can be so many barriers to movement: access barriers with equipment, guidance, or help figuring out movement that works for you and your body, as well as the needs, abilities, and limitations of both. A scarcity of time, space, or energy for movement is often in the mix, as is the pervasive feeling we're not wholly allowed to have *anything* for ourselves, movement we enjoy included. Psychological and emotional barriers.

If this is something already easy for you or something you already have good practices around, that's great. It will probably make a very positive difference with your menopause experience on the whole. Keep it up; adapt or adjust anything if, when, and as you want or need to. Watch that you don't overdo it: it may be easier to overdo it than it was in the past, particularly once you get near the end of perimenopause and joints and tendons are starting to become less lubricated than they used to be.

For everybody else, it may be more complicated. This is especially so if, as was the case for so many of us, we were taught to hate exercise and to hate ourselves and our bodies as our primary motivation *to* exercise.

In elementary school, my gym class often began with our gym teacher telling us all to get up and start marching as she put the needle down on a record. After an unnecessarily proud orchestral opening that never let up, as you'd expect from a team who brought you "Seventy-Six Trombones" and "Wells Fargo Wagon," came these booming lyrics:

> *Touch down every morning—ten times!*
> *Not just now and then!*
> *Give that chicken fat back to the chicken*
> *And don't be chicken again!*
> *No, don't be chicken again!*
>
> *Push up every morning—ten times!*
> *Push up starting low!*
> *Once more on the rise, nuts to the flabby guys!*
> *Go, you chicken fat, go away!*
> *Go, you chicken fat, go!*

"Chicken Fat" was recorded for a fitness initiative by then president John F. Kennedy. And it was indeed, sadly, created by Meredith Willson and Robert Preston, the composer and the lead actor, respectively, of *The Music Man*, who fell from grace to create this epic monstrosity. More sadly still, despite the fact that I've loved being active over my whole life, "Chicken Fat" and the many other cultural manifestations of "Chicken Fat"–esque dharma then and since really messed up my attitudes about movement. And I'm nowhere near alone in that.

I liked climbing, including things that aren't actually meant for climbing, which is how I lost two fingers. I was a roller skating superfan. I even got sneaker skates with tiny license plates on them that said "Heather." Fancy. I swam at the Y and the lake. My sixth-grade social studies teacher let me join her solitary morning practice when I was at school very early, and so was my very first yoga teacher (thanks, Ms. Miller). The mosh pit and other regularly scheduled 1980s urban adventures kept me moving in my teens. I got into bodybuilding in my twenties and played with kids outside every day at work. I still skated. In my thirties, I fell hard for boxing and kickboxing (aka punching the shit out of things to manage my rage during the second of the terrible Bush administrations). When I moved to the Pacific Northwest and had immediate access to trails, I hiked constantly.

There were times I wasn't active or enthralled with movement. There were times when the only movement I got was at work, which also often left me both too exhausted to move otherwise and with only a few hours for sleep until I had to go to the next job. Illness, including mental illness, injury, disability, poverty, and other kinds of lack of access—many of the usual suspects that create barriers

to enough, regular, and enjoyable movement for many of us—have created barriers for me too. The severe pain and loss of mobility that went from bad to worse over a decade or so sometimes made it literally *impossible* to achieve any enjoyable movement.

But I think one of the biggest barriers of all has always been the body-shaming, fat-hating, pleasure-defying, "Chicken Fat"–shaped garbage that took root in my big-thighed little psyche way back when.

That song made me feel lousy about myself and exercise. It presented exercise as urgent and militaristic work we had to do specifically to not be fat and flabby, *god forbid*. It presented bodies as enemies and moving them as something we **must** do to meet other people's standards. Since so much of the world at large and all its institutions and customs did and still do the same, it's been sticky as hell ever since.

Then puberty came calling and further amplified pressures to exercise. Once the scale and calorie counting were pushed into my equation, once "fat" (and its partner in crime, "ugly") made it onto the insult playlist, "exercise" was forever solidified for me as a soul-sapping drag.

LUCKY FOR ME, MUCH OF THE MOVEMENT I liked wasn't counted as (or as the "right" kind of) "exercise," so I managed to hang on to some movement that made me feel good. There are some kinds of movement I've temporarily or permanently lost the ability to do (also, buying yearlong gym access right before a pandemic started was hilarious), and I miss them.

It's semantic, I know, but as much as I can, getting rid of the baggage I will probably forever have around "exercise" by instead thinking about movement helps me out. It even helps me when I can't or don't get as much movement in as I and my body would like. It lacks the built-in shame that comes up for a lot of us from not "doing our exercise." You move, you don't move; you move more, you move less. None of that makes you a better or worse person, just someone who was able to move more or less on a given day.

MOVEMENT WE DO FOR OUR PHYSICAL and psychological well-being should be what we choose, based on what makes us *feel good* in all the ways that we can access.

Did you get that? Movement is supposed to be about feeling good, not about punishment, duty, or control. It can't always feel good in every way, like when movement involves recovering from injury, when we're sore after movement, or when we're working through emotional trauma that movement cues. But the aim is to have it feel good in most ways with great frequency.

Movement can specifically help with menopause by

- supporting circulation, which can counteract a bunch of menopause impacts

like cognitive issues, genital discomfort, headaches, skin conditions, foot pain, cardiovascular issues, and mood/ mental health impacts;

- protecting against bone loss, particularly when the movement is weight-bearing (including with our own bodies resisting gravity, which doesn't have to mean external weights or machines, though if that kind of weight-bearing movement works for you, go for it!);
- improving sleep;
- reducing stress and helping manage it;
- providing ways to feel good in our own bodies, including helping us to enjoy them at a time when we might be really uncomfortable in or with them;
- helping to increase or sustain sexual desire, primarily by helping with all that stuff above;
- providing opportunities for social interaction, if and when we want and have access to kinds of movement that are social;
- providing, if it's outside the house or *solitary* by design, an excellent way to get *away* from people and have some alone time.

Movement is anything where some or all of our bodies are moving, not just things we might have been taught were "exercise."

It can be a way or ways we move to do something else we like, like taking care of a garden or houseplants or playing with pets or kids. It can be something we do as a sport or with another kind of singular focus, rather than while accomplishing something else, like walking or stretching for the sake of walking or stretching, martial arts (assuming you're not also using it for fighting crime or vengeance) or dance. It can be something that's social, like softball or, hell, sex. If you aren't there already, you're probably getting on last call for your bones' ability to survive the roller derby, in case you had that on your bucket list.

The only "right" ways to move are the ones that ideally won't land us in the ER or otherwise cause us great pain, injury, and medical expense; the ways that feel good to *us;* **and the ways that we want to.**

Movement can help us even if we only do it (or only can do it) in a few different ways, infrequently, mellowly, or briefly. It's hard sometimes to get motivated for movement and often harder still if the ask seems daunting. **Any way we can get movement in benefits us.** Can it help us more if we do it more, with more intensity, and for longer periods? Yes, though only to a point. But if we want to and can do it in more ways, more often, more intensely, and for longer periods of time, we'll *be* doing it, and we'll know how we feel and that it helps us if that's right. That thing where we try and make the goal something far out of reach is so often the thing that keeps us from doing it or continuing to do it at all. It is not only

If you're someone who is already very active or highly athletic, you might find that some of your menopausal transition messes with your ability to stay active or train in the ways that you're used to, whether that's about fatigue, depression, stiff joints, changes in body composition, or vasomotor impacts. Anything you're using to manage your menopause might also impact your physical abilities. Know you're not alone in this: dealing with this transition as an athlete (whether or not that's a term you use for yourself) is something others have struggled with before and do now, but also something others have generally figured out. You probably will have to make some adjustments now and postmenopause, whether that's to your schedule, by changing up what you do or the intensity level, and to some expectations you may have about your body looking a certain way. If you're dreading the other side of things, don't; this *is* temporary, and postmenopause can actually bring some potential athletic perks, like increased energy and better mood. Thanks to your active habits up to now, you also likely already have better bone mass to keep you active through the rest of your life than you would have otherwise.

fine to start small; it is fine to stay small if that's all you can do or all you want to do.

When it comes to movement, do what you want and what you can that feels good to you. That's really it.

Even movement you like might still pull up poky feelings for you. You might have to do some (or some more) work to heal or let go of trauma or negative thought patterns and feelings you have around exercise or your body. A lot of us have that work to do or keep doing. How could we not?

It might feel daunting to engage in movement with or in front of other people, particularly if you already feel self-conscious. Menopausal or middle-aged people becoming active has not exactly been shown in the most positive light in pop culture: it's easy to feel shame or insecurity when we've seen ourselves made the butt (sometimes literally) of the joke. If we have social anxiety already, we also have that in the proverbial gym bag.

I asked professor, body acceptance activist, author of *Fat*, among other books, and also *tremendous* friend (some people are just better at it than the rest of us!) Hanne Blank about this.

Being worried about what you look like or how you appear to others when you're moving your body is normal, in almost exactly the same way as it is normal to believe that the zit on your chin is, in fact, the size of the Chrysler Building and *everybody* is staring at it. As you've probably figured out by now, the zit on your chin is just a zit, and we've all seen them before. Difficult as it can be to cope with the ways your own body changes, remember that perspective is key: you notice, and will always notice, far more than anyone else will.

You have the right to exist in the body that you have *right now*, whatever that body may be. You aren't hurting anybody by existing in the body that you have. You have nothing to be ashamed of by existing in the body that you have. It's the only one! It's unique and it's yours. Might as well do what you want to and need to do with it.

What she said.

"HYDRATE"

Estrogen and progesterone levels influence our levels of hydration. So do other things we are or may be dealing with during any part of menopause: stress, aging, irritable bowel syndrome, or medications that are diuretic.

Estrogen, in particular, has a lot to do with moisture: in joints and tendons, in our skin, in our genitals, and more. Estrogen helps us to retain moisture.

Once we're in the later part of perimenopause, estrogen starts to decline, so unless we do what we can to up it, our level of hydration will decline too. (For those experiencing sudden menopause, most of the moisture estrogen provides is lost very immediately.) More water can help keep joints more cushioned, tendons more stretchy, skin bouncier and more resilient, genitals moister and less prone to abrasions and infections. Staying well hydrated also can help with common menopausal miscreants like bloating and other digestive issues, headaches, cognitive issues, vasomotor effects, fatigue, and moods.

There aren't a thousand ways to get and stay hydrated. This is one of the few things in this book and menopause that just isn't at all complicated. There's really only the one way: water intake. You know this. To get and stay hydrated, we need to take water in, mostly by drinking it and by drinking (or eating) other things that have water in them.

EVERYONE'S FLUID-INTAKE NEEDS ARE different and fluid (no pun intended, for real this time). How much health experts tell us to drink as a baseline is also in constant flux and probably won't ever be right for everyone (for instance, this latest "drink as many ounces as half your weight" is potentially too much water for bigger folks to even *try* and drink in a day). You *can* drink too much water for your health, and when you do, it dilutes electrolytes, which can put stress on the kidneys and heart and make you feel tired, shaky, nauseated, and headachy. Hello from the time I thought I could cure a urinary tract infection by drinking gallons of water in one sitting. You don't wish you were there.

Health at Every Size dietician, *Body Kindness* author, and angel of diet-culture mercy Rebecca Scritchfield says that sorting out how much water is right for you can be something you try and learn to do more intuitively rather than by general directives. If you want a simple thing to measure or monitor to be sure you're hydrating enough, she says you can base it on thirst or on the quality of your urine: closer to clear is what you want; darker, murkier, or pungent is usually a signal we need watering. Headaches or muscle cramps are other signals of dehydration. Rebecca importantly wants to remind you that "water is in lots of things: fruits and vegetables, soups, smoothies, teas, hot chocolate—even things with caffeine are all ways to get water. Even if you don't love drinking water, you can still stay hydrated."

You probably know by now if you're someone who is and stays well hydrated or you aren't.

I personally suck at getting and staying hydrated, and I especially suck at drinking water.

If you're already good about this, keep it up, and so long as you're not concerned about overdoing it, you might want to increase it, especially if you're feeling thirstier or drier.

If you're not already good at it, it would probably behoove you to try and get better at it. If you want to try and improve at drinking water itself, you can start by just bringing a filled water bottle around with you. Even if you forget to drink it, you still have it to use for self-defense or a desperate shower.

"QUIT SMOKING"

Oh damn. We're here. I am about to be someone I cannot stand.

In my humble opinion, there's little in life more annoying than being told you should quit smoking. Especially because everyone tells you, all the time. I am now at least 25 percent more annoying by virtue of merely being a person who quit smoking. It's one of those things that comes with quitting that everyone knows but no one brags about.

If I wouldn't be a big asshole by *not* talking about this, I'd leave you and your smokes alone in peace. I swear.

The trouble is that smoking is one of the things consistently stated, in the whole of the menopausal canon, to be a thing that doesn't play nice with menopause. Even if there is a good deal of confirmation bias at play (and of course there is), as far as I can tell, they're right. In a whole bunch of ways, smoking—goddammit—makes us more likely to have some menopausal misery or makes certain things worse in some way.

I STARTED MENOPAUSE AS A SMOKER OF around thirty years. I started smoking when I was around eleven or twelve. I started drinking coffee next, wearing ties not long after, and quickly grew a loving

bitterness about everything and everyone. I was baby Fran Lebowitz.

Like Fran, I, too, loved cigarettes. Never didn't love them. Love them still. My relationship with cigarettes was one of the most stable, reliable, and supportive relationships of my whole life. If you're thinking something like, *Well, yes, but they were also slowly killing you the whole time*, you clearly know little about some of my other relationships.

Cigarettes kept me able to keep going when I was tired, post-traumatic, suicidal, depressed, angry, hungry, lonely, uninspired, or just lousy with lousiness. When people asked me how I did so many things (back when I did), and I said, "Coffee and cigarettes," they thought I was being cute. I was not.

I ONLY TRIED TO QUIT SMOKING IN EARnest twice. At neither time did I want to.

The first time I was in my midtwenties. I did not feel better without smoking. I did not have more energy. I did not breathe easier, feel calmer, or sleep better. I was in some of the best physical shape with the greatest physical ability of my life, and I was young, but I felt like the walking dead. I lasted nine months.

In 2017, to meet criteria for the surgery that gave me the ability to walk again, I had to quit smoking. My surgeon (Dr. Jayashree Srinivasan, in whose debt I forever remain) was clear: because nicotine inhibits bone growth, and I'd have to grow new bone to make the surgery anything but a waste of her time and talents and my risk taking, she would not do it if I hadn't quit for at least three months.

Damn.

I quit. I quit by doing many of the things you can do to quit all at once. I tapered down while using the patch. I got a vaporizer and eighty million bottles of vape juice and surgically attached it to my face. I was on an SSRI and gabapentin (both of which can potentially help with quitting and hot flashes, FYI). I had prescription inhalers and nicotine gum, herbal cigarettes, weed. I did just about anything within reach that wasn't more dangerous than smoking.

Even then, it sucked in the biggest way. I knew it would. It still blows sometimes, like when I'm writing a whole book without the comfort and speediness of even one freaking cigarette. But my chronic pain is so significantly reduced that I don't usually have to take any ongoing pain medications anymore, so long as I stay on top of what I do for prevention. My surgery gave me the ability to walk again and even feel the leg I had lost feeling in again. And I also never, ever want to have to go through quitting again. I am quit forever, for that reason above all.

I didn't know until after I quit that cigarettes were making menopause worse for me and probably had inclined it to be worse before it even started.

I didn't know (or didn't accept) that

❦ smoking is associated with hot flashes and with their being greater in intensity and frequency than for nonsmokers;

❦ smoking can make other symptoms more severe or frequent or bring them on earlier, like cognitive function struggles and vaginal dryness;

❦ smokers usually have lower estrogen levels than nonsmokers, a thing that might matter to you if you want to keep all the estrogen and the health protections it provides for as long as you can;

❦ smoking messes with sleep, especially when you have a smoke when you can't sleep, because there is no justice in this world;

❦ smoking makes some common menopausal skin issues worse, on top of setting us up for more skin trouble with aging, like collagen loss and dryness;

❦ smoking additionally increases some health risks that all of menopause and what comes after *already* increase, like lower bone density, bone loss, Alzheimer's, diabetes, stroke, and cancers.

Smokers also tend to start perimenopause one to two years earlier (though for some, as many as nine years earlier) than those who haven't ever been smokers. That can be great for ending painful periods or a reproductive option that wasn't wanted. That's obviously less great for people trying to conceive or those who want to keep their bodies' estrogen levels higher. Hormone therapy that includes estrogen also increases breast cancer and cardiovascular risks for smokers. Smoking may limit what MHT can be safely prescribed for you.

In case you're saying to yourself, *Self? Heather certainly didn't make a very good case for quitting with their story, though,* I will remind you that it's not my job to convince you to do anything. If you're a smoker, you already know, probably better than anyone, most of the risks it involves because everyone always needs to tell us about them, like we have never had anyone tell us about them ever before. You also know if you want to try to quit or not. If you want to, read on. If not, just don't forget what I said about how it messes up your ability to get back to sleep tonight.

WHY QUIT WHEN YOU'RE ALREADY IN HELL?

Quitting or cutting back in perimenopause can make some of the parts of quitting smoking that are tough even tougher. For a while you may, for instance, be about ninety times more irritable and angry than you already are. The upside is that because quitting smoking is considered virtuous, people will feel the need to be nicer to you than if your growliness were from menopause or something else.

Even though I'm still really crabby about my lost smoky love, I can see some benefits to my having quit, even *because* I did it during perimenopause. I can put a lot of my cancer anxiety and my growing concerns about losing my ability to sing—all of which amped up thanks to perimenopause anxiety—to bed. More anxiety I don't need. My circulation and teeth are in better shape. My skin started looking pretty fantastic. Cigarettes **always** set off hot flashes for me. Once I stopped smoking twenty cigarettes a day, I avoided around twenty hot flashes a day. My sleep improved.

The economic upside is huge. When I was a smoker, even in poverty I maintained a strong denial about what it cost. The app I used tells me that I would have spent over $10,000 on smokes over the last three years had I not quit. Some of that money has gone toward many a menopause comfort: my beloved cooling pillow, ice packs, massages, electricity bills (fans + AC = a financial house of horrors), well-engineered shoes, and even my workspace and tiny pied-à-terre pour *la ménépausie.*

In the event you aren't already sick of me and are curious about what I think helped me quit and stay quit, here are the highlights:

- **Find a real reason to quit that you really, truly give a shit about.**
- **Make a deadline to quit and try to stick to it.** Whether you're a cold turkey person or a tapering-off person, make a deadline and hold yourself to it. If you blow it, make a new deadline and try again.

- **Get any and all cigarettes out of your reach.** I wasn't lucky to be unable to get myself to where I could get cigarettes, but being stuck in bed in a rural place without transportation made it a thousand times tougher for me to break my quit.
- **Quit your way.** Try whatever you want to try and keep trying things until you find what feels like a fit.
- **Take advantage of cessation programs.** There are some programs that will pay for some or all of nicotine replacement therapies if you want them.
- **Don't be an ass to yourself.** If you fall back, you fall back. So what. Just say no to shame spirals. Sing yourself the rubber tree song from *Laverne & Shirley*. You might have to try and fail a lot of times, much like with the rest of life.
- **Don't try and have just one after you have quit.** You can't go home again. I'm sorry. But you *can* go somewhere else.

"GET SOCIAL SUPPORT"

In the *Golden Girls* episode "The End of the Curse" (1986), Blanche discovers she's in menopause after struggling with depression and sleeplessness. The discovery deeply upsets her: she feels less valuable and fears her sexuality and her gender identity will be over as a result. Her housemates help her arrange a therapy visit and go with her. Over the next few days, they talk together about their experiences in a supportive way. Dorothy talks about the positives she's found on the other side, and as Blanche shares more and more of her ickiest feelings, her friends are supportive and reassuring. She becomes more accepting of what's happening and tells her friends it was their support that helped her start to feel better about it.

The fourth season of Pamela Adlon's *Better Things* (2020) delivers a previously unheard-of whole *season* of television where menopause is a central theme. There are gems throughout, but the scenes of support and camaraderie from her also-menopausal friends are everything, as is the short video segment she makes at the end of the season about menopause that features a host of first-person menopause perspectives. When she shares the video with her family, you watch her daughters take it in, this thing they clearly hadn't heard of before, even though their mother has been in it for the whole season, and see newfound respect, compassion, and understanding happen around this and their mother.

Unlike most media portrayals of menopause, these depictions are sympathetic and set a positive example of how to care for and about people in menopause, not instructional segments on how to make us feel like garbage and make us objects of ridicule. We can find understanding, support, and care from others, and menopause tends to go a lot better for most of us when we do. This is one of the things that studies find again and again and that many a menopausal person's anecdotal stories hold up. Social support even impacts some of our health outcomes through and on the other side of menopause, like cardiovascular health, mental health, and longevity.

I hope this is obvious, but in case it isn't, I'm not just talking about support expressly about menopause. I'm also talking about all those other parts of life that may not even be connected to menopause directly.

Getting social support expressly about menopause is likely ideal, and I can't speak for you, but I sure wouldn't kick getting *any* kind of support I can out of bed. There's a lot I need support with during all this hormonal nonsense, and the same is or likely will be true for you.

For too many of us, collective responsibility, mutuality of care, consideration, and accountability are our hope, wish, or dream in our relationships and social settings instead of our expectation, insistence, and reality. Deeply sensible frameworks and social systems, as well as dynamics like the central theses of collective care and responsibility in Leah Lakshmi Piepzna-Samarasinha's *Care Work: Dreaming Disability Justice* or secure attachment, compassion, and empathy in Nora Samaran's *Turn This World Inside*

Out: The Emergence of Nurturance Culture, can look utopian even though they should be basic standards of social care.

It shouldn't be radical to suggest that we should all be cared for as much as we're caring for others or that our social relationships should act like the communities they are. It shouldn't seem weird to suggest that care should be a pleasure and a joy, not a burden, which is only possible in a sustainable way if it's mutual and equitable.

We know it's okay for other people to need help and care; it's also okay for us. We feel we should be reliable, that others should be able to count on us to care for them; the same should be true on the flip side. It shouldn't be radical to suggest we might need some help and that, when we do, we can ask for it and expect people to extend it to us.

Aida Manduley, LCSW, is a Latinx activist, trauma-focused clinician with a basis in liberation health and healing justice, and a human discotheque. They say,

The biggest lie that we're told—and I would say that this goes for everyone, just in different flavors—the lie that we're told is that we have to do it by ourselves. No one does anything by themselves. Any person who says they got to where they are by themselves is lying, either actively lying or deeply misinformed and spouting a lie. Look, find me any famous person, find me any philosopher, find me any person who's made it into the history books. A huge reason why they were able to is because they had people making their food and caring for their children, driving their cars, or horse buggies or whatever. None of these people did it by themselves. The fact that they got help was just erased. So now, other people think, "Oh, well, I gotta do it myself. This other person did it, so clearly, I gotta do it, too." That's not how it worked for them either. Actually, they got a lot of help.

These kinds of care, equity, and mutuality should be our expectations in all aspects of our relationships, not just with menopause. If they aren't yet, there's no time like perimenopause.

Please know this, too, is by no means something I have myself mastered. I've spent much of my lifetime providing a mind-boggling amount of one-sided care and life-transition guide labor for others and am only just recently starting to get the hang of setting up more mutual relationships and care webs. If chronic physical and emotional pain, disability, and menopause hadn't been part of my life, I'd probably be much further behind in this process than I already am.

WHAT'S SOCIAL SUPPORT LOOK LIKE?

I'm not explaining this because I think you're a dope. I'm explaining it because I think so many of us have so often gone without some of it that we might have forgotten all it can provide.

Emotional support is the kind we can get or provide through engaged listening and witnessing in a nurturing, validating, and otherwise supportive way. Physical care and comfort can be part of that too.

Esteem support includes things that affirm or otherwise help hold up or beef up our sense of self-worth and our confidence. If, for instance, we're feeling super insecure about things like body, gender, sexual, or cognitive changes, someone giving us esteem support can help us counteract or bludgeon those fears or insecurities with positive support for our general or specific awesomeness.

Tangible support can be everything from the gift of a cooling pillow (good for any occasion, for you menopause-support-people readers out there!), a new sex toy, help with childcare when you need to get some sleep, a ride to the market, doing some of the legwork to help you find other kinds of help you need, like a therapist or endocrinologist, or sitting down with you and helping you restrategize your life.

Informational support is what it sounds like: that's help by way of shared information, ideally when it's been solicited.

FINDING YOUR PEOPLE

Being willing to talk to people—or even just ask them for help—and then seeking out those people doesn't mean it's going to be easy to find support. Aida Manduley said that it's harder to find our people in crisis, and I think they're right.

Just finding other people who are or have been in menopause or who are willing and in some way capable of talking about it doesn't make those people the people we need; that doesn't make them **our** actual people. Some of them may share being in menopause but not share or understand something vital to our identity and experience.

To start, you can look to some of your existing interpersonal relationships, especially your more intimate relationships: your close friends, lovers or partners, whatever your version of family is. Obviously, here as anywhere, whom you ask for what is going to depend on any number of factors. You might have someone who is a great source of tangible support but not so great with the emotional support because they have biases or attitudes that don't work there. Everyone can't offer all the kinds, and you won't want them all from everyone. Plus, some of your family may be, say, three years old, a dog, in a crisis of their own, or just unable in some

other way. And some folks who might be great in other arenas of our lives may just suck at this and, for who knows what reason, just not be people we want to ask for support with this at all.

This might be one of those things where you find some of the best support about or during menopause outside your existing inner circle. Maybe someone at work is in it themselves and offers themselves up as someone to talk to; maybe your neighbor who has been there and has offered to watch your kid in the past is someone you ask for help now.

Support groups expressly for menopause are another option for emotional, esteem, and informational support. There are menopause support groups on all the talky platforms (Facebook, Reddit, etc.), including more specific subgroups. The bulk of those groups are often not very, sometimes not even at all, inclusive of queer, trans, and/or nonbinary people, and many also are places where there can be a lot of unchecked ableism and anti-fat bias. Weight loss talk is pervasive. There's also often a lot of normalizing of things that would ideally instead be challenged, like emotional abuse in marriage, body bashing, and some of the most toxic kinds of heteronormativity. However, if you poke around enough, you can find exceptions to all of those things.

When it comes to something still so unstudied as menopause and still so full of people trying to sell us things, good informational support can really come in handy. Sources of anecdotal hacks and other kinds of information that healthcare providers or other general sources of information might not offer can be super valuable. All the more so if you're on the margins, where queer, trans, and other gender-nonconforming people and people with disabilities, in particular, can find themselves in an informational void.

Leah Lakshmi Piepzna-Samarasinha said that she thinks "the time is really ripe for disabled and chronically ill folks who are going through menopause to really start pooling our collective knowledge: here's what we're experiencing and here's what's helpful. The vast majority of things that I use and practices that I have on a daily basis that support my body and mind didn't come from medical practitioners, but from other sick and disabled folks." I couldn't agree more, and that goes for a range of different communities with menopause. Micro–menopause community to the rescue!

ONLINE ISN'T THE ONLY OPTION. You can also create or find and join existing in-person support groups, circles, or care webs. Menopause mutual aid is absolutely a thing that we can organize or ask others to help us make happen if we don't have the spoons or ability to do that. You can check women's, queer, and trans healthcare centers or organizations, feminist bookstores, or other kinds of community centers. Menopause cafés—hosted coffee or tea klatches meant for menopausal people to connect—are another option, as is, for that matter, should you be so lucky, a local bar where all the old lesbians hang out.

Counselors, therapists, and other kinds of care providers are certainly also options. Honestly, I feel like the least any of us should get for just making it *to* menopause is at least six months' worth of the emotional support of our choice.

You can also find a sense of support in other ways. The menopause memoir—in books, articles, and now even podcasts and radio, film, television, and other media—can help you feel less alone and give its own kinds of emotional, esteem, and informational support. Babysitters can be hired or bartered, there are delivery services for the things you need but cannot drag yourself out of bed to get, and every kind of coach you can imagine is out there somewhere. We can also get some of the tangible or informational support we need from people and places that have nothing to do with menopause and, if we don't want to, without even sharing that's why we need help.

One of the ways partners, family, housemates, or anyone else who's a big part of daily life can support us is in accommodations, adaptations, or other changes we need in order to get through this or to adjust to the ways that we are just going to be different because of this from now on. That can be bigger things or little ones, but clear, tangible ways to help can go a long way for everyone and can be adapted for every age and ability.

I'm talking about stuff like

⚓ double checks of things like oven ranges, putting the dog back inside, locked doors, and other potential disasters cognitive issues can create;

⚓ adapting meals so that they're better for what you need right now, so multiple meals don't have to be made;

⚓ greater coparenting equity or shared childcare;

⚓ running errands: depositing a check, picking up a cat from the vet, getting your cannabis or other medicines from the dispensary and bringing it to you;

⚓ listen-and-validate-only (on their part) venting sessions for you;

⚓ a round of cleaning the bathroom before you take a self-care shower or bath so you don't have to clean up everyone else's leftover dirt first for a change;

⚓ a ride somewhere where driving yourself or taking public transit makes you homicidal;

⚓ getting you sex, massage, *and* power tools/toys for your birthday;

⚓ clean sheets;

⚓ a round of phone calls to help you try and find healthcare or other care providers for yourself *or* sitting on hold with your health insurance company and handing you the phone when the representative finally comes on the line.

You get to ask for the kind of social support you want and be as specific as you want to be, by the way. We're not begging for crumbs: we're asking for support we want and need and that people who want to support and care for us will be glad to offer if they're able. Being clear about what we do and don't want helps everyone: it helps us get what we need most expediently, and it helps the other folks who might be able to help us with whatever that is know if they're the right person for the job.

If you just want to vent and don't want advice, just say you are not interested in advice. If you want advice, but you're not interested in hearing about herbs or hormones or meditating or blue-green algae or whatever your particular nope in this is, say so. If you just want something very specific, like some weight-neutral cheerleading for body issues you're having or a referral for a particular kind of care provider, or you just need to know WTF to do when you get hives, just say so. Anyone or any community who gives you grief about those kinds of limits are *not* your people.

OH, ONE LAST THING: THE PERSON WE reach out to may not reach back or even see or hear us reaching. Or they may react with nonsupport, or worse, instead of support. One tip from my past experience is to stop knocking on doors no one is opening. I made so many bids for support with my ex—bids for affirmation of my value, my appeal, or my needs—that were rarely picked up, and the more ignored or unseen bids I made, the worse I felt. I also was inclined to project his disinterest onto others, which made it easy for me to get into a "no one is here for me" rut that was only a rut because I was mostly looking to people and places that were not going to be there for me instead of walking away and asking other people. I long needed a three-strikes rule for myself socially—and one of the good things perimenopause has done for me is give me the motivation to start.

I'D BE LAX NOT TO MENTION THAT supporting other people in their menopause offers benefits, too, and not just to the people we support. I've been thinking about it more and more like we're forming a union.

As an introvert and as someone who's had a long road to learning how to ask for help and still gets itchy just thinking about it, I was surprised to find that when I started talking to more people about all this, I really liked it. Most of those conversations have been both supportive and super interesting. It also gave me a better sense of what I actually needed—and could have!—and the more practice I get, the better I get at asking for and finding what I need.

Hearing and holding other people's experiences helps us feel less isolated and alone. When support is mutual, it can help us feel like less of a heel or a burden. Since it feels good to offer support when we can, it can get easier to ask for and accept help because we're reminded that providing it is *not* necessarily a burden. We can help each other to feel better able to insist on or negotiate for our needs, and if we're a support group in places where we share the same or similar needs—like a workplace, a board, or a community group—we can even do collective bargaining. We could even strike. Imagine the menopausal union songs alone.

CHAPTER FIVE

DOCTOR! DOCTOR! (OR ARNP! OR MIDWIFE! OR TCM PRACTITIONER! OR NOT)

"If they don't give you a seat at the table, bring a folding chair."
—*Shirley Chisholm*

Discourse about menopause often makes it sound like our choice in managing it boils down to whether we use hormone therapies or not. But hormone therapies are hardly our only management option—and for some, aren't an option, period—and even if we do use them, they can't often address all of our needs. How did we even get to the doctor's office, anyway? When did we decide we even wanted to go there in the first place? What happened to *that* conversation?

TO DOCTOR OR NOT TO DOCTOR? IT IS A QUESTION. AND IF YOU DO, HOW?

Seeking out any kind of care or intervention, medical or otherwise, is **optional** for managing perimenopause. It's neither a given nor a requirement.

Even if and when you do have access to healthcare for menopause, there's still the matter of if you *want* to seek it out. As with anything, the less you fit a given system, the less power or privilege you have within it or interrelated systems, and the more loaded your history, the trickier it all can get. Someone whose ancestry or life experience includes gross medical abuses like involuntary sterilizations, the Tuskegee study, medical sexual abuse, or nonconsensual intersex surgery will often feel different about even necessary medical interventions than someone whose heritage or experience is linked to power with doctors and humane treatment. There are many understandable and valid reasons why a person might be reluctant, or even outright unwilling, to seek out healthcare, particularly healthcare involving our reproductive systems.

Since *peri*menopause isn't something a doctor can often reliably test for or identify any better than you can yourself, no one needs to go for that reason alone.

Perimenopause, menopause, and postmenopause aren't illnesses, infections, diseases, or syndromes. They usually don't present any general additional health risks that require medical evaluation or care (and when they do, it's usually postmenopause). You don't *have* to "treat" them or their impacts: you don't usually *have* to do anything medically, or anything period, unless you want to.

But there are also lots of people who will want to seek out care and lots of people who will benefit from it. Just like seeking out healthcare for any part of or issue with menopause doesn't have to be the first thing you do or something you do at all, it doesn't have to be the last after you've exhausted everything else (and yourself trying everything else) either. There's no right or wrong answer here, just what you want for yourself. In the event you decide to look into medical or other kinds of healthcare with this, here are some ways to start.

WHICH KIND OF PROVIDER CAN YOU START WITH?

Depending on your unique needs, wants, preferences, philosophies, and access, any of the following kinds of providers could potentially work:

- OB/GYNs
- Nurse practitioners (RNs or ARNPs)
- General practitioners of traditional Chinese medicine (TCM), Ayurveda, Native American or Aboriginal medicine, or other indigenous modalities
- General practitioners of conventional Western medicine (aka family doctors or practitioners, GPs, or primary care physicians)
- Trans health providers
- Sexual or reproductive health clinicians
- Midwives
- Therapists or counselors
- Internal medicine providers
- Endocrinologists
- Nutritionists
- Physical therapists
- Massage therapists or other bodyworkers
- For just one impact, a specialist for that system, like dermatologists for skin issues, podiatrists or a pain clinic for foot pain, or substance abuse or eating disorder counselors if any part of menopause creates or results in a resurgence of those issues for you
- Neurologists
- The pizza guy

If you want someone who can be as all-in-one for menopause care as possible, you're going to want to try and find someone with that specialty who provides a wide range of kinds of care for people with menopause. Same goes for if you're looking to bundle as much care into one provider as possible for economic or other reasons.

Because menopause is an all-systems issue, theoretically that could be almost any kind of general practitioner. But in the present, few providers have sought out or received menopause education in medical school or in education for other modalities, like naturopathy, nutrition, psychiatry, or TCM.

While only about 20 percent of OB/GYN residency programs include menopause training, and it's often elective, this is the field where practitioners are most likely to have the most current menopause training or education. A lot of women and trans people use sexual and reproductive healthcare providers as general health providers anyway. So, if you want a place to start, this kind of care is accessible to you, and it's an arena of care or a particular provider you'd feel good starting with, it's a sound one.

If you can't access or don't want that kind of care provider, or the care the provider you see for that is limited to only obstetrics and sexual medicine, a general practitioner or nurse practitioner is another good initial choice. Even if the GP or ARNP you ask about this doesn't turn out to be the right person for you, they can often refer you to a specialist who is. Trans healthcare providers and/or endocrinologists—both experts at hacking hormones—are other potential good starting places.

The North American Menopause Society (NAMS) keeps a public directory of providers, some certified by them, who provide menopause-specific care. You can use their app or website to search that database. Telehealth and specialized menopause clinic options are also emerging.

As with any kind of new provider search, referrals from friends, family, or coworkers can come in handy. It may be helpful that those of us who suffer the most in this often lack the ability to keep quiet about our struggles, so if you know anyone who seems a lot better than they once did with menopause, you can ask if they got there with help and from whom.

Make sure a provider is right for *you*. If you're lesbian, a provider who cannot remember that lesbians exist is likely to make you feel worse instead of better. If you're trans or otherwise gender nonconforming, you need a provider who doesn't misgender you. If you're BIPOC and don't feel safe with a white doctor, you probably want a BIPOC doctor you do feel safe with. If you're asexual or a recent survivor of sexual assault, you need someone who respects boundaries you set about disinterest you might have in sexual solutions or discussions. If you have disability, someone who can't work with how menopause may interact with your disability is going to be of limited use to you, and someone who can't even talk about menopause without ableism isn't going to work for you at all. Even just intake forms—which you can ask to have emailed or may be able to view online before you even make an appointment—can tell us a whole lot about how inclusive or otherwise right for us a practice or clinic is. If big parts of our identities or life circumstances aren't even accounted for in intake forms . . . *well*.

If I've learned anything as the child of a nurse, it's to ask healthcare providers a ton of questions rather than assuming they'll offer things up or do all the asking. Whether we're asking in person or over the phone or reviewing their information online, we probably want to ask them or otherwise find out basics like the following:

◆ When was the last time they got menopause education?
◆ What did that education or training involve?
◆ How do they usually treat/advise their menopausal patients, and how do they decide what's best for a patient? How would they describe their overall approach to healthcare, to patients, and to menopause? How personalized is it?
◆ Do they work with any other providers? Who? What kind? Will they work in collaboration with your existing providers?
◆ How often will they want to see you, and how often will they check things like your labs or how you're doing with any given treatment or medication?

Another thing I've learned to do with healthcare, especially with new providers, is to bring a printout of what I feel is my most important health history, all current issues, medications, and supplements (you can take photos of supplement labels with your phone to keep info about them in easy reach), my pronouns and other things that matter to me and my care, my current questions or concerns, and anything else that may not be included on intake forms. You can keep that file on your phone or somewhere else in easy reach so you can always update, edit, or share it easily. If being in menopause is private information for you, I'd be sure to mention that. Because of the stigma that remains with menopause as well as health privacy regulations, it's unlikely someone will yell across the room about your menopause, but if it'd mess with your head if they did or endanger you in some way, let them know.

If you don't have many choices in care—like if your healthcare is through public health or the military or you live in a rural area without a lot of options—you can still ask to see someone with menopause education, training, or experience.

When to break up with or take a pass on a provider (if you have a choice):
◆ Because you want to. If you feel like someone isn't a good or the right provider for you, trust yourself.
◆ You don't feel safe with, confident in, or respected by them.

WILL YOU HAVE A HARDER TIME WITH PERIMENOPAUSE?

Statistically speaking, you probably won't have as hard a time as I have. But if you do, or might, I think it's helpful to have some ideas about why. That can make it easier to figure out what kind of care you might need or want to seek out, what you might want to be ready to do for yourself, and some of why you may be having the kind of menopause you are.

Who has a harder time and who an easier one falls across some predictable lines. It's often more difficult for marginalized people and more difficult the more marginalized someone is.

For all the times I read about Black women having more vasomotor symptoms, I saw almost no one *except* Black women consider that this might have more to do with the trauma of living under white supremacy than genetics. Some preexisting conditions, issues, or histories have been connected with a harder time of things in menopause generally or greater likelihood of some impacts. This isn't an exhaustive list, just some biggies:

- Cigarette smoking
- Caregiving
- Earlier onset of peri or experience of menopause
- Sudden menopause via oophorectomy or medical treatments
- Earlier first period
- Certain health conditions or issues including multiple sclerosis (MS), high blood pressure, fibromyalgia, migraines, back pain, and many other chronic illnesses
- Trauma survival, especially childhood trauma and sexual trauma
- Preexisting high levels of stress
- Previous or preexisting depression (including postpartum depression), anxiety, premenstrual syndrome, or premenstrual dysphoric disorder
- High sensitivity to hormones and hormone shifts

Suffice it to say, those who lack access or adequate access to needed care for perimenopause—be that self-care, social support, healthcare, or all of the above—will likely have a harder time with perimenopause.

In the event that you're reading this and you've got a level of privilege that allows you to help a peri-pal out who has need in any of these departments, I implore you to extend a hot hand their way, ideally before things get bad for them and they're in serious crisis. If you're the one with the lack of access, I encourage you to look for those folks who might be able to help bridge those gaps. There's no shame in asking for help that we need, and an ask now sure beats having to scream for it later.

They try and scare you or otherwise emotionally manipulate you into things they think are a good idea and you absolutely don't want. This is a lack of medical ethics, and that is very bad.

♦ They seem nonchalant or dismissive of your concerns or stonewall you when you voice them. They don't listen.

♦ Their medical education seems out of date.

♦ Their practice isn't inclusive of you in a major way, and no one is making any effort to change that and accommodate you. That may be about lacking tables that work for your size, a needed ASL translator, or the ability to stop talking about "your husband" when your wife is sitting right there.

Dr. Judith Hersh suggests three red flags to look for when screening healthcare providers to help you with menopause. If any of these come up, she says, you'll want to throw that fish back and try again. You can also ask a provider where they stand with these three things when you're screening them:

1. They order or suggest saliva tests for hormone levels and say they are accurate.
2. They say you need estrogen-level tests done to determine *peri*menopause (rather than to find out if you're

*post*menopause) in order to help you manage any impacts or issues.

3. They tell you bioidentical hormones are all safer (they're not) or prescribe topical bioidentical progesterone (which can't be efficiently absorbed through the skin).

Whether or not you seek out any menopause-specific healthcare, there are a few good reasons to mention menopause with existing healthcare practitioners or to make an appointment just to check in about a few important things:

♦ **If you're having a bad time of it, to screen for other reasons that may be happening.** Conditions that mimic perimenopause or menopause (and that also often do or can happen around the same time) include thyroid or adrenal conditions, diabetes, polycystic ovary syndrome (PCOS), MS, brain tumors or cerebral aneurysms, meningitis, high blood pressure, tuberculosis, HIV, and some cancers, particularly reproductive cancers.

♦ **If you're using medications for something else.** Some medications for other things can make menopause harder, while others can help. If you're already using any medications or thinking about coming off of or going on any, a conversation about your meds and menopause is a good idea.

- **If you have preexisting physical or mental health conditions or issues.** You can find out how they might interact with menopause so you can prepare yourself, or just know what might be coming, and what, if anything, you can do about it.
- **To get screened for nutritional deficiencies, allergies, or sensitivities.** These can all make a difference in your menopause experience. Allergies or sensitivities can play a part in vasomotor symptoms, gastrointestinal issues, and other impacts. Finding out if you have any can save you grief. If you're going to try and add new foods to help you with menopause, those screenings can save you an uncomfortable reaction and also might help you identify some foods already giving you grief.

HORMONE THERAPIES

Not everyone needs or wants to use hormone therapy in perimenopause or postmenopause. For some, the risks outweigh the benefits, so some or all kinds of MHT are an objectively bad idea. Many others can potentially benefit a great deal with little risk involved—and in most cases with added protections. What good or what damage it can potentially do varies depending on what MHT you're using and how you're using it, what you want it to help with, and your own unique health history and current circumstances. For more people than not, it's a safe and effective option.

IF THAT SOUNDS LIKE AN ODDLY RELAXED attitude, that may be because you've noticed that people, maybe even you, often have *very* strong feelings about hormone therapies, whether that's about using it for menopause, contraception, gender affirmation, or other reasons. Attitudes about hormone therapy can be downright evangelical, running the gamut from elevating it to sainthood to damning it.

Sometimes that has to do with known or assumed risks or dangers of hormones or of the Western medical system and its shitty history. Sometimes it's someone's feminism; feelings about the medicalization of menopause, reproduction, or gender; or larger issues with the pharmaceutical industry and capitalism. Those strong feelings can be based in bad personal experiences or outcomes with hormones or the bad experiences or outcomes of others. We may suspect or know hormone therapies were involved in the loss of someone we loved. Sometimes that's because they're not safe for us personally, and we inadvertently universalize. I can empathize with and relate to all of that.

People can also have strongly *positive* opinions. I come to most of my own thoughts, feelings, and ideas about hormonal medications by way of contraception and trans health and experience. So far, hormonal medications haven't been a good fit for me, period. My body does not like them, and estrogen isn't likely safe for me. However, I have a great and deep appreciation for what hormonal medications can do for many, many people. I know them to be lifesaving, like what they can do for some trans or otherwise gender-diverse people, how they provide relief for many health issues, and the massive job they've done to help millions prevent unwanted, unviable, or unsafe pregnancies. I also know them to help many people with menopause.

That all said, strong opinions of any stripe can feel like pressure to use or not to use and a lack of support for whatever is considered the wrong choice.

There's no universal right or wrong here. This should be up to *you*, ideally in partnership with caring, respectful, and highly qualified healthcare providers, based on an unpressured, informed process of decision making and consent. If you want to find out a little bit about it on your lonesome first, allow me.

AN EVERYTHING I THOUGHT I KNEW ABOUT MENOPAUSAL HORMONE THERAPY (MHT) WAS WRONG/ HORMONE THERAPY TODAY MASHUP

I thought hormone therapy for menopause was only about systemic estrogen. I thought it posed high health risks for everyone. I thought it was something you always had to keep taking once you started it. I thought that everyone who used it got a very similar regimen and that, at most, it varied only as much as different brands of birth control pills.

I was epically wrong about **all** of those things and more. Here's what I know now.

As you know too well, HT for menopause gained popularity in the 1960s, thanks in large part to Robert Wilson's scaring millions of women—and their clearly impressionable and probably also more than a little bit sexist doctors and husbands—into a desperate-by-design pursuit of lifelong estrogen therapy.

The hormone regimens that *Feminine Forever*, and, as a result, many doctors of that era, prescribed were different from what the Food and Drug Administration (FDA) had approved and vastly different from what, how, and for whom MHT is prescribed today. Wilson is also where the outdated framework of estrogen as needed hormone "replacement" (and thus, HRT) largely came from. Wilson very firmly and widely cemented the idea that menopause is a *disease* of estrogen *deficiency* and that when estrogen levels become lower, women must replace it or perish. And no longer even *be* women at all according to Wilson, lest you forgot, which you probably didn't.

The feminist health movement started waving red flags about the motivations and prescriptions of Wilson's work and that of his contemporaries in the 1970s.

According to *Our Bodies, Ourselves: Menopause*, "In 1977, Barbara Seaman's book *Women and the Crisis in Sex Hormones* alerted women to evidence that taking hormones could cause breast cancer, strokes, and blood clots and warned against the overpromotion of hormones for the treatment of menopause. Like *Feminine Forever*, Seaman's book became a best seller, educating a generation of women about the health risks of hormones." Concerns about known uterine cancer risks from unopposed estrogen use were also raised. That resulted in a change in prescribing recommendations: those who still had a uterus must use *combined* hormone therapy—an estrogen *and* a progestogen.

In the late 1980s and the 1990s, some observational studies (in which women who chose to take or not take HT were followed over time) suggested that HT prevented heart disease, while other studies suggested that HT increased the risk of breast cancer and blood clots. In 1990, the FDA found that the research done to date was not adequate to support adding heart disease prevention to the list of approved uses. But doctors are allowed to prescribe drugs for uses that are not approved by the FDA. Encouraged by the research suggesting that hormone treatment might be helpful for prevention, as well as by extensive drug company marketing efforts, many health care providers did just that.

This snowballed. More pharmaceutical companies and doctors promoted and prescribed MHT in a way that was, if not reckless, certainly not cautious. Despite a great deal of conflicting evidence and growing concern about its safety and the efficacy of its claims, Premarin was the most prescribed drug in the United States in the 1980s and 1990s.

Then a couple of things happened—a couple of studies, specifically: the Women's Health Initiative (WHI) study, launched in 1993, and the 1998 Heart and Estrogen/Progestin Replacement Study (HERS). HERS found that hormone therapy, as it was commonly prescribed and formulated at the time, was worse for those with preexisting heart issues, not *better*, as had been thought, and results from the WHI study backed that up. Even more impactfully, wide reporting of results from the WHI in 2002, mostly based on one press release, added that hormone therapy vastly increased *many* health risks.

Rose George wrote for the *Guardian* in 2015, "Compared with a placebo, the estrogen and progestin HRT was shown to cause 'increased risk of heart attack, increased risk of stroke, increased risk of blood clots, increased risk of breast cancer, reduced risk of colorectal cancer, fewer fractures and no protection against mild cognitive impairment and increased risk of dementia.'" The relative risk of getting breast cancer was given as 26 percent. The results were so shocking that the study was stopped in 2002. The press headlines were loud, immediate, and everywhere. The *Daily Mail* in 2002: "HRT linked to breast cancer." The *Guardian*: "HRT study cancelled over cancer and stroke fears."

KABOOM. Prescriptions for hormone therapy dropped by nearly 70 percent in some areas within a two-year period. The WHI study on a combined estrogen and progestogen regimen was stopped in its tracks.

THE THING IS, THERE WERE SOME BIG problems with what was reported and generally understood.

The WHI study didn't include anyone under the age of fifty. Those in the study were ages fifty to seventy-nine, and the average age of the participants was sixty-three, but the people who usually used the regimen were typically in their fifties, not their sixties and seventies. Generalizations were made for that younger group, even though they only comprised about 30 percent of those studied. The WHI study only studied *post*menopausal people, not people who were pre- or *peri*menopausal. The WHI study for the combined regimen specifically involved people who still *had* their uteruses, but the placebo group only included those who'd had hysterectomies. At least 15 percent of the subjects in the WHI study had a family predisposition for breast cancer. The participants in the

study had a statistically high incidence of preexisting health issues, and the results weren't adjusted for those or additional medications being used by the participants besides hormones. The WHI was also primarily about white women: only around 16 percent of its participants were of other ethnicities. None of these things were mentioned in the release or in most reporting on the findings.

George continues,

Some articles were better than others, but the worst ignored the fact that the estrogen-only HRT study was continuing. They also failed to distinguish between relative risk—the risk posed to that particular study group of women being given estrogen and progestin relative to the risk posed to those being given a placebo— and excess risk, the actual increase in risk between the two groups. In fact, as the WHI researchers wrote in the *Journal of the American Medical Association*, in terms of breast cancer and stroke, the excess risk was just eight more strokes and eight more invasive breast cancers per 10,000 person-years.

In fact, later results from the WHI and other studies show a *beneficial* risk-to-benefit ratio for the combined hormone regimen for those younger than the average WHI participant age and closer to menopause; they also found the specific progestin in the studied regimen was potentially less safe than other progestogens and progesterone.

The study also had participants start using estrogen therapies when it had already been a decade or more since they'd reached menopause, something we now know presents additional risks and dangers.

THE STUDY ON THE COMBINED ESTROGEN regimen was *not* discontinued because it found breast cancer and cardiovascular risks. That's what the press release stated. According to one principal investigator for the study, it was instead discontinued "based on a finding of likely futility." The problems with the initial release were apparently even known at the time, but the story is that reports had gone to print before corrections could be made.

In an NPR interview in 2013, Dr. JoAnn Manson, lead investigator of the WHI since 1993 and former NAMS president, said, "It was never the intention to deny hormone therapy to women in early menopause. We said hormone therapy shouldn't be used for chronic disease prevention. But many women and their clinicians were misinterpreting that."

In 2016, Dr. Manson, with Andrew M. Kaunitz, MD, also a member of the WHI team, published an article in the *New England Journal of Medicine* that included the following: "The WHI trial was designed to address the risks and benefits of **long-term** use of hormone therapy for the *prevention of chronic disease* in *post*menopausal women who were on average *63 years of age* at initiation of therapy**. . . . Its results are now being used inappropriately in making decisions about treatment for women in their 40s and 50s who have distressing vasomotor symptoms. Reluctance to treat menopausal symptoms has derailed and fragmented the clinical care of midlife women, creating a large and unnecessary burden of suffering." (The incredulous italics and bolding are mine.)

THE THING IS, IT'S NOT LIKE PEOPLE with concerns—or who immediately dropped their MHT use—were overreacting. The WHI study involved a total of almost thirty thousand people. Reporting came from credible sources. There are known risks and dangers of hormone therapies. Breast cancer and cardiovascular problems are hardly minor concerns. If you pile onto that any knowledge of or experience with how reckless the history of hormone therapy and Western medicine, period, is, *and* how the healthcare system tends to (mis) treat women and minorities, you can perhaps understand why so many people reacted the way they did and why those fears were so sticky.

It's reasonable to have concerns about medications and is obviously in our best interest to try and make low-risk medical choices when we can. The reporting and general understanding of the findings

A GLOSSARY FOR THOSE IN NEED (ESPECIALLY THOSE OF US WHO COULD NOT REMEMBER THE WORD "GLOSSARY")

Systemic: Systemic medication goes through the bloodstream and impacts all the systems of the body, not just one area or system. Systemic MHT is usually oral or transdermal, in the form of pills, patches, pellets, injections, creams, gels, sprays, or intravaginal rings.

Local: Local medication is not absorbed by the bloodstream in the significant way systemic medication is. It primarily impacts the area it's placed in/on. In this instance, that's typically going to be about uterine or vulvovaginal use, in the form of creams, tablets, suppositories, or intrauterine devices (IUDs).

Synthetic: Synthetic hormones are produced by synthesis: they're made in a lab, not by our bodies.

Custom compounding: Custom-compounded medications have been mixed specifically for a specific patient rather than commercially premade. Custom compounding is a very important option for those with allergies and sensitivities: a custom-compounding pharmacy can make a needed medication safe for someone it wouldn't otherwise be safe for. It also can make a big difference for people having a hard time fine-tuning some kinds of mass-market medications or finding medicines they need at all.

Custom compounding also presents some risks. NAMS makes clear custom-compounded MHT, specifically, is "not tested for safety and effectiveness or to prove that the active ingredients are absorbed appropriately or provide predictable levels in blood and tissue. In fact, they may not even contain the prescribed amounts of hormones, and that can be dangerous." Dr. Hersh adds, "I trust my pharmacist. He trusts the supplier he gets his ingredients from. But when studied, big quality problems have been found with suppliers. A pharmacist may think they're getting .5% of an active ingredient, but they get 200% instead, and they can't know that. There have also been problems with contamination."

That doesn't mean that custom compounding is all bad, or even mostly bad. You simply may want to be more vigilant if you use custom compounding when it comes to vetting your pharmacy. Just like it's always okay to screen your doctors for your safety, the same goes for pharmacies: you can always ask when a pharmacy's last safety checks were done, what the outcomes were, and any other questions you have to assure your safety.

Bioidentical: A bioidentical hormone has an identical molecular structure to that hormone produced by the body. In other words, bioidentical hormones are molecularly identical to our own hormones: those that *aren't* considered bioidentical have a *similar* molecular structure rather than an identical molecular structure. But being chemically identical doesn't mean they will necessarily act the same as our own do or would in our bodies. They also aren't, or aren't all, necessarily any safer, more effective, or better for you than hormone therapy on the whole that isn't bioidentical or that is but isn't advertised with that terminology.

They aren't more "natural." First off, the ingredients most often used for bioidentical formulations (like wild yam and soy) have to be made in a lab and made to *be* bioidentical. Hormones classified as bioidentical—a marketing term—are *also* synthetic. Both bioidentical hormones *and* those that are not may, and also may not, be made from "natural" sources.

Dr. Hersh says, "There has never been a study that's shown bioidentical hormones are safer. *All* hormone therapy is binding to the same receptors. If it's doing that, and having the same end action, who's to say one is better than another?" She also makes clear that topical bioidentical estrogen is well absorbed, but topical bioidentical progesterone is not. "It is virtually impossible to use enough topical bioidentical progesterone to balance any estrogen therapy, and that can leave people less protected from uterine cancer. In addition, there is [currently] no FDA-approved bioidentical transdermal progesterone on the market." Bioidentical hormone therapies are also usually custom compounded (but some premade bioidentical MHT is also available), so additional risks that custom compounding can pose can be in the mix as well.

Dr. Hersh says that *compounded* bioidentical hormones may be appropriate for topical vulvar use, but they should not be used for systemic MHT. Therefore, she doesn't personally prescribe compounded estrogen for systemic MHT and, again, advises against topical progesterone, period. But setting aside the matter of topical progesterone, possible quality-control issues with custom compounding and any dosage mistakes, misunderstandings, or misuse on the side of the user (which obviously also can be an issue with MHT that isn't bioidentical too), while regulated bioidenticals may not be *more* safe than synthetics, they also do not usually appear to be *less* safe.

of these studies weren't sound. But even when we know that, even when we know the past may have colored our perception of the present, it still makes sense to be cautious. There's nothing wrong with making health decisions carefully and mindfully. I recommend it.

HORMONE THERAPY TODAY

While we still need more and continued study, hormone therapy has come a long way since it started and is very different than it was sixty years ago or even just twenty years ago. It's difficult to sit with knowledge that came from bad outcomes for or harm to others, but a lot has been learned about MHT from past mistakes.

There's also been a lot more research done on hormone regimens thanks to not just the women's health movement and its influence but trans healthcare, cancer research, and endocrinology.

WHAT'S CHANGED?

We know much more than we used to. We have more diverse research and more options, and hormone therapy both as a whole and with menopause specifically is understood, considered, provided, and managed in very different ways than in the past. Currently, so long as it's being prescribed and monitored by a qualified provider, and the patient is following directions and communicating any changes or issues, MHT *is* safe for many, if not most, people.

MHT is safer now because the people for whom a given form or route of administration is most potentially dangerous are usually screened out and no longer prescribed it. Those using any form of MHT for whom it may come with more risk are also supposed to be more carefully and accurately monitored.

We have also different protocols, regimens, formulations, forms, and recommendations than we did in the past.

Much like with the estrogen amounts in early birth control pills, before, during, and for about twenty years after Wilson's era, systemic estrogen was also given at doses about **four or more times higher** than is usually prescribed today. Even though it's estrogen that got the bad rap from it, the problem child in the combination used in the WHI study that gave some scary results was the specific progestin, not the estrogen, and we know *that* now. There are more now-versus-then differences with these kinds of significance.

There are now numerous potential formulations of all kinds of MHT and many different ways to prescribe them, so they can—and should—be tailored to the wants, needs, body, and health—including the risks—of the person using them. If you see a qualified and quality healthcare provider about MHT, and it's safe for you, they're going to help you choose a regimen based on your needs, your health and health history, and your preferences. If what you're prescribed ever isn't working for you, they'll tinker with it: it's not usually MHT or the highway unless you want it to be. They'll probably tinker more than once just to adjust for hormonal shifts across the different phases of menopause.

Hormone levels and other important factors (like blood sugar, heart and liver health, and cancers) are now screened for in reliable, accurate ways and taken into account. More is also known about interactions with other medications and ways certain health conditions and MHT interact. Personalization alone has radically improved the risk-benefit ratio of MHT for those who use it.

WHY WOULD YOU WANT TO USE MHT? WHY WOULDN'T YOU?

Hormone therapies for menopause have been found to effectively help with hot flashes and night sweats, genital dryness, soreness or genital pain, urinary tract infections (UTIs) and other urinary issues, dry skin, joint pain, mood issues, cognition, sexual desire and other sexual response, muscle mass, and bone density. In the event you're someone who's interested in affirming or transitioning your gender with hormone therapy, some forms of HT can also help ease or counteract some of the impacts of menopause. Some forms of MHT can reduce some major health risks *post*menopause, namely, osteoporosis and related bone injuries, tooth loss, colon cancer, and diabetes.

What access you have to MHT and how consistent that access can—or can't—be is something to consider. MHT may also present some risks or dangers. What those are depends on the kind of MHT and regimen, your unique health history, and your current circumstances. Not using MHT can involve risks, though, too.

Hormone therapy is typically *recommended* for a few specific menopausal groups. For people who have had a total hysterectomy, the risks of breast cancer and osteoporosis are lower if estrogen therapy is used. Unless testosterone was being used before hysterectomy, estrogen therapy can ease what is usually otherwise a very sudden and intense transition. As much as a 90 percent drop in estrogen all at once is a massive systematic change. Estrogen therapy is also sometimes recommended for those who have bilateral oophorectomy *or* hysterectomy. It's recommended for those who experience early menopause (noninduced) before age forty-five, and even more so for those who reach it before age forty, primarily to reduce risks of genitourinary discomfort or pain, osteoporosis, heart disease, depression, anxiety, and dementia. Local vaginal estrogen is very often recommended for those over sixty-five and/or postmenopause.

HELLA BASIC MHT LITERACY

My aim here is just to give you enough to get a vague sense of what you might or might not want to consider and to give you some standard equipment for conversations with healthcare providers or anyone else qualified to actually prescribe you things that you want to talk about it with. This is my bicycle lane, and I'm sticking to it.

I DON'T LIST BRAND NAMES OR SPECIFIC MHT regimens. The range of options is vast (especially worldwide), ever changing, and constantly developing, and what's right for you is something only you or you and a care provider can soundly work out. Health information also changes superfast, especially with medications. Without further adieu—

Estrogen, progesterone or progestin, and testosterone therapies can potentially help with many impacts of menopause. Each or any of these three hormones are available as therapies, used alone or in combination. They won't be right for everyone, but they are both safe and effective for many people.

At the time of this writing, reliable, specialized healthcare organizations like NAMS, the UK National Institute for Health and Care Excellence (NICE), the American Society for Reproductive Medicine, and the Endocrine Society agree that estrogen-based systemic hormone therapy is safe for most healthy, recently menopausal people specifically for relief of hot flashes and vaginal dryness. Local estrogen therapies are also considered safe by these and other qualified organizations and experts.

The Endocrine Society, NICE, NAMS, the International Menopause Society, the Federación Latinoamericana de Sociedades de Climaterio y Menopausia, the Royal College of Obstetricians and Gynaecologists, and several other medical societies currently also support use of testosterone for menopause, particularly for low sexual desire.

All three of these hormones can potentially help with other menopause impacts too. As with any medication, they can be prescribed and recommended "off label" for other things they're known to help with but not yet specifically approved for.

None of us likely want headaches, but I'm not usually going to presume what's a wanted benefit or an unwanted side effect because that's personal. One person's unwanted facial hair is someone else's mustachioed dream.

ESTROGEN

Estrogen can currently be administered orally or nonorally (transdermally) via patches, pellets, gels, sprays, creams, injections, and vaginal rings, creams, or tablets. Transdermal estrogen has a safer risk profile than oral estrogen with respect to blood clots, strokes, and cholesterol changes because it doesn't interact with the liver. For those who have not had a total hysterectomy, it's currently most often recommended that estrogen therapy be used transitionally and for as short a time as possible. However, this can vary from patient to patient and is something that's in a bit of a state of flux at the moment.

Local estrogen—rather than systemic—can help where it's placed (usually vaginally) but can also sometimes help with some impacts in other systems of the body. Estrogen creams, gels, or sprays and local vaginal estrogen can be transferred to others, so handwashing is important with some preparations to prevent that; barrier use (condoms, gloves, or dental dams) can help limit a sexual partner's exposure.

If you're in perimenopause, still have a uterus, and want to do estrogen-based MHT, combined hormone therapy—opposing the estrogen with progesterone or progestin—is recommended to protect against endometrial cancer. That can be done via precombined medications (like combined hormonal contraceptives that contain a progestin) or by adding progesterone separately to an estrogen regimen via another pill or cream or progestin locally via an IUD. Systemic estrogen-*only* hormone therapy isn't likely to be advised for anyone who still has a uterus before they are postmenopausal due to uterine cancer risks.

The risks estrogen-based therapy poses have a lot to do with individual health history and age. Things that pose big risks at one age don't at another, and estrogen therapy can potentially offer protection in one situation and increased risk in another.

Like many other medications, MHT can be like the pumpkin carriage in Cinderella: the effects you get expressly from taking it won't continue when you stop using it. So, for instance, if it helped with hot flashes or joint pain, when you stop taking it, if those haven't ended for you independently of the MHT, they may resume.

Here's the quick lowdown about what estrogen therapies may do and some risks and risk groups. These are about either systemic or local estrogen or both. On the whole, local estrogen will do less (it mostly helps with genital effects), but it also poses far fewer risks.

Primary possible effects:

- May reduce hot flashes/night sweats
- May decrease vulvovaginal dryness and pain with vaginal sex (including for local estrogen, which is what it is often prescribed for)
- May help with cognition, and with digestive, mood, and sleep issues but may also have negative mood impacts
- May help prevent osteoporosis and decrease risks of colon cancer and diabetes
- May help keep skin thicker and more resilient
- May protect heart health if used soon after menopause

- May increase both "good" and "bad" cholesterol
- May help with incontinence and can also support bladder tissue and help reduce occurrence of UTIs

Possible risks:
- Nausea and indigestion
- Headache or worsening headache
- Bloating, vaginal bleeding or spotting, and breast tenderness
- Blood clots, deep vein thrombosis, stroke, or heart attack
- Uterine/endometrial or breast cancer

The breast cancer risk doubles if it is used for more than ten years. When used for less than one year, it is widely agreed, there is little or no increased risk of breast cancer, and estrogen-only MHT may even help *prevent* breast cancer for some. Again, uterine/endometrial cancer risks can be mitigated by opposing estrogen with a progestin or progesterone.

Folks for whom systemic estrogen is currently considered extra risky or dangerous:
- Smokers
- People who are currently pregnant
- People with or who have had breast or uterine/endometrial cancer, blood clots, heart attack, stroke, transient ischemic attack, liver disease or liver problems, undiagnosed uterine bleeding, untreated endometrial hyperplasia, any known or suspected estrogen-sensitive malignant conditions, or a known or suspected allergy or sensitivity to estrogen or other ingredients in their hormone therapy
- People with a family history or who are otherwise known to be at higher risk of developing breast cancer or heart disease
- People who are ten years or more postmenopause and/or over sixty and have not already started using it

SELECTIVE ESTROGEN RECEPTOR MODULATORS (SERMS)

The North American Menopause Society explains that SERMs

activate or block the estrogen receptors only in certain areas of the body and not others. That can make them safer than estrogen alone or result in fewer side effects. For example, a SERM that acts like estrogen mainly in the vagina and not the uterus helps avoid the risk of uterine cancer because it doesn't stimulate the uterine lining (called the endometrium) the way estrogen does. Because SERMs vary in

What about *phyto*estrogens? See the mini-herbal on page 279.

their activating (agonist) or blocking (antagonist) properties, they can be used to selectively target, prevent, and/or treat several diseases, including breast cancer, osteoporosis, and the genitourinary syndrome of menopause.

As of right now, there isn't a SERM yet found to work alone for vasomotor issues, but there is one FDA-approved combination of an estrogen *and* a SERM being used for this purpose. A SERM-estrogen combination can also sometimes be used instead of a progesterone/progestin-estrogen combination to protect the uterus like progesterone would.

PROGESTOGENS

Progesterone is the version of this hormone that our body makes. Progestins are synthetic versions that differ in structure from what the body makes. (There are also synthetic bioidentical progesterones that don't differ in structure.) Progesterone or progestin can be used alone or as a combined therapy with estrogen or testosterone.

A progesterone or progestin is commonly used either in combination with estrogen or by itself, especially in early perimenopause when estrogen is acting out. Progestin-only contraception methods—like a progestin IUD—or combined hormonal methods (like the pill, patch, or ring) are commonly used as

a form of MHT, especially in early perimenopause. That's often even accidentally accomplished by those who experience much or even all of their menopausal transition while already using those methods for contraception or another reason.

When used with estrogen therapy, progesterone or progestin reduces the risk of endometrial cancer by keeping the uterine lining thin (estrogen alone would make it keep growing and building up). Those who no longer have their uterus are not typically prescribed a progestogen since they obviously no longer need *that* benefit, but it is still often an option if other benefits it can offer are wanted.

Some people who may not be able to safely use a progestogen, or should use or be prescribed with caution include:
- people with bleeding or clotting problems, or undiagnosed vaginal bleeding;
- people with impaired liver or kidney function;
- people with depression;
- people with breast or reproductive cancers;
- people with some cardiovascular issues, asthma, or seizure disorders.

Primary possible effects:
- Helps protect the uterus
- May reduce or stop flooding (heavy menstrual bleeding)

- May help with hot flashes and night sweats
- May improve mood (especially the anxiety part of the mood spectrum)

Possible risks:
- Headache
- Breast tenderness or pain
- Muscle, joint, or bone pain
- Upset stomach, diarrhea, or constipation
- Increased depression, mood swings, irritability, anxiety, or fatigue
- Runny nose, sneezing, or coughing
- Breast and ovarian cancer
- Cardiovascular issues
- Worsened liver disease

TESTOSTERONE (T)

You might not even think about testosterone in this context. I didn't, and I'm even someone who's thought about using T for other reasons.

Testosterone does a lot of different things, but some of the biggest when it comes to managing menopause involve dopamine production, muscle mass and bone density, sexual desire, metabolism, mood, and cognition. Our bodies can even convert some of it into estrogen via the enzyme aromatase. Over the course of our adult lives, everyone's testosterone levels gradually decrease to some degree. By the time we're around menopause, many of us will have about half as much as we did in our twenties.

We have less data to work with regarding testosterone therapies for menopause than we do for estrogen and progestogens. As of right now, we know testosterone doesn't carry most of the risks estrogen-only or combined-estrogen therapies do, and it can be used by some people who cannot, should not, or don't want to use estrogen. The Testosterone Implant Breast Cancer Prevention Study, a ten-year study, has found that subcutaneous testosterone resulted in a *reduced* incidence of breast cancer compared to what studies of other kinds of hormonal treatment for menopause found.

Testosterone can be administered orally, transdermally, or intramuscularly. It can be used with other hormones as well. Prescribing testosterone for use expressly for menopause is currently considered off label. The amount of testosterone prescribed for menopause will vary, but unless someone is looking to also use it

Unless there are medical contraindications, if testosterone was used before or started at the same time, it's often continued lifelong after a total oophorectomy. Testosterone may also be suggested for those who have had a hysterectomy and are not having good impacts with estrogen or who don't want to or can't use it.

for gender affirmation, it will usually be low dose or microdose.

Possible effects:
- May reduce hot flashes and night sweats
- May help with sleep issues
- May help relieve muscle, joint, or bone pain and help maintain bone density and lean muscle mass
- May increase sexual desire or other sexual response
- May help with depression
- May suppress or stop periods and/or help with menstrual flooding
- May help with cognition, mood, and sleep issues
- May help with muscle mass, bone density, fatigue, and digestion.
- May result in weight gain
- May increase or change the texture, amount, or pattern of body or facial hair, including male pattern baldness
- May cause vocal changes (lowering voice)
- May result in clitoral enlargement

Possible risks:
- Acne or increased acne
- Cardiovascular disease or hypertension
- Increased risk of diabetes, hyperlipidemia, and elevated liver enzymes
- Sleep apnea or increased sleep apnea
- Risk of destabilizing psychiatric disorders
- Risk of thinning, less resilient genital tissue; increase in issues related to

genitourinary symptoms of menopause (see page 184)

People who should not use testosterone or should be carefully evaluated first:
- People who are pregnant
- People with unstable coronary artery disease
- People with a personal history of breast or other cancers or untreated polycythemia
- People who have PCOS

IF YOU'RE ALREADY USING T

As you may have already discovered, if you've already been using something more than a low dose of testosterone, and you haven't experienced menopause already because of oophorectomy or total hysterectomy, you won't likely experience menopause the way those who *haven't* been using testosterone often do.

If you've been using it in more than a low dose for more than a few months, your periods may have become lighter, shorter, more infrequent, or stopped. The hormonal cycling that happens with menstrual cycles and then does all the things it does in perimenopause (or sudden menopause) won't have the same patterns. You also may have already experienced a kind of half menopause and some of its impacts—like hot flashes—when you adjusted to testosterone. The good news is that your menopause transition may be a lot more gradual, with fewer estrogen spikes and, instead, a more gradual estrogen decline over a longer time than would otherwise be the case. T can be a way to ease menopausal chaos like estrogen can be.

If you haven't already, when you experience menopause, you may have genital issues—like dryness, soreness, or pain with some kinds of sex—earlier or more severely than others going through it around the same age who aren't using T. Local estrogen is one option for improving vaginal dryness or incidence of UTIs after hysterectomy or oophorectomy if systemic estrogen isn't wanted. Local estrogen will not have other effects some consider feminizing that happen with systemic use.

If you've been thinking about using testosterone for gender affirmation but have not yet started, and you are also having any menopausal impacts T can help with, it just might be kismet.

JUST LIKE WITH OTHER MEDICATIONS, you may not hit a home run with your first swing with MHT. You may need to work with your healthcare providers over time to make adjustments. If you're on other medications for other things, you might need to make adjustments with or because of *those* meds too.

HORMONES AND GENDER

If you decide to try or use MHT, which form of it you use is probably mostly going to be about what impacts you are looking for help managing, what forms of it are most likely to help, and what's safe, accessible, and works best for you. But how you feel about hormones and gender—whether that's about some of the effects MHT can have or about your feelings about the "gender" of hormones—might play a part too.

Again, hormones themselves do not have sex or gender. But as UK-based psychotherapist Tania Glyde, who's researched the experiences of LGBTQ+ menopausal clients in therapy and the healthcare system and is also just a magnificent human, says, "Society has pinned the gender binary on them to the point where just the idea of them can cause people to feel dysphoric, even when taking them supplementally could help with some issues."

As you no doubt already know all too well, if you experience these things, dysphoria and other big feelings like it are not, alas, often all that responsive to rational explanations. In the event that MHT is something you want to explore, but the kind of MHT that might provide what you want for your menopause feels at odds with what you want or what feels right for your gender, be sure to find an educated and supportive provider. A candid talk about this with them may help you find a kind of MHT that feels more affirming of your gender and can also help with the impacts you want help with. It may be that there's a way to take a kind of MHT you feel at odds with without it feeling so at odds. Whatever you do, rather than giving yourself grief for having feelings that may or may not be objectively "reasonable," my vote is to accept those feelings and ask to have them considered in your care and your decisions about MHT—and any other aspect of care.

CAN YOU JUST TRY MHT AND SEE?

Absolutely. It's okay to go on and then adjust as you need to or ditch it if and when you want. Unless you're a decade or more postmenopause, you probably don't have to make any now-or-never decisions about hormone therapy soon. The idea that we have to decide early and once and for all adds wholly unnecessary pressure.

It's generally considered best practice to start patients on the lowest doses, anyway, so you'll usually already be given a tentative start regardless. If you are going to use more than one kind of hormone, taking them separately rather than as a combined formula can make it easier to figure out what's working and what isn't and to make adjustments. It can also obviously make it easier to get rid of any one of them you feel like you don't like and still keep another. If your provider doesn't suggest that approach, it's something you can ask about. Ask your provider how long you'd have to take something to get past the side effects and get to the benefits, so you can get a good sense of when

you'll be able to really know if something is working for you or not and worth any lingering effects you don't want.

Be sure to also find out how to stop any MHT safely if you decide it isn't for you, rather than just stopping on your own without that guidance.

I WANT TO ECHO RANDI HUTTER EP-stein in *Aroused: The History of Hormones and How They Control Just About Everything*, when she says, "Those of us old enough to be in menopause can't help but wonder if the experts are going to change their minds again. Menopause choices highlight the ever-present uncertainty in medicine."

If and when you see a provider to consider or seek out any kind of MHT, make sure *they* have been doing their homework and *they* have been keeping up. Ask lots of questions. Ask them about the currently known benefits, currently known risks, and what studies have their utmost interest or concern lately. Ask them to explain why their approach for you is the approach they feel is best for *you*.

There's no forever-correct health information, especially in this still emerging arena. I've revised this part of the book several times during the course of writing and editing it, and by the time you're reading this, I'll probably have wished I could have changed it again several times since. This is why it's so important to find qualified care providers who keep up with

DOCTOR! DOCTOR!

the changing information and protocols, especially if we don't all want to have to do a ton of menopause homework of our own on the regular.

PLACEBO POWER

What works for people in any or all of menopause can be a whole lot of things, including things that technically (or based in the way we study them) aren't doing anything at all. Some commonly used and long-valued remedies for menopause have been found to have a placebo effect in studies. But that doesn't mean they aren't still effective for some people.

It may be those studies were flawed. Studies done on the herb black cohosh often used for hot flashes, for instance, have been criticized for potentially just not using the proper amount or formulation. Cannabidiol (CBD) is another example: at a certain dosage, it's definitely not a placebo, but at low dosages, it likely is. We know some modalities just don't mesh with conventional medicine or study methodologies well. It's also just as possible that some substances, medicines, or other kinds of treatments *are* a placebo and are *also* effective.

Many of us learned placebo means "not real" or "all in your head." That is absolutely not the case.

A placebo is something considered medically inert, something that, by itself, is not directly active. It can be a pill, the way we commonly think of placebos, but it can also be a kind of treatment, like cupping or Reiki. A *placebo effect* happens when what is considered a placebo still has an impact. The placebo effect is real. Those who study it are clear that it can even be **just** as effective as active substances and nonplacebo treatments.

The placebo effect isn't just about positive thinking or belief, but sometimes that's all or part of what's happening. As with a lot of menopause, it's neurochemistry. When it happens, the placebo effect works by engaging powerful neurotransmitters. Our brain, all its chemicals, and all the chemicals and pathways that interact with it have a lot to do with how we feel throughout our whole body and all its systems and everything to do with how we feel emotionally. The placebo effect illustrates what our minds and bodies can do when they're working really well together. A placebo effect is understood to happen for the following reasons:

1. **Our outlook and expectations are positive.** We expect to feel better when we take or do a thing, and that positive expectation nets positive results. Some of this also has to do with paying more attention to what's improved or improving rather than to what feels bad or hopeless.

2. **The mere mechanism of taking a medication (like swallowing a pill)**

or having a treatment has a positive impact. Positive associations, experiences, and beliefs can also create positive outcomes.

3. **We are engaging in or receiving care.** Our minds and our bodies tend to have positive reactions to things we recognize as care, whether that's external, like care from a bodywork practitioner or doctor, self-care, or both, like self-administering a pill prescribed by a care provider.

Any or all of those things can ping the reward centers of our brain, which then release endorphins. Just like we have estrogen and progesterone receptors, we also have opioid receptors. Endorphins, like synthetic opiates, bind to them and can result in relief, especially pain relief. It's even currently thought the more vulnerable we are to opiate addiction—which has a lot to do with how many of those receptors we have—the more likely we are to find success with placebos. One of the best-known studies of placebos showed that a placebo could, for some patients, do just as good a job in managing pain as morphine. Dopamine and dopamine receptors are also at play in the placebo effect, especially when it comes to our anticipation of positive effects.

Placebos don't have to be covert to be effective. Not only does the placebo effect still occur even with use of "open" placebos—where people are told a thing is a placebo right from the start—but pain researcher Dr. Luana Colloca found that placebos are *more* effective when the person using them *knows* they're taking them or that they are placebos.

The *nocebo* effect, which Dr. Colloca's lab also studies, is the antithesis of the placebo effect. When the nocebo effect is in play, belief in or expectation of a *negative* outcome results in a *negative* outcome. Again, the idea that our attitude *alone* is responsible for our experience of menopause is dismissive garbage that ignores or denies major players like genetics (which are involved in things like how many opioid receptors we have, no less), the past, and other giant and immoveable circumstances. That said, both the placebo effect and the nocebo effect can be at play with menopause to varying degrees and in a host of ways.

If you find something that may work for you via a placebo effect, that doesn't mean it isn't real or that you need to stop using that thing to find other help or treatment. A placebo effect is not just in your head: it can do some very real things, including in the menopause space, especially with sleep, pain, hot flashes, and night sweats. If you're happy with a placebo or a maybe-placebo, and it's safe and something that you can access and feel good about using, there's no reason to stop using it if you don't want to.

THE MENOPAUSE MARKET (THAT'S US)

A lot of people who want to make a lot of money are starting to pay attention to menopause. Menopause market projections suggest that within the next five years, even more people will be looking to strike it rich in the potential gold rush of our desperation and discontent. That attention may sound like good news to those of us who are members of an endlessly ignored generation. In some ways, it might be. In other ways, not so much.

It can be easy to assume the best of new companies or products when the people who own, run, or are presenting them either look like us or at least have themselves experienced menopause and are saying they just want to help us out. Since we very much were not born yesterday, we may be wary. On the other hand, I doubt I need to tell anyone my age that desperation can make us vulnerable: most of us have at least one job, apartment, or ex that taught us that already.

What newer and emerging companies or individuals want to sell us is all over the map: boutique healthcare or prescription subscriptions, supplements, CBD, lubes, lotions, skin potions, exercise regimens, diets, new brands or forms of hormone therapies, many of which are and will be advertised as safer or more effective without any substantial evidence of such. Even when they might be *less* safe. Some do and will continue to use fear-based or antihormone messages in their marketing. Given the fear and stigma attached to hormone use, even just saying something is "nonhormonal" (or "natural" for that matter) will play on fears about hormones.

These "just like us" founders or other salespeople are also often shitty to us in their apparent effort to help. They often use things that make us feel bad about ourselves, like ableism, ageism, fat shaming, and fears about our desirability, to sell their wares.

Big pharma, of course, is gonna keep big-pharma-ing. It's bullshit that it's for-profit, let alone the level of profit it involves. But that's just how it is for now, and some of us do or will need or want pharmaceutical medications, including for or during any part of menopause.

SOME OF WHAT IS BEING OFFERED *IS* useful, safe, and effective for plenty of folks. Telehealth services that specialize in menopause can provide that care to some people who wouldn't be able to access it otherwise. If that healthcare service insists you buy things from them that you don't need or want to or that aren't likely to be effective, that's an obvious problem. But if they are offering things you'd buy anyway, and they're as good and as affordable as the alternatives, so what? It can even be easier to get much of what you need in one place. Most of us already use or will need things later, like lube, genital moisturizers, or nutrition helps. Many of us buy rather than make those things. It's okay for us to buy them and for people to make and sell them to us. All the better if and when we can buy them from people we want to support anyway, like BIPOC women.

That all said, we'd be unwise to forget how much profit influences things, very much including people's care about our well-being, physically, emotionally, *and* economically.

By now, you likely also already know the basic rules of not getting scammed, wasting your own time, or just throwing money down the toilet, but when it comes to menopause, specifically, here are some red flags:

- Look out for keywords that play on ignorance or fear with menopausal therapies and other helps. "Natural" is one of the biggies, and "nonhormonal" is another, because so many people don't know that just because something isn't hormonal or is made from natural sources, that doesn't automatically make it better or safer.
- In order to access or continue to access a care service, do you have to also buy products from them?
- With healthcare, be on the lookout for things like those mentioned on page 94:

Are they doing saliva hormone testing? Is anyone certified by NAMS or another similar menopause-care accreditation body?
- Is what you're being offered in a healthcare membership worth it versus what you'd pay to get that care otherwise? Will you wind up having to pay for both the membership and outside menopause care?
- And that perennial favorite: if it feels too good to be true, it probably is.

Since a menopausal transition can potentially last many years and also potentially cause a lot of disruption and require ongoing management, it has the potential to get very expensive. I've always wanted to dramatically say, *"It's going to cost you,"* and it seems this is my chance.

Stuff we pay for that doesn't do any harm but also isn't actually needed or effective sucks for our budgets. And the more we're marketed to and the more there is to buy, the easier it is to really rack up a tab. You might want to consider setting a monthly menopause budget, organizing a menopause community care closet, or limiting your use of the internet to watching family members unwittingly reenact old *Jerry Springer* episodes.

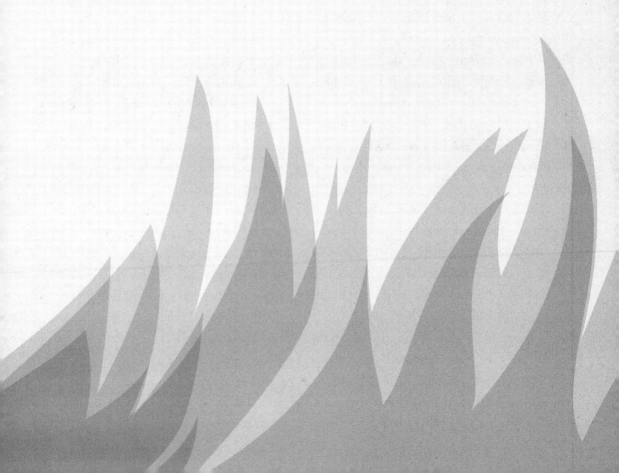

PART 2

BRACE FOR IMPACTS

SOME THINGS THAT CAN HAPPEN DURING PERIMENOPAUSE, WHY THEY HAPPEN, AND SOME THINGS YOU CAN DO ABOUT THEM

IN YOUR MANY MENOPAUSAL INTERNET-searching travels, you may have come across a list of the apparent and terrifying thirty-four "symptoms" of menopause, most often credited to uncited and unnamed "experts." I have both good news and bad news about that list.

The bad news is that all of the things on that list can indeed happen during some part or all of a menopausal transition, and some of them happen to more people than not and with some frequency. I also think they left some off. The good news is that none of this is likely to be as apocalyptic as that list—and even my own foul mood and impatience—can make it seem, even when you're having a not-wonderful time of things.

For one, those things do not all happen to everyone and also do not all happen at the same time even when they do. It is unlikely that you will find yourself in an epic battle with the worst of all of these at once, like that scene in *Jason and the Argonauts* where Jason is trying to take down all those skeletons by himself. Or in real life, harder still, where you've completely lost control of a classroom of thirty kindergartners after they all just had cupcakes and you have three minutes to get it back before all hope is lost.

Some of them that sound extra scary—like burning-mouth syndrome, electric-shock sensation, or loss of libido—sound that way because they have been named by people who clearly missed

their calling as horror writers. Many of the things that can happen during menopausal transition also resolve soon, or eventually, afterward. The people who make and distribute this list also neglect to mention how many of these things happen because they were already happening for people premenopause, are more about aging than menopause, and, most of all, can be managed and survived, if not always eliminated.

Menopause is a life stage. It's not an illness or progressive disease. "Symptoms," when we're talking about human bodies, are things we experience from illness, disease, or other health conditions. There are no "symptoms" of menopause in this respect, and I just don't feel like it helps any of us out to keep holdovers from Robert Wilson–era views of menopause.

Things happen to us in it, for sure: it has some *impacts* or *effects*, like puberty and pregnancy do. Parts of it or its impacts can also certainly interact with any existing disease, illness, or disability we might have. But unless it's part of a term currently used medically—because I don't want to confuse you more—like "vasomotor symptoms," I'll be talking about impacts and effects here, not symptoms.

What follows in the next seven chapters is information about the most common of those impacts or effects: what they are, why they happen, and if they happen and you want to try and do something about them, some options to manage them.

You Might Want to Write This Down

Logging your experience with a menopausal transition can come in really handy. Keeping track of the impacts and effects you're having can help you keep a bird's-eye view of what's going on. It's easy to lose track of how long or how severely some things have been going on—especially stuff extra easy to lose yourself in, like depression or fatigue—and to second-guess or downplay your own suffering. If you log it, you can see what's what to back yourself up if and when you want to seek out any kind of help.

If you do that, and you have logged known or possible impacts like hot flashes, fatigue, or headaches, anything over the next hundred pages or so, it's going to be easier for care providers to help you out and keep helping you fine-tune things, like MHT or other medicines or dietary or sleep-routine changes. I'd certainly also log dates of menstrual periods and how they go, when and if you have them, and any and all medications or supplements you're using, with dates, being sure to note any changes, such as in dosage or brand.

You probably want to keep this log on a mobile phone or in a notebook or bullet journal, but if writing it on a wall in blood with your fingernails feels more appropriate, that's cool, too.

CHAPTER SIX

VASOMOTOR CHAOS

HOT FLASHES AND NIGHT SWEATS

"Ask a burning question, get a burning answer."
—*Lynda Barry*

As if on cue, the very second I created a page for this section and typed in the title, I started to feel a hot flash come on. Some people apparently don't experience them. How nice for those people that must be.

Hot flashes (or flushes) and night sweats—currently clinically called "vasomotor symptoms" or "vasomotor disturbances"—are two of the most commonly reported and recognized indications of menopause. They're the wink of menopause media appearances: when a director wants to let us know someone's in menopause, they show us a telltale fanning of the face, soaked shirt, or sweaty brow for no good reason otherwise. Hot flashes or sweats often get patronizing laugh tracks, likely because people who haven't themselves experienced the worst

of them think they're funny or, for those who have experienced them yet still make jokes, maybe because they became delirious as a result *of* experiencing them, which is certainly plausible. What else *but* delirium could explain menopause in-jokes like "They aren't hot flashes, they're power surges!" or "I'm still hot, now it just comes in flashes!"

In reality, sudden, unexpected, and radical changes of body temperature can feel disturbing and disorienting, especially when they first start happening to you, you're not expecting them, and you didn't know what they'd feel like. Certainly, no one is laughing after weeks, months, or even years of interrupted sleep. Having to cycle between three different layers of clothing in a constant loop as you flash between hot and ice-cold, again and again, when you're just trying to get through a shift or a commute is really freaking stressful.

FLASHDANCE. OH. WHAT A FEELING.

Hot flashes are one of the most common impacts experienced by most folks at some point during a menopausal transition. While at least 25 percent of people apparently won't experience them at all, and some will but only rarely or for a short period, most of us—with either gradual or sudden menopause—will deal with hot flashes, sweats, or both.

They're more common when we're stressed; if we have certain medical conditions, including thyroid and autoimmune conditions, epilepsy, cancer, and leukemia; and if we have past or current trauma.

Not everyone feels the same way about them or has the same experience. I haven't yet heard anyone describe them as pleasant, exactly, but I did read someone who said that having been cold all their life, it wasn't terrible to feel warm. How disruptive or distressing you'll find them is probably going to have something to do with their severity or frequency—it's a lot easier to brush them off when they aren't happening that often or aren't that bad, obviously—and how you feel about them. If they or what they do—sweat stains, soggy sheets, a wet or red face, a need to pause or acknowledge to others what's happening—makes you feel shame, anxiety, or stress, they'll probably be more of a pain than if, even if the physical experience of them still isn't delightful, you can feel pretty relaxed about them as something that's certainly weird but usually no big deal and ultimately normal.

WHAT ARE HOT FLASHES AND NIGHT SWEATS?

What we know about **hot flashes** is that a body is seemingly minding its own business, when its blood vessels constrict and then expand rapidly in what are known as vasomotor spasms. Those spasms create a surface temperature change that causes the body to suddenly feel an intense heat, most typically on or around the face, head, neck, or chest and which might stop there or might quickly spread across or all through the whole body, like your internal thermostat is doing a sadistic version of the wave. If you prefer a more science-y explanation, they're "transient sensations of heat, sweating, flushing, anxiety, and chills lasting for one to five minutes, the basis of which is abnormal hypothalamic thermoregulatory control resulting in abnormal vasodilatory response to minor elevations of core body temperature."

Apparently, the temperature change that happens with hot flashes is minor, and even though it's mostly on the surface of the skin—if the body's core temperature changes at all, it's often a drop after a flash rather than a rise during—that's sure not what it can feel like. It can feel like you are literally catching on fire. Some people feel hot flashes in other areas of the body besides the face, neck, and upper abdomen. Some get a prickly feeling with them or even feel faint or dizzy. They may bring sweating with them (or not) and can leave the chills behind when they go (or don't). Some folks mostly or even only feel the chills instead of the heat. Sometimes they make you look red and flushed. They can bring about or happen concurrently with heart palpitations and panic attacks. Sometimes they can even bring feelings of severe dread or hopelessness.

Hot flashes generally last anywhere from seconds to minutes, but it can feel like longer. They can occur just once or twice in any part of menopause or happen throughout peri and even in postmenopause.

Night sweats are what happens when you have hot flashes in your sleep. That may sound like no big deal. However, if and when they disrupt your ability to sleep for days, weeks, months, or years, increase the amount of laundry you have to do, and bring you to your knees begging deities you don't even believe in to just give you ONE FREAKING NIGHT without them so you can get just a few hours of sleep uninterrupted, I assure you, they can be a very big deal.

Some people don't find them so at all, though, and may even just sleep through them, unaware they're happening at all.

They can be as short as hot flashes themselves, or the sweaty part can carry on for longer or hold on between hot flashes (like the not-at-all lovely time they and I spent together last night between 12:37 and 4:21 a.m.). Some people only experience hot flashes, some only night sweats, some both, some neither.

In perimenopause, both hot flashes and night sweats are often at their most frequent and intense the closer someone gets to menopause and usually when the time between menstrual cycles is getting longer. You might think that hot flashes and night sweats are not a bad trade-off if you get to stop having periods forever. Or not.

WHAT IS THEIR DEAL?

Most sources agree at the moment that the hypothalamus gets signals from variable or low estrogen, high follicle-stimulating hormone, and low inhibin B (a peptide hormone that declines through menopause, especially in later perimenopause), which effectively confuse it, and it sends our temperature regulation systems incorrect information as a result. There's less agreement about the why, from where, and how of those signals.

It's been long thought that fluctuating or very radically changing estrogen levels are the cause. Estrogen is a player in regulation of our body temperature. Higher estrogen levels are also generally associated with cooler body temperatures. So, it's no surprise that vasomotor instability happens when we've got fluctuating or decreasing estrogen levels.

Nina Coslov explains, "Recent research suggests that changing hormone levels cause a narrowing of the 'thermoneutral zone' (the zone in which we feel comfortable, not sweaty or cold) in people with hot flashes." People who experience hot flashes are thought to have a smaller thermoneutral zone between their own high and low temperature set points than people who don't and so are more reactive to minor temperature changes. Higher norepinephrine levels are another possible factor.

Hot flashes and night sweats are often set off by something environmental, psychological, gastronomical, or otherwise spark inducing. Because there is no justice in this world, some of the things that can often make them happen are some of the most wonderful things on earth.

Like so much of menopause and everything that happens (or doesn't) with it, the things that seem to bring on, worsen, or increase the occurrence of hot flashes and night sweats aren't universal, but some common culprits can be

- hot or warm weather or rooms;
- hot foods or drinks;
- coffee and other sources of caffeine;
- smoking (cigarettes)—both when it comes to having a smoke and being a smoker generally;
- alcohol;
- clothing around your neck or chest (turtlenecks, the iron maidens of menopause) or tight clothes (whose mother made this list, anyway?);
- spicy foods;
- stinky cheese;
- sugar;
- chocolate (I'm so sorry);
- anxiety;
- stress.

WHAT CAN YOU DO ABOUT THEM?

While this stuff happens primarily because of things that are or may be outside our control, we have some or complete control over some things that make vasomotor glitching more likely.

If figuring out which things those are for you isn't easy, you can keep a log (there's that log, again!) of your vasomotor happenings and include information that can help you find patterns of what seems to set them off for you: if you were stressed or anxious when they happened, what you had to eat or drink before them or while they were happening, what medications you're using, or what you were doing at the time.

What you do once you know those things is up to you. You may choose to cut out one or more of those things from your life completely. You may choose to limit or reduce those things instead or be pickier about where and when they're part of your world—say, by deciding that only drinking after five was obviously a rule made by people who weren't in menopause and swapping your drinking time to lunch so you can enjoy your hooch and still sleep. You may not mind having hot flashes at home but find them super irritating at work, so you might limit things that can bring them on at work but not worry about them at home.

You can also do what I most often do, which is to do or have some things that bring them on for me anyway, knowing full well they will make it more likely I get vasomotor symptoms (I can predict the hot flash that occurs with my first morning coffee with astonishing accuracy), then kick myself when they inevitably do. We may not want to avoid some of those things, because they may be what makes life worth living as far as we're concerned or what gives us the ability to write professional memos instead of deranged ransom notes. Some things are worth the heat.

Ya Basics (page 60) can help with reducing and managing stress; social support; quitting, reducing, or limiting smoking; hydration; breathing; and regular movement. So can better sleep, but that's obviously complicated here.

You're probably already doing these things because they are not particularly mysterious and you are grown. But in case they aren't already on your radar, it's generally helpful to do the following:

- **Keep rooms cooler if you can.** Other people can always put a sweater on, for crying out loud, a sentence with which you and yours may already be intimately familiar.
- **Avoid sweat-inducing man-made fabrics and heavy layers.** If you have to wear a work uniform that's made of either, see if there isn't a cooler or more breathable alternative. And all I can tell you about bundling up to go outside in winter is to try and learn to do it really freaking fast, because there are some deeply miserable minutes to be had in that process.
- **Keep an extra shirt (and/or bra, binder, tank, or other underthing) handy for occasions when you've soaked all the way through yours.**
- **Keep a fan handy too.** This is maybe the news the highest of femmes have been waiting for all their lives. For those of us who aren't into elaborate folding fans, one of those handheld electric fans, a menu, or a file folder will do.
- **Like your real or imaginary Bubbe, give your face, neck, and chest a cool rinse or a schpritz with some water.** A drop or two of peppermint oil added to a rinse, spray bottle, shower gel, or anything else you use to cool down can give some extra help too. But as a

125

fellow cashier working next to me in the 1980s reminded me after I asked why they were shuddering all day, don't forget that peppermint anything in or around your asshole or your genitals can certainly feel too refreshing.

◊ **Load up on ice packs and other cooling stuff.** The top shelf of my freezer currently contains an ice roller; three kinds of flexible, long, rectangular-shaped ice packs with stretchy straps and Velcro attachments; a couple small packs; two pillow-sized giant ice packs (Best. Things. Ever.); and plenty of ice cubes. You can also soak a T-shirt in cold water, wring it out, and hang it on your neck. I wholeheartedly recommend a cooling pillow, in case that wasn't abundantly clear by now. If you'd use a fan but don't want to broadcast what's happening to others, ice packs or frozen small water bottles can be slipped into all kinds of places where no one will see them or where anyone in their right mind isn't going to ask you why it's there.

◊ **For night sweats, do the helpful sleep things (see page 66).**

Feelings and attitudes *can* make a difference with this. If you feel ashamed about hot flashes or are anxious about them or the ways they make you feel, that stress and anxiety can make them more likely to happen or play a part in their happening more frequently or severely.

Stress-reduction techniques can be effective ways to manage hot flashes. Even when they don't prevent them, they can make them less severe, less uncomfortable, and less likely to bring panic attacks along for the ride.

Cognitive behavioral therapy (CBT) has also been found to help. This isn't about hot flashes or night sweats being psychosomatic. CBT won't necessarily *prevent* hot flashes or night sweats because they're physical. Instead, it and other kinds of therapy *can* help you prevent or manage stress around or with them, prevent or reduce any anxiety they cause, make that anxiety less impactful, and give you a tool to help calm yourself and your heart rate down quickly.

Plants or nutrition that might help:

◊ A lot of the herbs and other over-the-counter remedies that people suggest for these issues have been found in studies to be likely placebos or no more effective than a placebo. If you're still interested in them, you'll find a little list in the mini-herbal on page 279. Since stress and anxiety are such big players in vasomotor issues, supplements and herbs that may help counter those can also potentially help.

◊ Magnesium; vitamins B, D, and E; and melatonin are nutrients that may help you sleep through night sweats instead of being woken up by them.

Medications and other treatments that can help:

- **Hormone therapy (MHT):** Estrogen-based hormone therapy has been consistently found to help with hot flashes and night sweats for those who are *post*-menopausal or who have experienced sudden menopause, as well as, though less often, those in perimenopause, and testosterone has recently been found to be a potentially effective helper as well. Vasomotor symptoms are one of the things that estrogen-based MHT is apparently most effective at helping with during all phases of menopause. For those who can't or don't want to use estrogen, testosterone has also been found to help with vasomotor issues.
- **Gabapentin (Neurontin) or pregabalin (Lyrica):** For those not already on these medications, this is one off-label use. Other fibromyalgia treatments may be similarly helpful.
- **Selective serotonin reuptake inhibitors (SSRIs) or serotonin-norepinephrine reuptake inhibitors (SNRIs):** Some antidepressants can also help. Again, this is off label.
- **Clonidine and other blood pressure medications:** Also off label.

Some medications or treatments can cause or worsen hot flashes or sweating as a side effect, including tamoxifen, Lupron, and breast cancer medications, SSRIs or SNRIs, ropinirole, migraine medications, aspirin and other nonsteroidal anti-inflammatory drugs, opioids or tramadol (Ultram), diabetes medications, asthma inhalers, and heartburn and acid-reflux medications. And yes, some of these are, unfortunately, medications that some might need more during a menopausal transition, so it can be that something that helps one aspect of your menopause makes this one worse or even that you have hot flashes and night sweats during menopause, but because of these medications not because of menopause.

While the jury is still out on whether or not it's a placebo effect, recent studies have found that ongoing acupuncture can be effective at reducing the frequency and severity of hot flashes and night sweats. Studies have, however, supported the efficacy of herbal traditional Chinese medicine formulations with vasomotor issues for some time now.

HOW LONG WILL THEY LAST?

As is the case with so many things menopausal, resources vary. The best I can deliver is an unsatisfyingly vague anywhere from a few months to many years. The Study of Women's Health Across the Nation (SWAN) found that they *can* last for as many as ten or more years.

The median duration of vasomotor impacts with menopause is 7.4 years. They've been found to be at their worst for most folks in the few years before and after a final menstrual period. The SWAN study found that the median number of years they lasted following a final menstrual period was 4.5.

The SWAN study also found that for people whose hot flashes or night sweats started in early perimenopause, they tend both to last the longest, with a median duration of 11.8 years, and also to hang on the longest after the last menstrual period, for a median 9.4 years. Here's looking at me, kid. Damn. People (why can't I be you?) who *only* start having vasomotor issues after their last menstrual period apparently tend to have them for the shortest amount of time (a median of 3.4 years).

I know you want me to say these will, of course, stop. I wish I could. For *most* people, they will stop, or at least only happen very infrequently.

But for some, they won't and will be something to live with even clear on the other side, decades after menopause has ended. I can't tell you how sorry I am to tell you that, particularly since I already feel there's no goddamn end to them and the thought that this might be true for me really bums me out.

Be on the lookout: At the 2019 conference of the North American Menopause Society, the Study of Women's Health Across the Nation presented findings that those who experience frequent (defined as having them most days of the week) or persistent hot flashes may be considerably—about two times—more likely than people who don't to experience a heart attack, stroke, or other serious cardiovascular problems. The risks are also elevated for those experiencing hot flashes who are in their forties or younger. If this sounds like you, it's probably a good idea to be sure to keep up with cardiovascular health checkups. Changing behaviors that reduce cardiovascular risks generally—like reducing or quitting smoking, reducing or limiting alcohol use, increasing physical activity, reducing stress, and adapting your diet to be more heart healthy—can also obviously help.

CHAPTER SEVEN

MOODS, FEELINGS, MENTAL HEALTH IMPACTS, AND TRAUMA

"Evelyn stared into the empty ice cream carton and wondered where the smiling girl in the school pictures had gone."

—*Fannie Flagg*

Menopause was one of the things—like puberty, like sexuality, like not being a man—that would get you an instant hysteria diagnosis if it upset you, or your husband, enough to land you on a psychiatrist's couch in the nineteenth and twentieth centuries. Helene Deutsch, the first psychoanalyst to publish a book on the psychology of women who was herself a woman, and Sigmund Freud shared a mutual admiration society. If you are hoping she was a good, antisexist influence on Freud, you hope in vain. Most of Deutsch's general approaches and ideas *came* from Freud (no wonder he liked them). Deutsch's view of menopause was that, when it happens, "a woman's service to the species ends," a curious notion for a woman who kept doing her own work until she died at the tender age of ninety-seven.

Advertising for hormone therapies and sedatives in the twentieth century, particularly in and around the Wilson era, often represented those in menopause as hopelessly cranky, raging, nervous, weeping, nagging, exasperating shrills who drove husbands away, berated bus drivers for no good reason, neglected children, and otherwise ruined everyone's lives with their menopausal moods. Empathy for how mental health issues might be making the women *themselves* feel was largely absent, save to say it wasn't her fault; it was The Menopause. And medications can fix ~~her~~ it. So that ~~she~~ it can stop getting in the way of its host's ability to please everyone.

The cultural movement from treating menopause as hyster*ia* to viewing it as hyster*ical* wasn't an improvement, in large part because those making the jokes have, **129** until very recently, been almost exclusively people who haven't themselves experienced menopause and who are inclined to make those who are the butt of the joke, saving any real sympathy for—you guessed it—the tragically pitiable men who have to live with a menopausal person.

THE FIRST EXPLICIT APPEARANCE OF menopause on television appears to be an episode of *All in the Family* in 1972 called "Edith's Problem." It was groundbreaking at the time for mentioning menopause at all, and it did present some sound information and sympathy for Edith Bunker (from her daughter), who was having a difficult time with menopause without any idea that's what it was. Yet there's a *live* audience laughing while she struggles with intensely ricocheting moods and cognitive issues. They're laughing while Archie, her bigoted, insensitive husband—Edith's *real* problem—responds with verbal abuse, yelling at her to "Stifle!" (a running joke of the show, because silencing your wife as a habit is hilarious, apparently) and making sexist and ableist quips.

A 2002 episode of *That '70s Show*, "Over the Hills and Far Away," presented a menopausal mother with mood swings and cognitive trouble being cut off and dismissed when asking her husband, her son, and his friends for help and sympathy as high comedy. Her husband disparages her and menopause behind her back

to his son and his son's friends while the audience chuckles. The entire episode is centered on the suffering *she* causes this ring of overgrown man-children, with no acknowledgment at all that the person suffering most is her.

One of the rare sympathetic representations of a menopausal mental health struggle is the 2018 film *Pause* by Cypriot director Tonia Mishiali. The lead character lives a bleak life: her husband is abusive and self-absorbed, she waits on him hand and foot and is isolated from her family, and her best friend doesn't get it. The film opens with a visit to the doctor, who glibly lists every menopausal issue you have ever heard of, though there's no mention of the impacts of abuse or trauma. She's not asked how she's doing, what she might want or need help with, or given any information about when and how to seek help; instead, she is told it's all normal and summarily dismissed.

As a result, her sole coping mechanisms are growing periods of dissociation and escape into daydreams and sad, sometimes violent fantasy. A support group; recognition of her trauma, her abuse, her anger, and her severe depression; and treatment for it could have gone a very long way. As, of course, could radically changing her domestic circumstances. It certainly would have helped her to at least know that everything else she was already grappling with could be made more difficult with menopause and vice versa.

In a piece by Rhitu Chatterjee for NPR in 2020, Teri Hines, who suffered from severe depression during perimenopause and went a long time before recognizing it, said, "The physical nature of menopause consumes you. It's what we're taught to pay attention to."

The medicalization and capitalization of menopause in a sexist, misogynist world creates an environment where we're barely on the radar in this, period, let alone our mental health and how it impacts **us**, first and foremost, rather than how it might disrupt the otherwise peaceful lives of others. Mental health conditions and struggles are, in and of themselves, hard to recognize when we're in them, let alone when we're already in something where it can feel like our world and whole sense of self has gone topsy-turvy.

What can happen?
- Increased irritability and frustration
- Mood swings or more intense moods
- More trouble managing moods and feelings
- Impulse control issues
- Increased probability of addiction or more struggles with current or past addictions
- Anxiety and obsessive compulsive disorder (OCD)
- Depression
- Suicidality
- Changes to preexisting mental health conditions or mental states
- Interactions with past or current trauma, post-traumatic stress disorder (PTSD), and other effects of trauma

Most people who go through menopause will experience some mood issues, like mood swings, more intense moods, or increased sensitivity or irritability. For many, they'll be mild, infrequent, or limited to phases that last hours, days, or weeks, at most. I'm talking about things like crying more easily and getting frustrated or irritated sooner than usual or over small things (*while I'm on the subject, why* can't *they put the towel back on the rack the way they found it?*).

There's a moment in the "Is It Perimenopause?" episode of Canadian comedy show *Baroness Von Sketch* when a friend compliments a perimenopausal pal on her sunglasses, and she reacts by angrily tearing them off and throwing them out the window. That is **for real**. That stuff happens. And it *is* sometimes hilarious for everyone involved, including the person feeling and behaving that way (go figure: jokes made *by* us and *for* us are actually funny as opposed to when the joke is *on* us).

WHAT'S MOST COMMON WITH PERI-menopause and postmenopause is ***not*** developing a *new* mental health issue. The majority of people who experience menopause don't. Recent studies on mental health and menopause usually show only a slight increase in mental health issues like depression and anxiety for those in perimenopause (compared to those who are premenopausal) with the lowest rates for those in postmenopause. Getting to the other side of menopause can even resolve some mental health or mood issues for people.

But many people still *do* experience more challenging mood or mental health issues in menopause. Those entering a menopausal transition are at *least* two to three times as likely to develop depression as those the same age who are not yet transitioning into menopause or as they were in the years before perimenopause. About 20 percent of those in early perimenopause and 38 percent of those in late perimenopause experience symptoms of depression. Depression is more likely and often more severe for those who experience sudden menopause.

Anxiety is also more common during perimenopause but less studied than the connection to depression is. Panic attacks are part of that picture, and for those who also have hot flashes, they can happen together.

The Centers for Disease Control and Prevention reported in June 2018 that the largest increase in the number of completed suicides in America is among women between their midforties and early sixties. A recent study showed a 49 percent rise in emergency room visits for drug-related suicide attempts by women

Those Known to Be at Increased Risk for Mental Health Issues in Menopause

* People suffering or who have suffered with mental health issues like postpartum depression, premenstrual dysphoric disorder, PTSD, OCD, schizophrenia, or a major depressive disorder
* Black women
* Gender-diverse people
* Those with preexisting disability
* People with low incomes
* Those with low or no education
* Those with low social support (a group that typically includes those living with or who are survivors of abuse, disabled people, and trans people, among others)
* Those experiencing loss
* Those with a history of trauma or childhood adversity

in midlife. This isn't new: suicide peaked at menopause for those in the nineteenth century as well. If we're queer, trans, or otherwise gender nonconforming, we already came into this with higher suicide rates: some of us have survived previous attempts earlier in our lives, which three in ten young queer/trans/gender-nonconforming youth typically make.

Those who have vasomotor issues during perimenopause or menopause, sleep disturbances, or just a more disruptive menopause, period, are also more likely to experience depression and other mental health issues, which is hardly surprising.

WHY DOES ALL THIS HAPPEN?

The chemical aspects of menopause have an impact on moods and mental health. Because we don't experience menopause in a vacuum, what happens interpersonally, socially, culturally, and in the rest of our lives also has an impact on our mental health. Neatly separating which is which is often an exercise in futility.

FLUCTUATING LEVELS OF HORMONES can, as always, mess with our moods. Particularly in menopause, changes in estrogen and progesterone impact the production and receptors, and as a result the uptake and levels, of serotonin and norepinephrine—two of our biggest mood regulators and stress balancers—and dopamine, the MVP in our brain's reward system. This can be particularly

likely when estrogen levels are fluctuating, like they tend to be in the first half of perimenopause, and for people with greater sensitivity to fluctuations. Those who've suffered from premenstrual or postpartum depression or other related mental health issues are more likely to have similar issues during perimenopause (which I know is rotten news when you've been through those, and I'm sorry). Mood issues can also be associated with low estrogen levels, but not nearly as strongly as with fluctuating or *high* levels of estrogen.

One of the things progesterone does is help regulate our moods and keep us calm. In a specific balance, estrogen and progesterone regulate each other. When they're not in that sync—as they often aren't during perimenopause—they don't. We often feel those effects.

The changing balance of estrogen and testosterone can be another player. Testosterone doesn't spike or drop dramatically during gradual or sudden menopause like estrogen and progesterone can, but the levels of each relative to the other change, and that can have impacts on our moods and mental health.

THERE CAN BE A DOMINO EFFECT WITH other impacts of menopause: if we're sleep deprived and more stressed as a result, our mental health suffers. Our self-image may already be in a rough spot. We might be feeling the impacts of ageism. If, on top of those kinds of things, we also have common life factors during all this—coexisting health issues; crises or big changes with kids, parents, partners, or work; lack of adequate support—all that increases the likelihood of depression, anxiety, and other conditions.

Having a bunch of arghful or super-demanding life stuff, all while our biochemistry is flying up and down like a haunted elevator or radically changing to a kind of hormonal makeup we haven't had for more than a week at a time since we were kids—no shit that can have an impact on our mental health.

WHAT CAN YOU DO ABOUT IT?

First, Ya Basics: all the things that can help with sleep, stress, social support, movement, hydration, and smoking, goddammit.

If you're only having minor or occasional mood issues, on top of doing what you can with those basics, you may just need to let yourself feel your feelings, whatever they are, get whatever support you want and can, and process and express them. Minor mood stuff that happens during the menopausal transition most often is temporary and does typically resolve itself on the other side. And by all means, if it feels good to laugh at *yourself*, go for it. It's my religion.

Sometimes our increased intolerance in menopause is as it should be: it may not be that we're being too irritable about a thing now so much as that we probably should have been more irritated by it before. The answer to some of your mood issues may be changes you needed to make anyway in various parts of your life.

Just like with other impacts of or challenges during menopause, see if you can't make some room for the mood changes you're having. I know it might be easier to do that with more socially accepted, easier-to-joke-about parts of this, like hot flashes, and you might also have the idea that mood issues are always a problem that need fixing, not something to let be and accept. But since some mood issues and feelings in menopause have quite a bit to do with feelings we haven't made room for up until now or feelings that have waited far too long to be felt and expressed, this can be a good place to make the most of your menopause and

If you already have or have previously had a mental illness, be on the lookout as you enter perimenopause or menopause, as it might kick up again or take a turn for the worse. If you're not currently in the care of a mental healthcare provider, maybe pick someone reliable in your life to give you a heads-up if you seem to be struggling without recognizing it yourself.

let it be a vehicle or a motivation to make more room—and insist others do too—for those feelings.

WHEN IT'S MORE THAN A BIG MOOD

If mood or mental health issues are more than occasional, severe, or feel like they're going that way, and things like reducing stress, improving sleep, getting more support, or dumping that chump don't seem to be the fix, you've got some more options.

MENTAL HEALTHCARE AND MORE

Mental healthcare can involve different kinds of therapy or counseling, medicine (be that pharmaceutical or otherwise), or both. Which of those is best for you is going to depend on what's going on, what you have reliable access to and the ability to engage with, and what you want.

Mental healthcare is supposed to be for *you*. **Your** wants and preferences should rule this roost. If you don't want anything to do with any kind of social therapy and just want some meds, okay. If support groups make you want to crawl under a rock and you want one-on-one therapy instead, go for it. If you have a bad history with one kind of therapy, you are allowed to never try that kind again, and if you want to try something other people think sounds bizarre, so be it.

Just like with other kinds of care providers, you can screen care providers for mental health using the tools from Chapter 5. There isn't external certification or much specialization of any kind yet for mental healthcare providers in menopause, so you'll want to ask a potential provider some questions about it. *What's their experience with people in menopause? Do they have any specific education or training? If you aren't cisgender or straight, can they work with you with any menopause issues you're having inclusively?*

Tania Glyde says that if you're LGBTQ+ and seeking therapy when in menopause, it pays to look carefully for the right practitioner. "The way cisgender heterosexual women are treated when seeking therapeutic or medical help with menopause is too often inadequate; for LGBTQ+ people it can be much worse. Too many queer folks avoid seeking help because of anxiety about the way they may be treated. Knowing you may have to spend hours explaining, for example, your gender identity to someone is bad enough—having them potentially debate you about it is even worse."

You do not have to be at your wit's end to seek out therapy or other kinds of mental healthcare. Just feeling stuck and like you need a little help is enough. Just wanting it is enough. It's like a jack when you get a flat tire, some soap when you can't get a ring off, or a friend who'll help you pop a zit you can't reach. Mental health stigma can really mess up how we think about it. This is really all it is: a little help.

Cognitive behavioral therapy (CBT) in particular can help not only with a range of mental health issues, including depression, anxiety and OCD, and eating disorders, but also with vasomotor or sleep troubles. The long story short on CBT is that it's usually short-term therapy that focuses on changing thoughts and behaviors rather than, say, unpacking the history of your relationships. It's a practical, problem-solving approach that aims to teach you and your brain how to think about, react to, and handle things differently. If you're allergic to talk therapy, approaches like CBT or EMDR might be better fits.

JUST LIKE THEY CAN HELP WITH MENTAL illness or other kinds of mood dysregulation at other times of life, psychiatric medications may be of help now too. Selective serotonin reuptake inhibitors (SSRIs) or serotonin-norepinephrine reuptake inhibitors (SNRIs) can also help with vasomotor issues, so if you're asking about medications for depression and having vasomotor issues, that's something to mention. Similarly, if vasomotor issues and anxiety have been pairing up for you, antianxiety medications may help. If stress is setting off or increasing vasomotor symptoms for you, managing your anxiety can reduce that stress.

In some studies, those with schizophrenia, psychotic affective disorder, and delusional disorder have reported that psychotic symptoms worsened at menopause and that their medications no longer worked as well as before. If you're currently on antipsychotics, be aware that some of them can intensify menopausal impacts, so if you are having a bad time with things like vasomotor symptoms, sleep disturbances, or joint pain, you might want to check in for a possible medication adjustment.

Pharmaceuticals and other conventional approaches aren't your only options. Nutritional helps for stress may help, as might other kinds of therapies like somatic approaches, bodywork, meditation and mindfulness, or traditional Chinese or other indigenous medicine. Some people have success with cannabis for mental health support, particularly with anxiety, or with microdosed psychedelics (reminder: possession of these is usually criminal, sometimes feloniously so). Magnesium, omega-3s, folic acid, cysteine, 5-HPT, St. John's Wort, melatonin, valerian root, chamomile, and SAMe are effective for some people and some mental health issues. The study of the relationship between mental health, the gut microbiome, and probiotics is emerging and promising (and since probiotics can help with other menopause impacts, they might be a good can't-hurt-might-help). A recent study found a link between higher dietary fiber intake and lower rates of depression for those premenopause and perimenopause. Per usual, if you're taking any other medications, just be sure to check with your prescribing provider first before adding any new supplements or herbal medicines.

There's a troubling message that shows up in some menopause messaging: the idea that we are *only* having mental health issues because we're experiencing menopause within patriarchy. That sexism and misogyny are the only causes of our mental health issues, and we don't need mental healthcare or support, we need revolution.

There is a long history—*hystery?*—of pathologizing women and gender-diverse people and our feelings and moods that is absolutely based in misogyny and sexism. Because we experience menopause within all the conditions of our lives, those conditions *of course* deeply impact our feelings and our mental health. Some of the intense feelings people in menopause experience are absolutely cultural or interpersonal, and some mental health issues are totally made worse by life conditions. But some of them are not: some of them are genetic, some are based in our own past traumas and experiences, and many would likely be present for us right now no matter what culture we were living in.

Recognizing that anger or sadness, depression or anxiety can be about sexism, misogyny, and ageism—and that *those* are the problems, not us or our brains—instead of estrogen levels is important. I appreciate that. I also appreciate messages that a menopausal transition in and of itself is **not** an illness or disorder and that

the idea everyone going through it needs to be on psychiatric medication to manage it is *Stepford Wives*–level creepy.

Damn straight we need a revolution. However, even in a feminist Utopia, some of us would still have mental health conditions or issues as we went through this and would want, need, and benefit from some kind of mental health help. That doesn't make anyone who does some kind of hothouse flower, a bad feminist, or a whiner. Inequalities don't help any of our mental health, and they do all of us, to varying degrees, very real harms, including psychic ones. But even if those inequalities didn't exist or could be remedied, many of us would still have mental illness or other mental health issues and would still need ways to manage them.

HORMONE THERAPY

Whether or not MHT alone is very effective with mood and mental health issues is debated. Hormone therapies aren't as strongly linked to helping with mental health issues as they are with other impacts of menopause, though if mental health issues are in whole or in part a result of other menopausal impacts that MHT is effective at helping with (like genital discomfort or hot flashes, for example, or gender dysphoria, if menopause is amping that up for you), it can obviously help indirectly.

The combination of a psych medication like an SSRI, antianxiety, or antipsychotic medication *and* MHT has been found to be more clearly effective. In the event you're not into using estrogen but don't have the same feelings about progesterone, progesterone alone may be an option for you, especially in earlier perimenopause when estrogen is higher, and especially if your issues are more on the anxiety than the depression side of the spectrum. Studies done about the effectiveness of testosterone therapy and depression specifically for perimenopausal people typically show it to be no more effective than a placebo, but testosterone is well documented to improve depression for people whose testosterone levels are low, so it might be worth checking levels if use of T is something you want to explore.

Of course, if gender dysphoria is the mental health issue at hand, hormone therapy may be able to as effectively help with that as it can at any other time of life.

YOU WILL SURVIVE (BUT IT MIGHT NOT ALWAYS FEEL LIKE IT)

As little as we're prepared for the physical impacts of menopause, we can be even less prepared for the emotional ones. We might expect or have heard about mood swings or even "rages," especially since both are the source of many a demoralizing jibe at menopausal people. And as little as moods or expressions of our feelings are taken seriously, our *feelings* themselves are rarely taken into account at all.

If we had it in our heads that feelings in menopause were the usual clichés—a certain kind of suburban prickliness or a trivial, surfacey sorrow—we're likely to be surprised. We might not be expecting that "rages" can have a basis in very real anger and that our tears might spring from shame, self-loathing, hopelessness, or deep grief. A lot of managing our moods and mental health in menopausal transition is about making room for our feelings, very much including some that might scare us.

Hot flashes and irritability are a walk in the park compared to some of the rough feelings or dark mindsets we can experience in a menopausal transition. I think I had it in my head that because my period's stopping was going to mean an end of pain, because I could care less if men find me attractive or not, and because I'd already resolved any feelings I had about reproduction, I wasn't going to have any big feelings to contend with in this. I was wrong.

A COUPLE YEARS AGO, I GOT THE MOST horrid of haircuts. It'd be a compliment to that cut to say Florence Henderson would have loved it. My partner did that thing partners are supposed to do when presented with a partner's bad haircut bravado, which is to say he lied very sweetly. Come bedtime, I tossed and turned, between bad-haircut stress and night sweats. I finally gave up around 2 a.m., when I went into the bathroom and experienced a carnival of all my worst agonies over the last handful of years, re-enacting the face journey Florence Pugh took in the last twenty minutes of *Midsommar* in the mirror at myself until I lay down on the cold floor and sobbed until dawn.

Some of it was the haircut. My gender identity is effectively Doobie Brother with hips, and I'd already had to cut a bunch of my shaggy mane a couple years before because I couldn't care for it properly with my disability. I was trying to grow it back out, and now it was shorter than before and also hideous, all when I'd gone to get it trimmed to try and *up* my self-esteem. But that haircut grief was only a surface reflection of my bigger, rougher feelings, the kind you can't just grow out. In hindsight, it was emblematic of the loss of control I had been experiencing in every corner of my life, and when I'd always had so little to begin with, no less. From physical pain to lost opportunities to the political landscape to the betrayals and loss of my previous relationship and home to unplanned teenage children and *other* people's awful exes to eldercare strain to goddamn perimenopause: you name it, I felt it acutely in those hours.

Lucky for me, I have a great therapist, a very emotionally supportive partner, good friends and coworkers, my fair share of creative outlets, and a whole lot of practice managing trauma and big, rough feelings. If you don't have it already, once you're in perimenopause, you're probably going to get some of that practice too.

People talk about postmenopausal IDGAF. Perimenopause, on the other hand, seems to be a space my genius friend, coach, personality theorist, and Unitarian Universalist minister Leela Sinha described as "when fucks come home to roost."

Ze said that, "It's not that all of a sudden you have these feelings. It's your tolerance for them that changes. What you're going through, how you're feeling about it, the support you need and aren't getting: all these things can stop letting you tolerate what you did before. I think what happens is your fucks come home to roost. They've all been out there like laying eggs and doing whatever they are doing, and now they're like, nope. They don't float away. They come home."

Even though we've likely been having and brewing them for years, maybe even the whole of our lives, big feelings can come up on us like a tornado in menopause. Sometimes we're the sister the tornado drops a house on. Sometimes we're the tornado.

ANGER, RESENTMENT, AND OTHER KINDS OF BIG GROWLY PAIN

The feeling both the most mocked *and* the most feared in menopause is anger. It is feared because anyone with half a clue who sees how we have to live in the world already knows full well we keep anger locked inside of us, though they don't likely know how much. It's mocked because mockery can hide that fear, enable mockers to recuse themselves of any responsibility to take it seriously, and diminish us all the more, which makes us feel like our anger would be ineffectual and probably only hurt us more if we *did* express it. It's silencing. I find the term "rages" and the way it's used for anger that happens in menopause to also be silencing, diminishing, and patronizing, much like I do when it's used about adolescent anger. Anger doesn't start with our hormones. It's usually been simmering throughout our lives, often based on the experiences and conditions of our lives. Hormones just help blow the lid off.

As *Rage Becomes Her* author Soraya Chemaly said,

One of the top three reasons women report getting angry is the lack of reciprocity in relationships. They feel taken for granted, uncared for, unloved, even as *they're* providing care to parents, to children, to spouses, to friends, to coworkers to neighbors, whoever it may be. Being exhausted and fed up at the same time accumulates. I think a lot of the rage people feel is because for the entirety of their lives their needs were not being addressed or met fairly. But now, with the added stresses and exhaustion of this physical transition, that situation is not tenable. This—a lack

of reciprocal care and attention—is not about hormones.

Those who express anger in menopause are often portrayed as themselves unbalanced, rather than as expressing feelings about imbalances that they have often been living with lifelong and that can't even take a pause for a few years during a challenging phase of life where we just need five goddamn minutes to take a little care of ourselves. If we're angrier in and around menopause, it might be because those imbalances may even get worse thanks to losing privilege, be that youth, fecundity, or both. It's also probably because after a lifetime of holding, managing, and making room for other people's giant feelings, to discover many or even all of those same people not only won't do the same for us but refuse to acknowledge even the validity or mere existence of our own feelings really pisses us off.

If menopause makes it harder to keep anger inside, it might help save our lives, not just our spirits. Soraya says,

What happens if people suppress or repress anger and strong negative feelings is that it degrades health in many, many ways. If you look at illnesses in which the majority of people experiencing them are women—autoimmune disorders, chronic pain, eating disorders, anxiety, other mental health distress—a lot of those involve this quality of mismanagement of emotion, and of this emotion in particular. It's not a causal relationship. It's not that you repressed anger, so you're going to have an autoimmune disorder, but there is a relationship, though it's not well understood at the moment. The thing that connects all of these predominantly quote unquote female ailments is often that people are not expressing anger.

loss and grieving for that loss: that can be about the end of periods, cycles, fertility, or childbearing, changes in our bodies or parts of them as we knew and were attached to them, the loss of some kinds or parts of our identity or of some kinds of power or privilege, or grief as we close chapters of our lives, even if we're glad or even excited to move on to the next.

> "I rarely cry. I save my feelings up inside me like I have something more specific in mind for them. I am waiting for the exact perfect situation and then BOOM! I'll explode in a light show of feeling and emotion—a pinata stuffed with tender nuances and pent-up passions."
> —Carrie Fisher

Unexpressed anger, resentment, and other big, hard feelings we're often expected to keep to ourselves, even in our intimate relationships, make us sick or sicker, keep us unwell, and amplify our physical and emotional pain. I'm an unfortunate expert in this.

SADNESS, LOSS, AND GRIEF

With or around menopause, there are loads of reasons we might feel sad aside from depression. People often treat us differently (including discounting our feelings as "hormonal," "just a phase," or "in our heads"). We may see ourselves differently. We may feel overwhelmed or scared about changes in our abilities. We may feel isolated, lonely, unsupported, or abandoned. We may be dealing with

As with anger, these feelings are often dismissed as merely hormonal, which can be exceptionally invalidating as well as dangerous. Deep sadness, loss, and grief plus depression form one of the most common routes to self-harm and suicidality. I'll talk more about feelings of loss and sadness in Chapter 14, but since it can come up before we get to actual ends, I wanted to be sure to bring it up early on too.

One of my least favorite popular menopause narratives is "Menopause isn't about loss, it's about positive change!" Just as there are no universal *physical* experiences of menopause, there are also no universal emotional ones. It may be that menopause feels wholly positive for some. But given that most of us are complex people with layers and long and complex life histories, it seems more likely that even with whatever we gain and whatever change we feel happy about, we may still experience some feelings of sadness, loss, or grief.

Aida Manduley said,

One of the forms of grief that is important is disenfranchised grief. Disenfranchised grief comes when, societally, you're told that the thing that you're sad about, you shouldn't be sad about, or that it's not a loss, and that you should just shut up and move on. A lot of people have fears, worries or grief about their changing body. We may be sad about the reproductive stuff, too. We can be sad about a lot of things. Not having room to express it or thinking or being told that it's taboo messes people up. We need more opportunities to talk about the grief that may come with menopause, not just the benefits. We can't rush it and just be like, "Let's be positive!" We can't have a holistic approach if we're not looking at both.

SHAME

I like to think of myself as shameless.

I've worked in sexuality for a couple decades. I spent several years of my life being naked on the internet, and I won't say I invented TMI, but I added a good deal to the canon. I testified in federal court for an American Civil Liberties Union case where a giant photo of my breasts was put in front of the whole courtroom, and the lawyer for the George W. Bush administration pointed to them and said to me, "Do you recognize this?" (Every day since I was eleven, yep.) I've been out for as long as I've known there was an out to be, public as an abuse and assault survivor, an abortion-clinic worker and an abortion haver, a dropout, a suicidal person, a hot mess. I kept an earnest online journal for around ten years, and boy, if you're not ashamed of *that* level of cringe . . . well, surely you *must* be shameless.

And yet, in much of perimenopause, I did what a lot of people do—I made self-effacing wisecracks but shared few deep, dark fears or even more garden-variety types. As much as I hate to admit it, shame has clearly been part of my own perimenopause picture.

Shame is good at hiding in some corner or another and sneakily infecting everything while we've got our attention elsewhere, thinking we're doing just fine. And it can be a goddamn killer with menopause. Shame runs like fever through support groups, memoirs, and social circles with appearance changes, sexual changes, temporary or permanent loss of abilities, mental health struggles, relationship conflicts—even with something as human and benign as hot flashes, sweating, the need for rest, or simply experiencing menopause at all.

We're all experiencing this within an overarching culture that has baked and is still baking thousands of years of shame into anything and everything that has to do with having the kind of body, and the sex usually assigned to it, we have if we're going through any kind of menopause. In the world we live in, it's made shameful both to be fertile and not to be, to be sexual and not to be, to be young *and* to be old, so long as we are girls, women, or have a body that has included a uterus.

Some of us have been warned that difficulty would happen to us as deserved punishment: for enjoying certain kinds of sex, for being queer or trans, for not getting married or having babies, for getting married too *many* times or having too *many* babies, for being fat, for being the wrong color, the wrong religion, the wrong nationality, for having the audacity not to have been born male. We may have been told we'll experience more pain for being who we are and that we'll deserve it, too—that because there's something "unnatural" about who we are, our bodies will punish us. Just as they have about menarche, pregnancy, and sex, puritanical and evangelical warnings have long been issued about menopause. The idea that if we don't "live right" sexually

and reproductively, we'll pay for it later—including that we'll one day find ourselves barren, shriveled old hags (and apparently none of us lives right, since if we live long enough, we all wind up shriveled, old, and barren)—remains pervasive.

THE GREAT UNKNOWN

Mona Eltahawy, an Egyptian feminist activist living in New York, is one of my favorite people on the planet. She's the author of *Headscarves and Hymens: Why the Middle East Needs a Sexual Revolution* and *The Seven Necessary Sins for Women and Girls*. We learned last year that accidentally crashing dates might be our favorite thing to do together. Mona said,

> Perimenopause during this particular time has me feeling like I'm going through the micro the world is going through the macro of. I feel that this pandemic is like the world going through perimenopause. In that sense, I connect very personally with it. I feel, in perimenopause, there is Mona over here and Mona over there. I'm in this

Not all the big feelings we may experience in this are negative: some can be big and *positive*. I'm only focusing on the hard ones because positive feelings might surprise us, but they won't usually fuck us up. Some positive feelings seen on the menopausal horizon include relief, gratitude, happiness, courage, anticipation, desire, fascination, ease, curiosity, content, liberation, receptiveness, amazement, resolution, rebelliousness, satisfaction, excitement, and a deep self-love. And of course, sometimes we might not have big feelings at all. We can feel apathetic with some or even all of any part of menopause too.

transition period where that Mona, who I used to be, I'm moving away from, but I'm not really sure who the Mona is yet that I'm moving towards. I really feel this is what the world is going through right now. I see us as standing in a corridor, a long corridor, where that world that we've come from, we are never, quote unquote, going back to that. There is no going back to normal, quote unquote. That is done. We're along this corridor now, and it's not really clear what kind of world we will emerge through at the other side of the corridor.

There's obviously no one way to feel about this kind of epic uncertainty, but suffice it to say, you are probably going to have *some* feelings about it. In fact, I think it's fair to say you're probably going to have a whole bunch of ways you feel about it, because it entails potential uncertainty about a whole bunch of parts of who you are and your body and your life all at once, some of which may be in conflict with each other—like, for instance, feeling thrilled about moving into a time of your life when you can move away from reproduction and into professional interests but full of rage and sorrow at the encroaching ageism you're already dealing with in that pursuit. It can be a lot. Just even the not knowing can be a lot.

YIKES TO WATCH OUT FOR

I've had a hard time, but so far I've been mercifully spared some of the most devastating, debilitating, dehumanizing head trips, fears, and feelings that can do a real number on you during any part of menopause. These—far more than physical discomfort—seem like the real soul squashers to me, especially if they wind up piggybacking onto depression, anxiety, OCD, or other mental health conditions.

I'm talking about objectively false, effed-up, yet common ideas like these:

- If you can't do all the things anymore or lose any abilities or ease in any abilities, you are or will be broken, useless, and no longer vital.
- If you don't look young, your love, sexual, or social life; your professional success; and/or your own positive body image are doomed.
- Any iteration of "old"—like looking old, sounding old, feeling old, getting old, or just plain being old—is bad.
- We, our bodies, things that happen to them, and menopause itself are disgusting.
- If you didn't reproduce, you wasted your life or your body. If you're no longer (or were never) able to reproduce, the thing that made you and your life valuable is gone.
- If you or your body look or feel differently, particularly if you're femme, and in ways that don't fit within hegemonic definitions of femininity, you aren't a "real" woman or femme anymore.

- If you aren't able or don't want to do as many things for other people as you did before, you're cold, uncaring, selfish, or a bitch, and you must still do all you can for everyone else, even if it means sacrificing needed self-care.
- If you can't or don't want to have sex in the same ways or at the same frequency as you did before—or even at all—or if your genitals or other parts you consider sexual look, feel, or act differently than they did, your sex life, sexual relationships, or sexuality are over.
- Your value to men, for a whole range of reasons, is at risk, will soon be gone, or is gone already, and if you lose value in any men's eyes, it's your fault, not theirs.
- Menopause = the end.

If any of these kinds of ideas or beliefs are canoodling around in your psyche, I cannot encourage you strongly enough to start recognizing them as false and toxic and making your way to the rubbish bin with them as soon as you are able. You'll probably need help doing that if any of these have their claws in you. The sooner you get it, the better.

Do other people believe these things are true? Do all of them appear in many forms in our culture and our lives? Will you have to live with some or all of these beliefs even if you stop or have stopped believing them or never did? Yep, yep, and yep. Most of these are based in deep-seated, widespread cultural bias and bigotry. But they can't mess you up as deeply if you don't let them take root in you or if you start working on finding them and weeding them out. I don't mean to go third-grade teacher on you, but I think this is what then fifty-one-year-old Eleanor Roosevelt was talking about when she said, "No one can make you feel inferior without your consent."

Taking an inventory of your own emotional land mines and other thought-and-feeling danger zones about any part of menopause can be helpful. Get cracking on any you can vanquish. Cultivate an awareness of the places where you're extra resilient and where you're extra vulnerable. Be ready for them to change, as they often will as you pass through different phases of menopause and life lived throughout it. This isn't about trying to fix yourself where you're "broken." Rather, it's about seeing where you might need to better protect yourself or give yourself care, and where you can be less vigilant; where you might need to make some extra room for yourself and your feelings, and where you won't.

THE TEMPTATION TO TRY AND SHOVE hard feelings back in, dismiss them, or try and deal with them all RIGHT THIS VERY MINUTE is often great, especially if they make us have to look deeply at ourselves, our relationships, or other parts of our lives in ways we'd really rather not. Especially now, of all times. But as Aida

Manduley says, "When you ignore feelings, they don't go away; they go underground. When they're buried, they don't stay buried forever. Once they've gone under, they often come back in even more confusing, less recognizable ways." (My Florence Henderson 'do sends its best.)

"There is no magic one-size-fits-all recipe for how to shift your relationship with your feelings and create more space for them, but it's key to go slow rather than trying to rush it. Self-compassion as you figure out this new path is also essential, because you're doing something pretty damn hard—figuring out how to change the wiring you've been building for years, and even decades. That's no small feat."

I know it sucks to have to do more work when we already have so much on our plates, especially with menopause now on the pile. At the same time, it might be that now is actually a great time for it. We're already in flux. We're already having to make some adjustments. We're already changing. What's a little more? If we don't let ourselves at least feel the feelings that come up, getting through this is going to be a lot harder, and we also might be missing out on some of the good stuff menopause can offer us.

Allowing ourselves to feel and express hard feelings like our anger, sadness, or shame is in the best interest of our health and well-being, especially when we're going through something that has additional whole-body and life impacts and,

on the other side of it, can leave us with some increased health risks. Feeling and expressing these feelings may save our quality of life, too, giving us an escape hatch from locking our feelings inside where they can keep us from the kind of life we want to be living and that may well be within our reach.

In *Body Kindness*, Rebecca Scritchfield talks about how negative feelings can be useful because they offer us guidance in decision making. If we want to get better at nourishing ourselves, we might have to dig deep into our shame to better our relationship with food. If we let ourselves feel our sadness and grief about losing what felt like the better times of our lives, we might better see the road to making the rest of our lives just as, if not more, fulfilling. If we don't let ourselves feel anger about being taken for granted and not cared for in our families, we can't even see that to try and change it.

It's not super complicated: you'll probably have some hard feelings. Let yourself have them. Let yourself feel and—in healthy ways, of course—express your anger or sorrow, grieve as you need to, and drag any shame that shows up out into the light. Get help doing that—from therapists or counselors, books, or supportive people in your life—if and as you need to.

If menopause is what finally takes our foot off the brakes on our hard feelings so that we can give them some gas and move forward, well, thank menopause for that.

MENOPAUSE AND TRAUMA

The more digging I did on menopause, the more I discovered some of why I've had a harder time with it than some other people do.

There was *nothing* in the giant pile of menopause books spanning over one hundred years that I read about trauma. That's not surprising with the older ones: trauma is a newer framework. But I didn't find it in current resources either: I only found it when pouring through studies. And, of course, in firsthand experiences. That's also not surprising: those with trauma are more often marginalized people with marginalized voices.

OMISADE BURNEY-SCOTT TALKED about some ways that menopause and trauma have collided for her:

My brother died unexpectedly, and then Hurricane Florence came through and all but destroyed my hometown. Then I got fired from a high-profile job. Of course, it's just our luck that just about the time that menopause happens to us, our garbage fires come on. It is reductive and dismissive to say, oh, you're just going through menopause. *Am I really?* I also may be going through a divorce or separating from partnership. I may also not be satisfied with the work that I've dedicated the last twenty-five years of my life doing. I may still be trying to parent children. I may have aging parents or I may have

peers who are deceased. Oh, I forgot, and they're also killing Black people all the time. So, it could also be I can't sleep more than four hours in the night because Breonna Taylor's murderers are still walking in the street.

If you've already been living with trauma, it's not going to come as a shock to you that just as trauma—and post-traumatic stress and more of trauma's by-products—tends to play a part in everything else in our lives, it can play a part in menopause.

STUDIES SHOW THAT TRAUMA AND ITS effects influence impacts of perimenopause or postmenopause like hot flashes and night sweats. If we have trauma history, we tend to experience hot flashes and night sweats more often and increasingly or with greater severity, all the more so with childhood trauma.

We may have body or sensory memories that some menopausal impacts or changes really mess with, like genital discomfort, anxiety, or heart palpitations. Ways that our bodies and minds feel with menopause—whether that's about the whole overall lack of control or about things like stifling heat or panic—can cue or bring us to otherwise reexperience or revisit trauma.

A recent cross-sectional analysis found that those in menopausal transition who'd experienced or were experiencing emotional interpersonal violence (IPV) or abuse were more likely to report difficulty sleeping, night sweats, and pain with intercourse. Those who reported physical IPV were more likely to report night sweats. Those reporting a history of sexual assault were more likely to report vaginal dryness or irritation and pain with intercourse. Symptoms of PTSD were associated with all menopause symptoms, including difficulty sleeping, hot flashes, night sweats, vaginal dryness, vaginal irritation, and pain with intercourse.

Trauma and PTSD can clearly play a part in what impacts we experience and at what rate or severity, *and* our experiences of menopause and its impacts can cue our trauma or PTSD. And much like trying to untangle which stress or hard feelings come from our lives and which come from menopause, it can be difficult to separate what's coming from menopause and what from trauma.

The immediate and lifelong impacts of trauma often increase our stress—which always tends to make menopause more difficult—and can keep it high. Hypervigilance or hyperarousal, intrusion (intrusive memories or re-experiences of trauma), or constriction (dissociation, numbing, or shutting down), all common effects of trauma, are themselves stressors and can affect how we experience menopause.

If trauma is attached to events like puberty or pregnancy—whether that's about trauma that happened during those times or about some part of those experiences, like gender or body dysphoria or heavy bleeding that was part of miscarriage—some or all of menopause may remind you of or otherwise bring up some of those feelings for you.

Trauma survivors often already have to deal with memory lapses, difficulty focusing, and other cognitive issues as a result of our trauma: if menopause piles more on, this increases our burdens and can also pull us back into our trauma, since it can be impossible to distinguish what's because of menopause and what's because of trauma.

THERE ARE SOME OTHER SOCIAL AND emotional parallels that can happen.

For most of us, menopause is not consensual. No one asked us or got our permission to do this thing that impacts the whole of our bodies and selves. Even if it's not something we would otherwise mind, even if it's something we want, it still is not consensual, and that can link up with quite a lot of trauma.

If feelings of shame cue your trauma, any shame you feel with or about menopause may as well. If any part of your experience of menopause feels like something you need to hide or if you experience diminishment or gaslighting during menopause—à la "It's no big deal," "It's just something women have to go through," or "It's all in your head"—that can bring back memories of abuse or experiences of disclosing or reporting abuse. As trauma survivors, many of us will have experienced stigmatization and marginalization simply by virtue of being survivors in a culture that blames victims instead of protecting them, often with the accompanying discrimination, aggressions, or microaggressions. That can make any and all of those things that come with being someone in menopause—ageism, often paired with sexism and misogyny and/or transphobia, ableism, anti-fat bias, misgendering, and other kinds of additional bias—extra awful.

Having to experience, survive, manage, and work to heal from trauma already asks so much of us and all feels like such a raw deal already. Something (or some*things*) bad already happened to us, and as if that didn't suck enough, we have to deal with the range of often lifelong impacts it has *and* do a ton of work, often at our own expense and with little cultural or even community support, to cope and heal. Finding out there's one more thing it can have a negative impact on stinks. But I've found it is, at least, helpful to know, especially if we already have at least some tools, practices, or other helps for managing trauma that work for us in our tool kits.

WHAT TO DO ABOUT THIS SEEMS TO ME to be the same things we do about managing trauma and any of its impacts, paired with managing menopause in all the ways we can.

Finding out what can happen in and around menopause—or what might be worse or more likely for those of us with trauma—can give us a heads-up about what, based on what we already know about ourselves and trauma, might create issues for us. If we know to be on the lookout for those things, we're better able to distinguish them from our trauma and plan how to manage them. Grounding, mindfulness and breathing practices, journaling, self-soothing, body scans, and emotional support are all things that can help with managing both trauma *and* menopause. If you're already in some kind of counseling or therapy, you can talk about menopause and any of the ways it is or might be interacting with your trauma.

If you're not already in some kind of counseling or therapy or haven't done any work for yourself to heal from trauma, now might be an ideal time. Not only will you have some options if your trauma and menopause wind up a bad mix, but this might be one of those places where menopause can help give you the nudge you need to make caring for yourself a priority. If menopause winds up being a trauma-healing helper, that's certainly likely to improve your attitude about menopause, which, all by itself, can improve your experience.

All of the usual things we can do for ourselves to take good care when dealing with trauma apply here. We can ask for help when we need it and set whatever limits and boundaries we need with whomever we need or want to set them. We can do what we need to feel safe. We can be patient and gentle with ourselves and our bodies.

WILL MOOD AND MENTAL HEALTH ISSUES IN MENOPAUSE END?

If they're just or mostly about menopause, then yes, probably. Data and anecdata both generally reflect that mood issues and mood disorders that only showed up during a menopausal transition resolve soon on the other side.

Studies of mood during menopause have usually found an increased risk of depression during perimenopause with a decrease in risk postmenopause. Those improvements are likely about hormone fluctuations (and all the neurochemical chaos they cause) resolving and our brains getting used to our "new normal," as well as menopausal impacts ceasing or, at least, considerably chilling out.

If our mood stuff or the degree of our mental illness is related to *feelings* we have *about* menopause, and we can resolve or make peace with those feelings, we'll also likely experience improvements. For instance, if depression or anxiety during menopause is about fears related to aging, and you can work some of those fears out, you're going to feel better. If your flares of anger are often based in getting to the end of your rope with having the lion's share of work in your household, then if that situation can be changed to be more equitable, you aren't going to get so angry or as angry as often. And if the way you felt in menopause is what got you to realize that you probably always needed medication or other kinds of treatment for a given mood issue, then yeah, you're likely to stay feeling better.

WHEN MY OWN MENTAL HEALTH TOOK A major downturn during perimenopause, it took me a while to take extra steps. I was already in therapy. I was already doing things that I know help me. But I got to a point where I was weeping all day for a couple days a week for months and clearly needed something else.

For starters, it was hard to tell it was happening. As it was for Teri Hines, the physical impacts were far more on my radar than the psychological and emotional ones. For the longest time, I thought if it was this bad, it surely was about the gazillion hard parts of my life and the greater horrors of the world at large, not menopause. The extra vulnerability and decreased resilience I'd been feeling, the way menopause stigma adds to mental health stigma, and my own bravado also undoubtedly all played parts. I also felt so overwhelmed trying to manage everything else already—including my growing depression—that trying to find a new prescribing psychiatrist in a pandemic felt like a bridge too far.

Thankfully—especially as a person with suicidal ideation, which can make it extra easy and extra dangerous for me to get lost in my own darkness—I have the benefit of some people and communities in my life who pay attention to how I'm feeling, who take my feelings seriously, and who also either deal with mental health issues themselves or are supportive and accepting of those of us who do and what we do to manage them. I also don't have shame around needing or getting this kind of help. Thank goodness for all that, because getting back on antidepressants and recognizing that depression was simply going to be an issue I needed to vigilantly manage in my menopause turned out to be one of my biggest saving graces in all this.

I think it's likely that the numbers we have on mood issues, disorders, and mental health struggles in and around menopause are lower than they should be. Between the cultural joke made of menopausal mood issues, the mental health stigma that permeates our culture, the fear of being pronounced the current version of hysterical, and how raw and vulnerable all of this can already make us feel, not to mention how many of us are so focused on the moods of others that we barely check in with our own, any expectation we're all going to stand up and raise our hand with this seems preposterous.

I figure that if someone like me, with a long history of mostly positive experiences with mental health help and care, surrounded by people well educated about mental health, took that long to get more help, you have to know how many people with radically different circumstances and experiences may never get there. We already know that some people don't survive the mental health struggles they have in this.

My best advice in this arena is that it doesn't hurt to err on the side of yes-I-am-probably-depressed or yep-I-think-these-panic-attacks-are-happening-more-often. Once we're in a mental health crisis, it gets harder and harder to see it and sometimes also harder and harder to climb out and back to the surface, especially when we're already so exhausted and overwhelmed. If in doubt, I say get checked out.

P.S. KEEP AN EYE ON YOUR MENOPAUSAL companions and their mental health, wherever it is you find them: in person, online, at work, or in your intimate relationships and family. We all could use more spotters to just let us know if we look like we're struggling and to check in to see if we want or need any help. You might even make agreements among one another to be each other's mental health security guards and let each other know if and when you think you're spotting what looks like a psychological rough spot.

(prefix)_____

(first name)_____

(type of pasta)_____

(adjective)_____

(noun)_____

(plural noun)_____

(noun)_____

(adjective)_____

(plural noun)_____

(name of Disney princess)_____

(adjective)_____

(verb, past participle)_____

(noun)_____

(adjective)_____

(noun)_____

(proper noun)_____

(type of fruit)_____

(kind of sex)_____

(adjective)_____

(adjective)_____

(noun)_____

(adjective)_____

(noun)_____

(plural noun)_____

(noun)_____

(noun)_____

(adverb)_____

(name of body part)_____

(verb)_____

(verb, past participle)_____

(name of medication)_____

(name of punk band)_____

(plural noun)_____

(noun)_____

(noun)_____

(plural noun)_____

(adjective)_____

(adjective)_____

(adjective)_____

(plural proper noun)_____

A Victorian Menopause Psychoanalysis
Case Study (Mad Lib)

When I began to analyze _____ _____ Von _____,
(prefix)   (first name)   (type of pasta)

the idea of a _____ neurosis on a hysterical basis was far from
(adjective)

my _____. But when I today review my _____ on this case,
(noun)   (plural noun)

there is no doubt I have to consider it as a severe case of _____ neurosis
(noun)

with _____ _____ and _____ phobias,
(adjective) (plural noun)   (name of Disney princess)

which was due to the climacteric, _____ abstinence and
(adjective)

was _____ with hysteria.
(verb, past participle)

Physical symptoms included paralysis, convulsions, hallucinations,

auto _____ cism, latent _____ _____, and vivid dreams
(noun)   (adjective)   (noun)

of _____, _____, and _____.
(proper noun)   (type of fruit)   (kind of sex)

It is a _____ episodic hysteria based on an _____ _____
(adjective)   (adjective)   (noun)

etiology.

I find it _____ to separate the hysterical _____ in
(adjective)   (noun)

the _____ of the mixed neuroses from _____ asthenia, _____
(plural noun)   (noun)   (noun)

neurosis, etc., for after this separation I can express _____ the
(adverb)

therapeutic value of the cathartic _____. I would venture
(name of body part)

to assert that it can readily _____ of any hysterical symptom,
(verb)

whereas, as can be easily _____, it is powerless in the
(verb, past participle)

presence of an _____ complex, and can only seldom, and
(name of medication)

through _____, influence the psychic _____ of
(name of punk band)   (plural noun)

the _____ neurosis. Its therapeutic _____ in the individual case
(noun)   (noun)

will depend on whether or not the hysterical _____ of the _____
(plural noun)   (adjective)

picture can claim a _____ and _____ position in comparison to
(adjective)   (adjective)

the other neurotic _____.
(plural proper noun)

CHAPTER EIGHT

BRAIN! (COGNITIVE IMPACTS)

"One of the keys to happiness is a bad memory."
—Rita Mae Brown

For as far back as I can remember (always a moving target), my intelligence has felt like the one thing people almost universally valued about me. I've heard people who I know didn't like me very much still talk about how smart I was, how creative, how witty, how literate, how sharp, how insightful: all the stuff of cognition. When other things about me would fail to be valuable to people—my personality, how I looked, my heart, my dedication, my care of or service to other people, my talents, my so-called charm—my brain could often be my lone saving grace, giving me at least enough redeeming value to get by.

When you grow up in this world raised as a girl, it's harder to feel valued without giving a lot of yourself up: being a "smart girl" can be one of the few ways it feels like you can get value without having to completely sell out.

My mind has often been my life raft. It's helped me avoid or escape abuse, figure out creative ways to keep myself fed and housed, and react quickly, usually, during almost every kind of shit totally hitting the fan.

I also love my brain: it's one of my favorite parts about myself. I love how weird and busy it is, the quick connections it makes even when it loops over itself too fast, as it often does, its lyrical, sensory, musical memory, its own strange genius. Even the ways it can be considered dysfunctional or atypical feel essential to my own cognitive brand and how I experience the world through it.

Memory isn't always a benefit and is sometimes a burden. I've never been good at avoidance or compartmentalization. My memory has been very sharp for a lot of my life, which has resulted in me being the friend, the child, the partner who remembers exactly what terrible thing the other person said or did, that they promised, what I asked them to do that they forgot, and certainly all the lies. Many of my memories are painful. Cumulative trauma and chronic pain have already challenged my mind and how it works. It's not like I wouldn't benefit from forgetting some things—from some haziness to soften the edges. Yet the experience of losing memory—words for the most basic things, appointments, someone's name I feel terrible forgetting, lyrics, how to do things—deeply scares and frustrates me.

It's impossible for me to identify the isolated impacts on my brain of trauma, pain, illness, injury, neurodivergence, drug use—medical and not—menopause, and aging. They're hopelessly tangled: there's just no way to pull them apart. But right about the time my perimenopause was likely just getting started, someone named nominal (or anomic) aphasia for me, the inability to retrieve the right—*wait, what was that again?* Oh, right: **words**. I couldn't recall the word for something incredibly obvious but could describe what it was in great depth and with my hands, the way of my people, the way it usually goes with this kind of aphasia. Only now do I know that aphasia and other cognitive issues aren't just part of aging; they're also part of menopause.

The prospect, the inevitability even, of losing more memory makes me feel some

kind of way. I worry it's too late to write some stories down because the changes have already happened: How much of my memory is reliable anymore? (Is *this* why the memoirs older people write are so juicy?) How much of it will be on the other side of this?

I USED TO BE ABLE TO FOCUS SO INTENTLY that someone could come stand right behind me and even talk for a while without my noticing them at all. That kind of hyperfocus—as well as the massive spurts of energy that sometimes went with it and could result in absolute magic—jumped the shark a few years back. Now I seem to only get the ADD downfalls and none of the benefits.

The differences between the last time I wrote a book and this time couldn't be clearer. This time it's often felt like my brain is trying to swim through mud to get from one thought to the next. Keeping up with all the things I have to do in a day without missing anything is impossible. Any of us going through menopause right now have also likely had bigger struggles with this than we might because of the impacts of the pandemic—the stresses and strains and, if you've contracted it, even the additional cognitive issues some with coronavirus are experiencing.

SOME PEOPLE CALL IT BRAIN FOG. SOME people call it cognitive decline or dysfunction. Some of us aren't going to remember what we call it, so we don't bother calling it anything. Whatever you call it, some common cognitive impacts seem to happen to many people in perimenopause and postmenopause. Higher numbers of people self-report it anecdotally than tends to be found in studies, but studies usually still find cognitive impacts in menopause common for a lot of people: about 60 percent of us. Mind, self-reporting has value, all the more so with things like this that are hard to quantify, and I also want to know if those studies account for everyone who didn't remember to show up for the study in the first place.

WHAT CAN HAPPEN?

◊ Changes with memory, be it difficulty with word retrieval and other verbal memory and articulation issues like nominal aphasia or more general forgetfulness, like losing your keys for the ninety millionth time or spacing an appointment.

◊ Decreased cognitive flexibility, including difficulty or increased difficulty with attentiveness, focus, processing, and concentration. You might feel like your processing speed or your ability to problem-solve is decreasing. Learning can be or feel more difficult or slower to cement, especially in later perimenopause. If you have ADD/ADHD or other similar issues, you may struggle with them and with executive function

more than usual or find you need to adjust any medications you take for them or other ways you manage them.

◊ Difficulty regulating emotions. For more on that, see the mental health and moods section on page 129.

How subtle or severe any or all of these changes may be is highly dependent on a range of factors. As you'd expect with a more dramatic and sudden change in estrogen levels, cognitive effects are often more prevalent and severe with sudden menopause than with gradual menopause. They are also more common for those who have preexisting issues with executive function or other concurrent or past issues that can impact memory and other parts of cognitive function, like head injuries, neurological illness or difference, adrenal or blood pressure conditions, alcoholism or other substance addiction, medical treatments (like chemotherapy), or medications (like pain medications or tamoxifen).

Changes to cognition are stressful for everyone. But if you already have cognitive difficulties or differences, they can be extra stressful.

WHY?

When they're happening at the same time, as they will most often be with gradual menopause, cognitive impacts of aging and menopause are difficult to separate. There's also been long argument

How Do I Know This Isn't Alzheimer's or Other Dementia?

It's probably not if

* you're under sixty-five;

* it isn't severe: if you struggle with verbal memory, thinking fast, or managing or organizing your life some, but those things aren't unmanageable or progressive, and you're not struggling a lot with memory of recent events, disorientation (like not knowing where you are) or deep confusion, major language difficulties, difficulty doing common daily tasks, hallucinations (even though you might *feel* like you must be sometimes), apathy or aggression, basic hygiene, severe mood swings, or deep suspicion of other people. "Behaving inappropriately" is also on that list, but what that means at this time of life is incredibly nebulous.

If any of the above *are* happening, and you don't already know the cause, it's probably worth a checkup with a care provider.

about whether cognitive issues that occur during or with menopause are really about menopause, aging, or both, and we're still without a strong consensus. However, recent studies suggest that at least some of this is about menopause, due both to the chemical changes of menopause itself and to some of the other things that often happen during menopause, like vasomotor issues and sleep disturbance and deficit.

It's well established that dropping or declining estrogen creates cognition issues. Estradiol enhances the growth of new neurons and neuroplasticity. Dopamine plays a big role in executive function. Declining estrogen levels can increase metabolism of dopamine, which

results in lower dopamine levels. Changes in estrogen also create changes in how we process serotonin and norepinephrine: that impacts cognition too. Estrogen also influences blood flow to the brain, so changing levels of or drops in estrogen change how vasodilation and vasoconstriction work in our brains, something anyone with migraines already knows all too well. *Fluctuating* levels of progesterone and estrogen, like during early perimenopause, also likely play a part. In fact, some may have experienced similar cognitive impacts before in life during some phases of menstrual cycles, with pregnancy or post-pregnancy, too.

Higher levels of stress during perimenopause have been associated with greater incidence of cognitive issues. Just as unsurprisingly, links between depression and anxiety and cognition issues during the menopausal transition have also been found. It can feel like cognitive issues and hot flashes are linked, and people who experience hot flashes more tend to also report cognition issues more as well. Sleep deficit and disturbance has a huge effect on cognition, and hot flashes and night sweats that interfere with sleep have been linked to executive function troubles.

WHAT CAN YOU DO?

Ya Basics can help.

Movement gets blood to our brains. Movement where you really engage your mind and your senses brings extra cognitive benefits, one of many reasons to pick movement you actually like and that engages you rather than trying to dissociate and forget you're doing something you hate.

Dehydration messes with cognition both in the present and the long term.

Social support can help. It's less of a big deal if our brains aren't operating like we're used to if we're not trying to run the world on our own, so tangible support, in particular, can be extra helpful here. Social engagement—even the little stuff, like saying hi to your dog-walking neighbors or waving at your neighborhood postal worker—also supports cognition.

Smoking, at the time, can improve cognitive function. That sharpness you feel when you smoke is real. Unfortunately, it's also real that over time, it contributes to more cognitive fuzziness than nonsmokers or quitters experience.

Sleep and stress are often the biggest of biggies here. Sleep deprivation and low-quality sleep mightily mess with brains. Unfortunately, sleep medications can have impacts on cognition too, so if you can improve your sleep without them, or at least without regular use of them, that'll serve you better here if you want to be less fuzzy. On the other hand, if the choice is sleep medication or no good sleep, your brain is likely to do better if you get sleep that way than not at all.

Stress—especially when it is or has been chronic—often plays a big role in cognitive function, and when gonadal hormones are chaotic or shifting, that impact can be even greater, another very frustrating thing you may recall from adolescence. Stress is also linked to higher risks of Alzheimer's and dementia, so if you already didn't have enough reasons to work on reducing and better managing stress, add protecting your brain and its functions in both the short and long term to that list.

Chronic stress, traumatic stress, or both can actually rewire our brains and are associated with more trouble with executive function and other kinds of

BRAIN! (COGNITIVE IMPACTS)

cognition for those of us in menopause with trauma history.

Some things have been found to help with those impacts, including help with the formation of new neurons and pathways in our brains and rewiring some of how they work.

Antidepressants are one possible helper, as is cognitive behavioral therapy, both things that can help with other menopausal impacts as well. If your cognitive issues have something to do with existing anxiety, depression, or other mood issues or disorders, as they can be for many during menopause, treating those issues will also help with cognition. Talk therapy and other kinds of help and support to help you heal from trauma can also help with any cognitive impacts it may be having or upping now.

Just FYI, clonidine and gabapentin, two nonhormonal medications that may be prescribed to help with vasomotor disturbances, are associated with *adverse* cognitive effects.

The Food and Drug Administration hasn't yet approved any kind of hormone therapy for cognitive issues with menopause, but people who go on MHT for other reasons often report improvements with cognitive function. A recent study has found that MHT for *post*menopausal people does likely have cognitive benefits. Specifically, the study found that longer lifetime exposure to estrogen (be it

through what our bodies make, MHT, or both) is associated with "better" cognitive status. I'd also be willing to bet that anything, MHT included, that helps reduce menopause impacts can help with cognition by virtue of reducing the stress those impacts can cause.

This is hardly news to the existing coffee or tea drinkers among us, but caffeine is linked to cognitive sharpness. The amino acid L-theanine can apparently reduce some of the jitters caffeine can deliver and enhance the cognitive effects of caffeine. It also raises dehydroepiandrosterone, serotonin, and dopamine and can help you sleep better to boot. Nice. Green tea offers both of them, some mushrooms have L-theanine too, and it's available as a supplement. Refined or high amounts of sugar are associated with cognitive fogginess, so how you take your coffee or tea might change how much it does for your brain.

NEUROPLASTICITY!

Everyone around me is no doubt tired of my too-cheerful "It's good for your neuroplasticity!" chirps, but (1) they just don't understand how exciting it is for me that I can remember that word, and (2) neuroplasticity *is* very cool, especially if you, like me, are a big nerd.

For those who haven't had to listen to me or anyone else drone on about this, neuroplasticity refers to our brain's ability to reorganize itself. Keeping up our neuroplasticity is maintaining our brain's ability to stay flexible; to grow, maintain, prune, and adapt neural pathways; to learn new things; and to stay sharp. Think of it as limbering up for your brain. The extra cool part is that much of the stuff we can do in the service of that is already good for us in other ways and/or is stuff we want to do. The positive feedback loop we get from doing things we enjoy is a big part of the neuroplasticity picture. So is repetition, which means that you get to do things you like over and over again and help your brain in the process.

The good-for-you things you already know about that help include Ya Basics. Also helpful is learning or trying new things you're interested in! Both novelty and new challenges increase neuroplasticity (aka how to rationalize going all in with the most ridiculous of hobbies, adventures, or geekdoms!). Feeling rewarded while doing a thing that matters to you is an important component of neuroplastic change. So is giving something your whole attention. In other words, you now have another very good reason to ask other people to leave you the fuck alone for a bit. Reading fiction is something else found to specifically help, as is traveling or moving to a new place.

In my humble opinion, one of the benefits of learning new things in menopause

is that it can be a lot less frustrating and heartbreaking than trying to do things you already knew how to do, maybe even well, but suddenly seem to really suck at or be unable to do at all right now. Even if we suck at the new thing, we were never good enough at it to know how *much* we suck.

TAKE A MEMO

s.e. smith did me the kindness of gently reminding me about staying organized on paper a few years back: specifically, about how much something like bullet journaling can help when you're grappling with executive function. It's helped me a ton, and when I fall off the bullet journal wagon, it's always readily apparent in the myriad of things I lose the plot with entirely.

If paper and handwriting aren't your bag, technology probably has you covered. There are a gazillion organizational apps—calendars, habit helpers, alarms and countdown clocks, journals—to pick from. Too, if you have the economic (or barter) access, there are people whose job it is to help folks with this. Getting the help you need to keep your various kinds of shit together is absolutely a form of self-care.

My label maker is also my pal in this and is especially fun for bad puns—*you don't bring me flours anymore*—shade—*I know you know pasta is not legumes*—or—

NEVER GONNA GIVE YOU UP
NEVER GONNA LET YOU DOWN
NEVER GONNA RUN AROUND AND
DESERT YOU

WILL COGNITIVE CHANGES END?

The Seattle Women's Midlife Study (508 participants, run between 1990 and 2013) and the Study of Women's Health Across the Nation both appear to show that cognition changes that show up in peri-menopause often don't continue at all, or aren't as frequent, constant, or severe in postmenopause. It's entirely possible that if you have cognitive changes in peri, they may be temporary. That said, aging brings changes in cognition, whether those are the more drastic changes senility and de-mentia can bring about or the subtler and more gradual cognitive changes that hap-pen for most people over time.

WHEN I TALKED WITH PROFESSOR, AU-thor, psychologist, and feminist human-development whiz Sharon Lamb about this, she gave me a reminder I clearly needed. She said, "That language you're using about you being less smart or losing your brain? It's really just different, not a loss. You're still smart, you just can't access things as quickly or make fast connections. But I bet you can step away, think things through, and let things come to you. It's a transition to a different way of thinking."

I feel ridiculous that Sharon had to say that, but I'm so glad she did.

I feel like it echoes so much of how we frame and think about all of our bodies and ourselves and menopause and how often we and others can make a mess for ourselves and everyone else with our ableism. Leah Lakshmi Piepzna-Samarasinha said some of my favorite things about this when we talked:

Menopause is something bodies go through. There's disabled wisdom we can draw on to help listen to and learn from and hold those changes in the best way possible. Not only celebrate them but learn how to be with the parts that are hard or challenging.

What if we looked at menopause as a life cycle transition that many kinds of bodies are going to go through in a million differ-ent ways? Even if someone is able-bodied and -minded and is going through meno-pause, they might experience some body and mind conditions that are disabled body and mind conditions. "Oh, I've got mobility challenges," or "My memory is different," or "My chronic illness poked up," or "I'm having what you'd call clerical body trouble."

There's the implicit, common idea that disability is bad. I've heard it in the same breath as "Menopause is not a disability" and "Menopause is a natural process that we all go through!" What I want to say is, well, so is disability. Disability is part of the natural range of ways there are to be human. There's not all the normal people and the defects. There's no one way to be human. Nobody (and no body) is a defect.

With cognitive impacts or changes, as with any part of menopause, aging, or both, I get to have what feelings I have, including feelings of frustration, grief, loss, or fear. But I also need to learn to accept my changing brain just like I've done with changes to my abilities due to my spine or migraines, just like I'm trying to do with my changing body shape, digestion, and sexuality and my changing needs for sleep and care. I also need to have some more faith in my body, including my brain, to adjust to these changes as it has to every other throughout my life.

I'm starting to see that I might also have some things to gain with these changes. My brain has always been a frenetic, blinky, 24/7 switchboard: it might be nice if it chilled out a bit and moved more slowly. I might come to thoughts and ideas I wouldn't with the brain I had before. My experience of life might be gentler if the edges of my memories got softer. I might be able to understand some things, some people, differently than I could before. As a creative person, I'm curious to see how this new brain might come to making music, visual art, or writing and to educational and other kinds of theory. If my brain is changing, I have the literal ability to perceive and process things differently than I have before: there's bound to be a lot of discovery there, which might turn out to be a tremendous gift. For all I know, I might even turn out to like this new brain better than the brains I've had before.

CHAPTER NINE

PAIN! (AND OTHER NEUROLOGICAL IMPACTS)

"Pain, pleasure and death are no more than a process for existence."
—*Frida Kahlo*

None of the menopause reference books or other general resources I've read have much to say about neurological issues and menopause, including pain (unless it's vaginal), despite the fact that people in menopause have been found to be twice as likely to experience chronic pain as the rest of the population. There appears to be an even higher pain burden for people having a more difficult time of menopause. Never you mind that one in every four people in the United States alone has disability, so a lot of people who experience menopause are also people experiencing disability at the same time.

This likely has a lot to do with the invisibility of disability and disabled people in menopause, as in so much else. Normalizing menopause is obviously positive, but lazy approaches to that further render disability, those with it, and those for whom menopause causes it, or more of it, even more invisible than we were already.

Some of us come to menopause with neurological disabilities or diversity, including pain, and menopause or some parts of it can impact those (sometimes for the worse, sometimes for the better). The same goes with trauma—often a player in many kinds of physical pain or chronic pain. But while we're lacking a lot of information, we do know that menopause often doesn't help with pain and other challenging aspects of neurology.

If you already have pain due to any preexisting conditions or variations, I think your best bet is to talk to specialists in your particular condition(s) or variation(s). Even if there isn't specific study of or information on it (or them, if you've got more than one source of or player in your pain) and menopause yet, given how many people are usually in some phase of menopause at a given time, they probably have knowledge from working with other menopausal patients.

WHAT KINDS OF NEUROLOGICAL OR PAIN IMPACTS OR INTERSECTIONS CAN BE PART OF MENOPAUSE?

If you already have pain from preexisting injury or illness, including neurological conditions or variations, it will likely be part of your menopause experience. I say likely because sometimes pain and other neurological conditions can reduce or even resolve in some phase of menopause, like some pain from endometriosis, menstrual cramps or ovulation, estrogen-triggered migraines, and some kinds of seizure disorders. With things that are directly linked or highly impacted by estrogen or fluctuating hormone levels, even if menopause itself ultimately resolves or reduces them, things may get worse before they get better, especially in early perimenopause.

Our nervous systems make up and manage a lot in our bodies and our experience of them—our sensory experiences, our cognition and communication, our movement, our internal homeostasis. With both menopause and our

neurological system having so much impact on our whole bodies, there are a lot of paths where they can cross.

Potential neurological impacts of the menopausal transition or menopause:

- Joint, tendon, and muscle pain and more of these kinds of pain with any preexisting pain disorders, like arthritis
- Foot pain or restless leg syndrome
- Low back and other spinal pain
- Headaches, particularly migraines and tension headaches
- Increased or resurgent allergies, sometimes with sinus headaches
- Changes in seizure patterns or frequency
- Increased spasticity
- Vision changes
- Dizziness or vertigo
- Vulvovaginal or uterine pain (see pages 189 and 179)
- Autistic people, those with ADD/ADHD, or both, may experience an amplification of their experiences, particularly with sensory, cognition, and communication issues, with any or all of these, and increases in a range of challenges (very much including social and support challenges—research on menopause and autism is particularly scarce, which obviously really sucks for people with autism). Much like during adolescence, since menopausal transition can amplify these experiences, it

can be a common time for a first diagnosis of autism, ADD, or ADHD.

- Body memories from trauma
- Increased or worsened symptoms, impacts, or relapse with neurologic or neurologically impactful conditions and their effects, like multiple sclerosis, fibromyalgia, Parkinson's, cerebral palsy, or Alzheimer's, and all the more if certain impacts are happening—like sleep disturbance—that, by themselves, can make things worse with a given condition

The why for some of these issues usually depends on the specific what. For example, increased pain because of body memories and trauma could happen because of pain increasing due to hormonal changes or because of something like genital discomfort or anxiety cueing trauma.

Common factors at play when it comes to neurology and pain broadly:

- Fluctuating hormone levels and, depending on the issue, high or low estrogen, high or low progesterone, and low testosterone, too, if that's happening
- Impact of hormone fluctuations and changes on dopamine and serotonin uptake and levels and, when relevant, on the effectiveness of other medications or dosages
- Impacts from the stress often involved in menopause, including elevated cortisol levels, especially when that's frequent or chronic (which can do everything from increase inflammation, thus pain, to cueing trauma that brings painful body memories up, to lowering pain thresholds so that we're more likely to feel pain or more pain in the first place), and muscle tension
- Low-quality sleep or not enough sleep
- Some pain, increases in pain, or development of pain disorders during or after menopause caused not by menopause but by the aging process

WHAT CAN HELP?

If you're already dealing with pain, you probably are already doing what you have access to, can, and want to. If you're new to dealing with pain or other neurological issues, here's some news.

For starters, Ya Basics:

- Dehydration, stress, sleep trouble, inactivity, and smoking can all amplify or trigger neurological events and pain, make us more neurologically reactive and sensitive, and just get in the way of our neurological system doing its best. Any improvements you can make to those should improve any pain and neurological impacts to some degree.
- Social support can help because pain and other neurological wonkiness can suck and be very isolating, and having someone to complain about it to or a

The Strange and Unusual: Creepy Crawlies, Tingles, Sparks, and Other Neurological WTFs

I know you're dying to know. I like weird body stuff too. In the immortal words of Lydia Deetz, I, myself, am strange and unusual.

Formication: Not as fun as it sounds. As nerve endings in the skin deteriorate, it can feel like bugs are crawling on or under your skin. This is probably more about aging than menopause itself, and there's really nothing to do about it but know what it is and that it is **absolutely not bugs**. I repeat: it is **not bugs**.

Burning-mouth syndrome: A burning or stinging feeling in the mouth—the roof, tongue, or lips—that can happen once, sometimes, or chronically. It can happen for a number of reasons, but low dopamine and dropping estrogen levels—and the changes in saliva those create—are two. Hormone therapy might help, and other medications used for it include gabapentin and other anticonvulsants, clonazepam, and some kinds of antidepressants and antianxiety medications. Pay attention to anything that seems to bring it on (like foods, drinks, toothpastes, or mouthwashes), and if you find anything, avoiding or limiting that thing may help. If and when it happens, sucking on ice chips or drinking or eating something cool can provide relief.

Tingling in extremities, electric shock sensations, sparks, or zaps: If your foot's ever fallen asleep, you know what this kind of paresthesia can feel like. It can also feel like weakness, cold, or burning, not just sparky. It's probably about fluctuating hormones but also can happen with aging and our nerves, like formication. But since it can also happen with things that require evaluation and treatment, like vitamin deficiencies, spinal issues, multiple sclerosis, kidney or liver disease, thyroid problems, brain tumors, Lyme disease, or rheumatoid arthritis, if it's happening often, it's a good idea to get checked out just to be sure it's only happening because of menopause or aging.

Pain medications help a lot of people, and there's nothing wrong with using them when we need to so long as that's what we want and know is okay for us. When we're talking about medications that can become addictive, just a heads-up that addiction is a higher risk during menopause, a lot like eating disorders are something we're at greater risk of. If you're someone who knows their risk of addiction is already elevated, you might want to consider other options.

shoulder to cry on that isn't your steering wheel for a change is really nice. Bonus points for social support that's also disability community, whether everyone in it shares your same issues or not. Care webs are everything.

What else might help?

◊ Vitamins (A, the Bs, C, D, and E), minerals (zinc, selenium, and iron), and omega-3s can help support the neurological system and supplementing them may help with pain if you're deficient. Magnesium can be a big helper, especially at bedtime. Glucosamine and chondroitin can also be of help.

◊ Anti-inflammatory eating—some foods are associated with inflammation and some with helping to prevent or reduce it. Polyphenols (particular kinds of micronutrients)—also helpful for heart health—are one group of foods particularly associated with preventing or reducing inflammation. Some common and fairly accessible foods rich in polyphenols or that are otherwise anti-inflammatory include almonds, apples, avocados, beans, berries, broccoli, cherries, citrus, coffee, dark chocolate, grapes, green peppers, hazelnuts, mushrooms, olives and olive oil, onions, peppermint, rosemary and other herbs (fresh or dried), sesame or flax seeds, sweet potatoes, tea, tempeh, turmeric, and (red) wine.

◊ There's increasing evidence that our gut microbiomes influence our neurology, including pain, so prebiotics and probiotics may help.

◊ Massage and other kinds of bodywork or physical therapies.

◊ Topical pain treatments, like numbing or warming muscle creams, magnesium or arnica cream, or prescription pain creams.

◊ Cannabis, systemically or topically, as THC, CBD, or both.

◊ Acupuncture. Extra bonus: if you seek out traditional Chinese medicine for pain and you also have hot flashes or night sweats, you can try one of the herbal medicine formulas also found to help with those while you're at it.

- Selective serotonin reuptake inhibitors (SSRIs), serotonin-norepinephrine reuptake inhibitors (SNRIs), gabapentin, and other medications that can sometimes help with vasomotor impacts may also help here.

If you have preexisting conditions and are using any medications for them, keep your prescribing provider in the loop when it comes to your menopause and any changes in pain. Sometimes menopause changes how your body responds to medications or treatments.

CHAPTER TEN

GUTS TO GONADS

DIGESTIVE, URINARY, AND GENITAL IMPACTS

"We could certainly use a detective!"
—*Carolyn Keene*, The Secrets of Shadow Ranch, *Nancy Drew Mystery Stories #5*

The Trotula, a group of texts about women's medicine from twelfth-century Italy, held a positive view of menstruation but a negative view of anything that stopped it from happening, including menopause. The Trotula held with the views of Galen: that menstrual flow is necessary for the health of the whole body and that when flow isn't happening, this is very bad, and so one has to induce periods or find other ways to "release" blood from the body via everyone's favorite Middle Ages pastime: bloodletting.

Galen also believed the uterus to be a "wandering womb," the notion (and also the name of my new Sarah McLachlan cover band) that it can travel to various parts of the body—the lungs, the liver—by following the *smells* of things, causing all kinds of ruckus with its strolls.

The uterus and its ovarian companions can't go for evening constitutionals, but as you may already have experienced, they can certainly cause some mayhem, including for their immediate neighbors.

DIGESTIVE IMPACTS

Monstrous belching was the rage at my middle school. All the kids were doing it. My *dog* was doing it. I couldn't do it.

My preschool-age stepsister, a champion belcher, tried to teach me. I was a failure. When I have burped, it's generally been embarrassingly demure. My gastrointestinal (GI) system has always gravely disappointed my machismo.

This is no longer an issue, to say the least. What started as tiny, louder burps has, over the course of the last couple years, evolved into full-fledged frat-party-of-one belches. I never would have thought menopause would have any impact on my digestive system, but I could probably perform this next section for you in burps.

WHAT CAN HAPPEN?

Mostly, everything that can already happen, or may already have been happening, with your digestive system throughout your life up until now. Digestive upsets can start for the first time if they're new to you and can get more frequent or severe if you're already familiar with them.

Those can be

◊ bloating;

◊ indigestion or nausea;

◊ heartburn, acid reflux, or gastroesophageal reflux disease (GERD);

◊ difficulty or increased difficulty with digestion and slower digestion;

◊ increased or new food sensitivities or allergies;

◊ bowel movement changes, including constipation or diarrhea;

◊ gallbladder issues or liver disease;

◊ gas, belching, or farting;

◊ new irritable bowel syndrome (IBS) or IBS made worse or more reactive, especially if it was linked to menstrual cycles in the past.

WHY?

Stress—and the Clyde to its Bonnie, cortisol—is often the biggest culprit in digestive issues during menopause.

Lowering and, eventually, low estrogen is another why for cortisol increases that happen with menopause and can wreak havoc on our digestive systems. Adrenaline also goes up when estrogen goes down, and it's no friend to our guts either.

This is also one of those things where it can be difficult to separate what's about menopause and what's about aging. Aging slows the digestive process, especially when circulatory systems start to slow down, and creates changes in some of the enzymes and other fluids our bodies make and need for digestion, as well as changes to the esophagus, the colon (including slower or longer "colonic transit time," aka your daily bowel movement commute), and the organ mass and mucous membranes of the intestines. Age-related tooth loss or other dental changes may affect or start to affect our digestion during some part of menopause but aren't because of or directly related to menopause.

The reduction of moisture in our bodies, including less saliva and fewer secretions in the GI tract, that menopause (by way of lowering and low estrogen) brings can play a role, as can changes to our metabolism or body shape and size that might come with it.

IT TAKES A VILLAGE (OF MICROBES)

Dr. Siri Carpenter explained for the American Psychological Association,

If aliens were to swoop in from outer space and squeeze a human down to see what we're made of, they would come to the conclusion that cell for cell, we're mostly bacteria. In fact, single-celled organisms—mostly bacteria—outnumber our own cells 10 to one, and most of them make their home in the gut. . . . The human gut is an amazing piece of work. Often referred to as the "second brain," it is the only organ to boast its own independent nervous system, an intricate network of 100 million neurons embedded in the gut wall. So sophisticated is this neural network that the gut continues to function even when the primary neural conduit between it and the brain, the vagus nerve, is severed.

I'm writing this in the midst of a gut microbe renaissance: there's a lot of emerging information about gut microbiomes—the diverse community of microorganisms that live inside our GI tracts—from scientists, doctors, and people selling things.

So far, we know that the bacterial environment of our gastrointestinal system is a big deal and has an impact on our overall health and well-being, especially our digestive, neurological, and immune systems. When it comes to menopause, specifically, how our gut metabolizes estrogen is also in play. The "estrobolome"—which is not the Thunderdome of menopause my imagination wants it to be but the subset of the gut microbiome that specifically metabolizes estrogen—works to help us balance estrogen levels.

Doing the things we can to help our microbiome out during menopause (and at any other time of life) is objectively a good idea. Go figure: a lot of the things that help our GI systems also help *all* of our systems, at any time of life, including during and after menopause. Our digestion matters to our well-being way more than most of us know. When it isn't working well, we're likely to suffer more than just stomach upset, because digestion is how all our nutrients get—or don't—to the whole of our bodies. Issues with digestion can impact everything from our skin to our stress levels to our immune systems.

WHAT CAN HELP?

First, most of Ya Basics:

❧ Reducing and managing stress—a biggie with digestion
❧ Improving sleep
❧ Getting regular movement
❧ Not smoking, dammit
❧ Getting and staying hydrated

Also:

❧ Getting more fiber in your diet, especially *pre*biotic fiber, which can be found in dark greens, beans, whole grains, nuts, seeds, and some fruits
❧ Adding *pro*biotics, whether that's with a supplement (be sure it's fresh) or via fermented foods that are good sources

of probiotics, like kimchi, yogurt, kefir, pickles (pickles!), miso, tempeh, sourdough bread, and kombucha

♦ Sugar, alcohol, caffeine, and fried foods may be our friends, but they aren't our *gut's* friends, so do with that information what you will

♦ Our BFF magnesium and its pal zinc

♦ Herbal GI helpers like turmeric, ginger, and milk thistle—which you can have via teas, smoothies, or lattes—digestive enzymes, or digestive bitters

♦ Anti-inflammatory foods (listed on page 169)

♦ Over-the-counter stuff (used in moderation): antacids, proton-pump inhibitors, histamine (H2) blockers, bismuth and other antinausea medications, laxatives, and antidiarrheals

♦ If you're having frequent GI issues, and it's okay for you to do, you might use food logging and experimentation to see if removing, adding, or differently combining or timing what or when you eat makes a difference (you can also get checked for food allergies/sensitivities/intolerances, as new allergies or sensitivities can happen during menopause)

♦ Limiting antibiotic use to only what's necessary (as antibiotics mess with our gut and genital flora)

♦ Improving *how* you eat (not what, **how**)

HOW TO EAT

Almost everything I learned well into adulthood about *how* to eat was focused on losing weight, being thrifty, or not throwing food at people. That last lesson has yet to stick, so watch your back.

It's alarming to consider how little I was taught about how to eat to actually support my digestion and to help my body be better nourished. I sure would have been better off knowing about it earlier, but it really matters now that my body—as is often the case for all our bodies in and around menopause or with aging—lets me get away with even less than it did before. Love that hot sauce and your ability to eat while running for the bus if and while you still can, friends.

With menopause in mind, kiran nigam filled me in on some basics.

Schedule time for meals, as you would for a meeting or a date. Regular mealtimes set the body up to anticipate—and thus, ready itself for—meals.

Relax before and while eating. Learning that digestion is a parasympathetic body state made my brain do a Bill and Ted "Whoah." Even though I had learned that before, I don't think it had ever sunk in. Eating is supposed to be a state of *rest and relaxation*. The phrase "rest and digest" is representative of the parasympathetic nervous system, much as "fight or flight" is of the sympathetic nervous system. That's extra brain 'splody, because, honestly, the way I have been eating much of my life has usually been fight *and* flight. But if we're not relaxed before and while eating, our bodies can't digest, assimilate, and metabolize what we're eating as well as they would otherwise.

To chill yourself out before eating, you might take a walk, stretch, grab a disco nap, meditate, or just sit down and listen to a song that relaxes you. To integrate this kind of practice into my life, I'm having to learn to let go of a genetic predisposition to everyone eating before food gets cold and to slow down the frenetic ballet that is my cooking style.

Before and while eating, take some slow, deep breaths. Take a moment to pause before eating and effectively Be Here (at Lunch) Now. If you already say a blessing or grace or have some other kind of gratitude or spiritual practice before eating, you already got this. For the rest of us godless heathens, there's always "Rub a dub dub, thanks for the grub" or, what I like to think the Ramones say before dinner, "Hey ho, let's go!"

Eat sitting down. We know this already, but maybe some of us need a reminder and maybe we even need that reminder every single time we're going to eat.

Eat your meals slowly and chew like nobody's business. kiran says that, ideally, we'd be chewing each bite about thirty times, until food becomes the consistency of a smoothie. When we eat too fast, without chewing properly, food is in larger pieces than our stomach is designed to handle, and we also tend to swallow air with our food. All of that causes digestive stress and can lead to bloating and gas. And perhaps even hysterical flatulence.

Drinks. kiran suggests a little warm liquid before meals, like warm water with lemon, bone broth, or miso to wake up digestion. She also suggests a couple sips of apple cider vinegar at the beginning or in the middle of your meals to help increase the acidity of your stomach, which can help activate important digestive enzymes. Fizzy water can neutralize stomach acid we need for digestion, and too much of any kind of water around or with meals can water down digestive juices and make digestion harder, rather than easier, just so you know.

HOW MANY ANTACIDS IS TOO MANY?

As Claire Maldarelli wrote in *Popular Science*, "If three work, the entire box will probably work better, right?" Claire couldn't understand my antacid habits better. *Alas, no.* As others have as well, Maldarelli determined there's no one right answer for everybody, but, as with proton-pump inhibitors, we really should be aiming to only take them as directed. If we have issues for more than a couple weeks, we really should see a care provider if possible to find out what's up. Otherwise we risk potential impacts like constipation, kidney stones, milk-alkali syndrome (a breakdown in the stomach lining), and osteoporosis, already a bigger risk for us once we get to the other side of menopause, on top of potentially trying to treat something with antacids that simply needs a different means of management.

kiran encourages eating and drinking foods and beverages that support the liver and gallbladder, which collaborate to help our bodies regulate hormones. These might be an extra good idea if you're using systemic hormone therapy, since they make your liver do some heavy lifting.

Those foods and drinks include dark leafy greens and fresh green herbs, beets and beet greens, artichokes, endive, broccoli, seaweeds, avocado, turmeric, garlic and onions, green juices, beet and carrot juice, dandelion root, milk thistle, or holy basil tea and filtered water.

Some things that support those organs include saunas, steam rooms, exercise, and other things that make you sweat (yes, I'm laughing too), body exfoliation or dry brushing, massage, and Epsom salt bath soaks.

When should you get checked out by a care provider?

- If you're living on antacids (or a prayer) or other over-the-counter medications or treatments
- If, no matter what or how you eat, or what other practices you pick up to best support your gastrointestinal system, it's just regularly bad news
- If you have difficulty swallowing or other throat problems with or after eating
- If you're frequently having IBS, constipation, diarrhea, stomach pain, gas, or other digestive maladies that don't resolve, including any signs or symptoms of liver, gallbladder, or other digestive disease or major problems, like jaundice, body swelling, frequent nausea, vomiting, superfunky urine or stools, or new skin conditions like psoriasis or eczema

WILL DIGESTIVE PROBLEMS GET BETTER?

The aging stuff is the aging stuff: if it's happening because of aging, we can do the things we can do to best support our bodies and their systems, but so long as we're still alive, we can't just not age. But if you can make some digestion-supporting changes and work on the basics that help with all of menopause, they'll usually help. The digestive system of our youth is in or heading to the past, and what worked—or didn't but the issue wasn't as hard to bounce back from—just might not work anymore. If you're having issues, you probably have to change some things up.

If you're having gastrointestinal issues during a menopausal transition, it's almost impossible for it not to have at least *something* to do with stress. Even for people who aren't having a hard time of it, what's going on with our bodies causes them stress, and that puts a strain on our digestive system. Same goes with sleep disruptions. Once our hormones stop wildly swinging on chandeliers and we and our bodies can literally relax more, we *are* likely to feel at least a little better.

Some gastrointestinal issues are specifically known to resolve postmenopause. If you experience IBS that's specifically triggered by estrogen, progesterone, or both, it should resolve when you're on the other side and have little of either. Same goes for bloating and gas. Here's hoping I can still burp on the other side, because it really is impressive.

THE UTERUS AND OVARIES

The biggest changes happening to both, especially the ovaries, are why we're all gathered here in this book today.

PERIODS AND MENSTRUAL CYCLES

For the longest time, I had this Utopian notion that what happens with periods is that you have them like you have them and keep having them until you just stop

having them out of the blue, and then they're done.

That is not how it usually goes.

The one thing about menopause just about everyone already knows is that it means the end of menstrual periods. What everyone doesn't always know is what the unpredictable and sometimes rocky road to that point can look and feel like.

WHAT CHANGES?

If you have already forever stopped having periods for other reasons or never had them in the first place, nothing should change about that during any part of menopause. They'll stay stopped.

Once periods are supposed to be over for good, we shouldn't have anything happen that looks or feels like a period. If you find yourself having vaginal bleeding postmenopause or otherwise after your periods are supposed to be all the way over, and you don't already know why, you should seek out healthcare. There's a very clear consensus that postmenopausal bleeding or bleeding long after removal of the uterus—even spotting—should not go without evaluation. It *could* be minor and benign—like bleeding due to vaginal tissue thinning or because of an abrasion with sex—but it could also be a signal of something more dangerous or that needs care, like polyps, fibroids, or reproductive cancers.

If you don't currently have menstrual periods due to use of certain contraceptive methods or other medications, nothing will likely change for you either.

If you have had and are still having menstrual periods, menstrual changes in perimenopause may look a whole bunch of different ways, all for mostly the same reasons.

Changes to the length of each cycle:

There can be more time in between periods, less, or a mix of both. A common pattern in early perimenopause is cycles first getting shorter for a while—that could be months or years—sometimes even to the point where there are only a couple weeks between cycles and occasionally even less time than that. In later perimenopause, they often stretch out and get longer, eventually with missed cycles in between, until you get to the place where it's been a full year without any periods and you get to cross the menopause finish line. Like anything that's an average, there's a whole world of variation with all that, so that doesn't guarantee that's how it'll happen for you; it's just what's most typical. Cycles change up like this first because of higher estrogen and fluctuating levels of estrogen and progesterone, and then, later, estrogen getting lower and lower, but

follicle-stimulating hormone still stubbornly trying to make ovulation happen.

Shorter or longer menstrual periods and lighter, heavier flow or otherwise plain old different flow: I think it's fair to say many people won't often be concerned about or have an issue with lighter or shorter periods (which will usually happen later as estrogen gets lower because it's building up less uterine lining as a result). It's another story when they're heavier, longer, or both. The heavier and longer a period is, the more work—and stuff that costs money to buy, and work missed that would give you the money you need to buy the stuff, argh!—required to manage it. If your periods make you feel in any way less than awesome or downright awful, that's longer that you have to feel the way you feel.

Some people will experience menstrual "flooding," a term that, for a change, seems undoubtedly to have been coined by someone who themselves experienced it. It's less colloquially called hypermenorrhea or menorrhagia, if you like those better. It is what it sounds like: **super-heavy menstrual flow**. It likely happens because of high estrogen or big fluctuations that are common in early perimenopause, but it can also happen because of abnormal cell growth, fibroids, or endometrial polyps—which can increase or grow during peri—or endometriosis.

Don't just scream; take good care of yourself if it happens for you. *Our Bodies, Ourselves* says that if you feel faint when sitting or standing while flooding, "this means your blood volume is decreased; try drinking salty liquids such as tomato or V8 juice or soup. Taking an over-the-counter NSAID such as ibuprofen every four to six hours during heavy flow will decrease the period blood loss by 25 to 45 percent." Nonsteroidal anti-inflammatory drugs (NSAIDS) can help because they inhibit prostaglandins (lipids that control blood flow, inflammation, and uterine contractions), which is also how they help with cramps. Bumping up your iron intake is also a good idea, especially since it's common to be iron deficient in perimenopause anyway.

What you usually use for managing menstrual flow might not cut it. Time to build that ark. Things made for postpartum bleeding may work better than stuff for menstrual periods. Both disposable and washable pads made for this purpose exist, as do disposable and washable undergarments for this level of flow.

If it's not so occasional (and you don't already know why), if it's scary-major, or both, check in with a care provider if you can. Heavy vaginal or uterine bleeding can occur for a few reasons, and some of them—endometriosis, bleeding disorders like von Willebrand disease, pelvic inflammatory disease, an issue with an intrauterine device (IUD), or reproductive cancers—require care. Polyps or fibroids may or may not, but it's smart to get them evaluated. If flooding happens often, is very severe, or is paired with a level or kind of pain that's unusual for you, I vote to get checked out. Plus, even if flooding is happening for nonworrisome reasons, you can find out about more options for managing it, like some kinds of hormone therapies (or changing yours up if flooding is only happening once you got on it), including some hormonal contraception methods, a progestin IUD, or uterine ablation.

A standard when it comes to figuring out if you need medical care or not based on heavy flow is this: if you're filling more than two heavy-flow pads for more than two hours in a row, seeking out care is advised. If you're seeing big globs, anything larger than a quarter, it's worth making sure everything's okay.

MENSTRUAL FLOW CAN ALSO LOOK DIFferent in perimenopause in terms of color or texture. It may be more globby or thin than you're used to. Spotting may also happen more often or in place of a period.

Menstrual pain and premenstrual syndrome (PMS): These should resolve once you're postmenopausal and no longer having cycles. No more menstrual cycles almost always = no more pain related to menstrual cycles. There are a few highly ginormous upsides to menopause, and this is one of the biggies. Even before you get past menopause, if you skip cycles or have shorter ones en route, that's usually less times you'll experience whatever comes with your periods.

What happens with either or both *during* your menopausal transition, though, is mostly anyone's guess. For some people, they get worse; for others, they get better; others go back and forth unpredictably. You might also experience PMS for the first time in your life, or you may experience it at different times in your cycle or feel it in different ways. It absolutely can get worse, just so you're aware, but it also absolutely can get better. And don't forget, once you get to menopause, it most assuredly **will** get better.

If you're using testosterone, sometimes menstrual or uterine pain may increase.

IF YOU ALREADY TREAT ONE OR BOTH OF those kinds of pain, you can still keep treating them. Depending on your particular source of that pain and your unique psychological maelstrom, there are some treatments you might want to consider, especially those that can potentially help with other impacts of menopause, like progestin IUDs, antidepressants, acupuncture/traditional Chinese medicine, or hormonal contraception methods. If

you're having a great deal of pain or severe PMS or premenstrual dysphoric disorder and are already close to menopause anyway (or even if you're not), you may even want to have a talk with a provider about hysterectomy or oophorectomy.

If you start to have pain you never had before, check in with a healthcare provider to screen for fibroids, polyps, a burst or problematic cyst, or other possible issues. New pain won't likely start *just* because of menopause.

WHAT CAN HELP?

If you've made it all the way to perimenopause and had periods along the way, you either already have things you do that help you with any issues, or you've given the hell up and accepted your fate. If you're in the former group, you'll probably just do those same things.

If you're in the latter, I propose it may be worth one more try so you don't have to go down suffering needlessly. It might be that something you haven't tried before helps, that something that didn't help in the past helps now, or that just giving yourself more care than you have in the past does the trick. If ever there were a time to give yourself some extra TLC, this is it. On the other hand, you may just be sick of even trying at this point, a feeling I wholly understand. With threadbare heating pad and world-weary uterus, I raise my empty bottle of Vicodin to you in salute.

In case you want to try a thing:

⚱ All Ya Basics can help: all the sleep, stress, movement, not smoking or smoking less, hydration, and social support stuff.

And also:

⚱ Acupuncture

⚱ Heat packs or hot tubs (if you can stand it)

⚱ Massage or other bodywork

⚱ The chiller-outers in the mini-herbal on page 280

⚱ Orgasm

⚱ NSAIDS and other analgesics

⚱ Prescription pain medications

⚱ Hormone therapy/progestin-based contraception methods like an IUD

⚱ B vitamins, vitamin D, calcium, and—wait for it—magnesium, which may help with PMS, pain, or both

LA GRANDE FINALE (OOH LA LA)

Menstrual periods and menstrual and fertility cycles are over after menopause.

That's supposed to be a complete stop. Another period two years later, unexplained spotting, or what still very much feels like your same old cycle shouldn't be happening postmenopause. If you go a full year without periods because of menopause, you are now on the other side, a place where a bunch of other things may still be going on, where you and your body may still be adjusting to changes, but *not* **periods**. Again, if you have *any* vaginal bleeding after menopause, best to get it checked out, and I'd say the same for anything else that just feels like your menstrual cycle still isn't over, even though it's supposed to be.

Of course, if this wasn't the case for you already, you will also no longer be able to reproduce once you reach menopause.

The physiological and psychological (and social!) issues not being able to become pregnant can cause are the same issues menopause can cause. There can be, however, a lot of *feelings* very specific to this. I talk more about those and the feelings about the end of periods and cycles on page 141.

I want to be sure you know that if you're having or are going to have the kinds of sex that can result in pregnancy, this is very much an "it ain't over 'til it's over" situation. Unless you already can't get pregnant anymore or never could, until it has been at *least* one year since anything even remotely resembling a menstrual period, you're going to want to assume that you can still potentially become pregnant and use reliable forms of contraception consistently and correctly if you don't want to become pregnant. Pregnancy can and does still happen for people in perimenopause, even at the often bizarrely unnoticeable end. Some forms of contraception can also provide vehicles of MHT to help with other impacts. In the event you're looking for something new and natural, the Trotula of Salerno suggested fresh weasel testicles tucked into the bosom, a method probably really effective at keeping people not just far enough from your nethers to make reproduction impossible but would likely always assure you your own seat on the bus to boot.

GENITALS AND THE URINARY SYSTEM

"Genitourinary syndrome of menopause" is the most current medical term for the group of different possible impacts of any part of menopause on the vulva, vagina, and lower urinary tract.

It's unwieldy as terms go, and "syndrome" definitely implies something is wrong rather than simply *different*, as is often the case. But it at least beats others, like "vaginal atrophy," "senile vagina," or what sounds like the annoying tagalong little sister of the Roman goddess-y sexually transmitted infections (STIs) chlamydia, gonorrhea, and syphilis: "atrophic vaginitis."

I FEEL LIKE SO MANY OF US LEARN TO live in fear of vulvovaginal changes, specifically, and have been conditioned to assume that (1) whatever we consider to be the worst will happen, (2) that anything that happens must be a *bad* thing, and (3) that any vulvovaginal changes that do happen will be tragic and unmanageable. The way that postmenopausal genitals

have been talked about historically certainly doesn't help. That fear has been and is still exploited to promote therapies, surgeries, and other for-profit approaches to these changes.

Of course, we've *never* been able to win in this world when it comes to our genitals.

Few of us have missed out on en masse cultural mockery about inner labia that are "too big"—that are "meat curtains," or other terms that make you wonder how the trash who came up with this stuff was able to get close to them in the first place—a mons and/or labia majora that are "too" puffy or fleshy; vaginas that are purportedly too "loose" or even too well lubricated and otherwise comfortable for the person whose body part it is, like that's even possible. The Venn diagram of those voicing all these kinds of complaints is a circle, by the by, and doesn't include anyone we would likely want *near* those parts. Even if you keep those folks away from your own parts, that stuff can still make its way into all our internalized body negativity and fears.

In case you had the optimistic idea that all this would die down once you made it to a certain age, I'm sorry to be the bearer of bad news (again). Now too big becomes too small; too loose, too tight; too wet, too dry. Cisgender women and other folks who try and meet these standards are often mocked for doing so by the same people upholding them, and trans women's vulvas and vaginas can, of course, never be perfect in this system, no matter what. (People with penises and testicles aren't spared either. Scrotums stretch out over time, and penises look, feel, and behave differently as people age, too. But those changes aren't and can't be weaponized the same way and are rarely as impactful.)

There's just never a "just right" for *anyone* in this mean, demented, and seemingly never-ending version of Goldilocks.

SMALL WONDER SOME OF US LIVE IN fear and dread of what might happen to our genitals with and after menopause. I'd love to say I'm not a member of this group. I shouldn't be, right? I'm a queer sex educator. I know from a lifetime of enjoyable field research that my genitals aren't required for me to experience and take part in sex and other kinds of pleasure. I have seen way more genitals than the average person: I know how incredibly diverse they are. I know there's no "right" way they have to be, look, or feel for them to bring me pleasure and for me to accept them. I coach other people through this. I am also someone who cares a lot about disability justice and access, who knows how to make adjustments and accommodations for others and to ask for them for myself, and who thinks those things are liberating, not shameful or humiliating. I shouldn't have any issues with this.

And yet, I do. I've internalized and do battle with my own fear and dread about vulvovaginal changes already happening and coming for me down the road too.

Last year, I was given three rounds of antibiotics in a row (to go with another of the joys of midlife: not-a-baby's first root canal) and wound up with the **mother** of all yeast infections. It hurt like hell. There were tears. There were sores. I knew how Swiss cheese felt. It was only the third yeast infection I'd had in my whole life, and boy, was it ever trying to make up for lost time.

My partner was out of town at the time and came back before it had resolved. I said I was in the mood for sex but that my cunt was way out of commission and had to be benched for that game. Trying to find some things that I might enjoy, some topside action was suggested, as well as a little "It can't be that hideous, can it?" I appreciated the try, but it really could be, and it really *was* that hideous.

It dredged up my hidden fears about vulvar and vaginal changes. I felt afraid this was the beginning of the end, a sneak preview of how my vulva was going to always be eventually, that I'd lose the ability to have it be part of my sex life or to feel okay with someone else looking at it without worrying they'd run from it as from the walking dead. Again, I know better: I am very familiar with this anatomy, in all the ways a person can be. But, as is so often the case with all things aging, I knew far less about it in menopause and beyond.

W E'VE ALL HAD TO DEAL WITH MES-sages from our cultures, communities, and maybe even our families, friends, and sexual partners about the apparent right and wrong ways to think and feel about our genitals. I'm sure we've all had enough of that. You're going to feel how you feel, and when you read or experience some or all of what I'm about to discuss, you might have some challenging feelings. (Or not!) I want to give you permission to have your feelings, whatever they are.

I also want you, and me, to know that it'll be okay, regardless. Even if anything in here freaks you out big time, the "worst" that could happen, in my humble opinion, is if you got it in your head that these parts of your body, like any others, are only right or ideal at one time of life and broken or defective otherwise. People can usually do fine with vaginas or vulvas or bladders that need extra TLC, daily regimens, adjustments, treatments, or medications. People can also work out how to have a life when these body parts don't operate at all how they did before, no matter what: we are adaptable. People usually *don't* do so fine when they decide and dig into the idea that their bodies, or any parts of them, are just no good.

POTENTIAL (AND SOME CERTAIN) GENITOURINARY IMPACTS WITH MENOPAUSE

- Dryness, burning, or irritation of the vulva, vagina, vestibule, perineum, or rectum in (most commonly later) perimenopause or postmenopause. For some people this can result in pain, either with things like sexual activity or in daily life, like when sitting.
- Decreased genital elasticity.
- Decreased vulvovaginal secretions, lubrication, or intensity of genital sensation.
- Pain or discomfort with vaginal sex or speculum or bimanual exams.
- Changes to the appearance of the vulva, most often reduced labial size, thinning of the vaginal walls, vestibule, labia, perineum, and rectum (and thinning of the lining of the urethra, as well), and color changes. The tissue of the vulva may look less vividly colored than before (just like the rest of us): paler, darker, or both.
- A shortening of the vaginal canal and a gradual smoothing out of the rugae, the ridges inside the vaginal canal. There are usually changes to the texture of the inner labia too: they often start to become smoother in late perimenopause.
- Thinner pubic hair or a change in hair patterns. It appears my inner thighs made some kind of deal with my mons because my pubic hair swapped spots.

- Increased or new urinary tract infections (UTIs), yeast infections, bacterial vaginosis (BV), or other genitourinary infections or imbalances.
- Genital fissures or tears and skin issues or disorders, like lichen sclerosis or hyperkeratosis.
- Changes in scent.
- Urgency, incontinence, or other urinary issues.

OY, WHY?

It's mostly about estrogen. Estrogen helps keep the whole body moister, genitals very much included. The thickness of genital tissue and the urinary tract also has to do with estrogen.

Fertility cycling also produces cervical mucus that impacts the pH balance of the vagina: the acidity of that mucus helps prevent imbalances and infections (and also provides extra lubrication). With menopause, what's considered "normal" vaginal pH changes from a 3.8–4.5 range to higher, usually between 5 and 6, the same level it usually is before puberty, too. That's okay, but it can change our vulnerability to imbalances and infections.

Vaginal pain or discomfort with sex or changing sensation can also be influenced by your stress levels and your sleep. Hydration—or more to the point, dehydration—also plays a part in genital dryness, just like it does with the rest of the body, as well as with vaginal infections,

especially UTIs. Some of this can be about aging or habits that are common for people in midlife or later, like reduced physical activity (so less circulation) or less frequent genital sexual activity.

You may not experience these impacts—or experience them in any major way—until late perimenopause or postmenopause. Unless they're things you're already dealing with or otherwise predisposed to, they rarely show up in early peri.

INCONTINENCE, BLADDER ISSUES, AND OTHER GENITOURINARY DELIGHTS

If you have a bladder and you have (or had) a uterus, you may already know that bladder issues—urgency, frequency, incontinence, UTIs—are common at any age in people born with those organs. You may also already be quite aware it's common to experience an increase in some or all of these issues after pregnancy and childbirth and with aging. All of those things and changes in estrogen levels can change the muscle tone of the bladder and the surrounding muscles, like the muscles of the pelvic floor. The thinning of the urethra plays a role here too.

WHAT CAN HELP?

- **Pelvic floor muscle training (PFMT) aka kegel exercises:** Squeezing your pelvic floor muscles—the same muscles you may squeeze as a habit to get rid of the last drops after you urinate—on the regular can strengthen the pelvic floor. That can help with prolapse prevention and incontinence, as well as how the vagina and genital sexual response feels, and help keep circulation moving in the whole pelvic area. You can do them in the elevator, you can do them during sex, you can do them with any of the many kegel exercise gadgets that currently exist for this purpose, and your body will usually do them involuntarily with orgasm and after you urinate, so if you don't want to bother yourself with doing them on purpose but still want to do them, well . . . there you go. (They write themselves, I swear.)

◊ **"Double voiding" and other bladder retraining:** Double voiding is just a fancy term to describe peeing and then waiting a bit to try and do it again not long after. Bladder retraining, like double voiding and extending times

between toilet visits, can also help strengthen those muscles and help with bladder leaks and urgency.

◊ **Pads/absorbent underpants:** As with anything else in life, if you need them and they make your life easier, I think you should use them. If you need to hear this: try not to get into a shame spiral about these or to think about them any differently than you'd think about things you've used for menstrual flow. This is just an accommodation or assistive device, like a cane, a wheelchair, an ice pack, a service dog, a cab, a sling, or a translator: it's about providing you and your body with what you both need to live your life. There's no shame in that.

◊ **Medications:** There are numerous medications for different urinary issues. Systemic estrogen hasn't been found to help with any, but topical estrogen can help with some kinds of incontinence,

Pelvic organ prolapse: Prolapse of the bladder, uterus, urethra, vagina, small bowel, or rectum can happen at any time, especially for people who've carried pregnancies to term or late into them and have had vaginal deliveries. Once estrogen starts going and stays low, those risks can increase, particularly postmenopause, because estrogen helps keep the connective tissues of those organs strong. Estrogen therapy can also potentially help with or prevent it. If you think you might be experiencing a prolapse, seek medical attention. While we're here, risks of breast, cervical, vulvovaginal, endometrial, and ovarian cancers also increase once we're over fifty. It's ideal to get or keep in the habit of health screenings for those at least at the minimum suggested, which is about every three years. Pap smears can often be done less often than that.

as can some tricyclic antidepressants and serotonin-norepinephrine reuptake inhibitors (SNRIs) prescribed off label.

UTIs, BV, and yeast infections: Treatments and preventions for these are basically what they've always been.

There isn't much scientific evidence that diet impacts UTIs or vaginal infections, including yeast infections. However, it's not like taking care of our digestive systems isn't good for us anyway. And if you find, as some folks do, that yeast-fermented or other foods seem to make you more prone to yeast or other infections, I see no reason not to trust what your own body is telling you.

Planning ahead with probiotics if and when you have to take antibiotics could help you keep from winding up with a zombie vulva like me. UTIs, BV, and yeast infections are easier to avoid if you avoid or quickly tend to exposure to bacteria or conditions where they thrive. You probably already know this stuff: I'm talking about urinating before and after genital sex of any kind (masturbation included!), wiping from front to back, not sitting around in sweaty, tight gym clothes and the like, claiming your birthright of comfortable underpants, and hydration, hydration, hydration.

Douching is just bad news. On top of changes from menopause itself, douching makes BV more likely—and is absolutely, positively *not* a way to treat it. You just want to do whatever you can to avoid anything unnecessarily disruptive to the bacterial environment of the vagina. Keeping the peace as best we can is the name of the game, and douching is the equivalent of declaring war.

For UTIs, BV, and yeast infections, if you get them often enough that you know what they are when you get one, you can talk to a healthcare provider and see if they'll give you an open prescription for the treatments you use so that you don't have to go all the way in and pay for a visit when you both already know what you've got going on. We all know how much fun a bus ride isn't with a UTI.

Vulvovaginal helps: Genital dryness and inflexibility can feel very uncomfortable—sometimes even when, or especially when, you're just sitting around. They can also play a part in issues like UTIs and BV. You'll find specifically sexual adaptations and helps with these in the next section. These next helps are more general than sexual.

Most of Ya Basics: Smoking, dehydration, and lack of activity are all associated with greater dryness and inflexibility, having them happen earlier rather than later, or having them be more severe. Emotional support—both with vulvar and vaginal issues but also with bladder and urinary impacts—can go a really long way, and improving sleep and reducing and managing stress can also help you out, especially when this is part of your stress.

Vaginal and vulvar moisturizers: Dr. Judith Hersh agrees with me that if you're thinking it's time for moisturizing around your eyes or neck, it's probably also time for vulvar and vaginal moisturizing. If you're not thinking about any of those things, but you're reading this book, it's probably time to consider all of them, as your skin is going to start getting thinner and less resilient in all three places around now if it hasn't already. It'll feel better and hold up better if you moisturize. You're welcome.

They're not the same thing, by the way. *Vaginal* moisturizers are used inside the vagina, usually every few days. Vaginal moisturizers are usually suppositories, liquids used with an applicator, or liquids you use with your fingers. Some common ingredients in many of them right now include hyaluronic acid, vitamin E, cannabidiol (CBD), aloe, and flax. You can use lube you use for sex or other purposes as a vaginal moisturizer if you like; it just might not be as effective or long-lasting as options made expressly for this purpose.

Vulvar moisturizers—usually creams and balms—are used daily or as often as you want. They usually have an oil base, like olive, coconut, or vitamin E oil, with something else to lock the moisture in, like shea butter, honey, or beeswax. So if you want to get thrifty, crafty, or both, or you just want to be able to have something that's just right for you, it's simple enough to make your own. Or you can just use any of those oils by themselves.

Dr. Hersh said that she's found that there are few people who *don't* need something for vaginal and vulvar health in later perimenopause and postmenopause. She tells her patients in their forties to tell her if they experience any genital discomfort so it can be addressed before it winds up resulting in fissures, tears, or vulvodynia, a chronic pain condition.

With vaginal or vulvar moisturizers or lubes, just be sure to be on the lookout for and try to avoid known harmful ingredients like parabens, petroleum products, propylene glycol, and sodium hydroxide. If you're prone to yeast, you likely want to avoid glycerin, and if you're prone to any kind of infection, silicones might not be a great choice since they can hang around for a while.

Much like with the tissues of the rest of our body, maintaining circulation, moisture, and resilience of the vulva and vagina is important. It obviously matters if you want to engage in genital sex, but it's also important to be able to continue to get healthcare like speculum exams. The rest of the genitourinary system is impacted by vaginovulvar changes too. Dr. Hersh makes clear that "vaginal health goes hand in hand with bladder health, as the two are intimately connected: the bladder is directly above the anterior vagina. Keeping vaginal tissues healthy can also help with bladder control." She adds that even sitting or wiping can result in vulvar tears for some people postmenopause.

She says that doesn't have to be medications or hormone therapy: vaginal and vulvar moisturizers, used regularly as a practice—not just when or after there's pain or discomfort—often do the trick. She's a particular fan of hyaluronic acid suppositories or gels.

Hormone therapy: Topical estrogen, in the form of a ring, tablet, cream, or gel, applied directly to the vulva and vagina is the kind of MHT usually prescribed with vulvovaginal issues rather than systemic estrogen. How often you use it depends on the specific vehicle for it and how it's uniquely prescribed for you. The Food and Drug Administration has approved bioidentical options for those who prefer those, and a daily oral selective estrogen receptor modulator has also been approved for this purpose.

Intravaginal dehydroepiandrosterone (DHEA): Newer on the scene, DHEA, a hormonal precursor of estrogens and androgens, is another option that's been found to be effective for local (not systemic) vaginal therapy.

Surgical and other medical procedures: There are also medical procedures and treatments, from fractional CO_2 lasers to radio frequency waves to fillers, that are currently being offered as options for some vulvovaginal and other genitourinary issues. If you get to the point that you're considering any of them, you're hopefully already working with a qualified reproductive menopause healthcare provider who can give you the most current and specific information about any of these and all of your options. If not, that's whom you'd want to talk with to find out more: most of this stuff isn't supported as either safe or effective with research to date, and those that are or might be both should still be approached very cautiously to assure you don't add both insult and injury to your existing problems.

VAGINAL OR VULVAR PAIN

If you experience vaginal or vulvar pain, I'd encourage you to see a vulvovaginal pain specialist. Do **not** keep doing anything that hurts if you can avoid it. It won't help. If a healthcare provider or someone else tells you to have sex to help things even though it hurts, not only should you ignore them, but if they're your healthcare provider, you should dump them. That is terrible advice far outside best practices with vulvovaginal pain. Having sex or doing anything else when it hurts is the surest way to make it keep hurting and often progressively worse each time. This is an area where a lot of providers don't know what they're doing because it's highly specialized. Do all you can to find care from someone who specifically works with genital pain.

"USE IT OR LOSE IT"

This is said often about the vagina, sex, and menopause, sometimes even by healthcare providers. I think it is deeply icky and even a little rapey, honestly. I hate it. But you're probably going to hear it, so I want to talk about it and be less gross.

What is ultimately meant by that phrase is that just like the other muscles and tissues of your body, the vagina tends to stay more elastic when you stretch it on the regular. What that phrase unfortunately says as well is that (1) the only reason that matters is sex, and (2) you better keep having sex with your vagina, or you—or any partners—won't get to have your vagina to *have* sex with anymore.

I hope we can just agree that this framing is objectively terrible for more reasons than any of us has or certainly wants time for. For those who cannot or choose not to have this kind of (or any) sex, being told they need to be sexual in this way to keep a body part functional can feel dismissive, othering, and invasive. Others may feel like suggesting sex as prevention interferes with the way they want to think about or engage in sex or their sexual relationships. As Leah Lakshmi Piepzna-Samarasinha said, "What if you don't *want* to use it? What if you have pelvic trauma? What if you have scars? What if you're asexual?"

It's also really freaking vague. What's "it"? And how did we get back to sixth grade, where that's a question again in the first place?

I'M GOING TO PUT MY SEX EDUCATOR HAT on and answer this based on what I know, which, in this department, is a lot. Any kind of targeted stimulation of the vulva and/or vagina that gets some circulation moving in that area should help keep those tissues more pliable, or at least pliable enough that you feel comfortable in your daily life.

Additionally, anything that can help keep the vagina in the habit of being flexible—if it is in that habit in the first place or is something a person wants to continue—can help the vagina retain its flexibility, as is the case with any other kind of muscle. Because of heteronormativity, this is often said or assumed to require vaginal intercourse of some kind. I don't see why it would need to.

That kind of sex—be it with a toy, a penis, or fingers or hands—can be one way to make those things happen. But it's not the *only* way, and the way anyone goes about this also doesn't have to be sexual.

Vulvovaginal stimulation to help with circulation and flexibility could be genital sex with a partner or masturbation, with or without toys in either case, or you could just hang out watching a movie holding a Hitachi wand on your mons or doing kegels around a small dildo or vaginal dilator—progressively sized devices made expressly to help people retain or expand vaginal elasticity and/or comfort with having something inside the vagina—and whether any of that stimulation is sexual for you or not is up to you. Riding an electric bull could probably also do the trick, in the event you have access to one of those and excellent health insurance.

The genitals are interconnected, so if you're someone who does not want to involve their vagina when it comes to direct stimulation, stimulation of the vulva is still likely to help some. Whether or not you are having sexual feelings or a sexual context when you do this is likely to be irrelevant, unless you are someone who needs to be feeling sexual for any of this kind of stimulation to feel good or okay. Certainly, if you're doing anything with vaginal *insertion*, feeling sexual often helps a lot with flexibility, but just getting deeply relaxed—like with a yoga practice, for instance—and/or engaging with pleasure in other ways can often accomplish that too.

Neither sex nor other kinds of genital stimulation are required to keep those tissues healthy, but that ooky phrase sure doesn't make it sound as consensual as it absolutely should be. If you don't want to do any of this, you do not have to, and you also shouldn't feel like you have to. It may not always still *feel* like your body as you're going through perimenopause, but it very much still is. If—for whatever reason, be it sex, pap smears, a safe place to keep your cash—you want to do what you can to maintain vaginal flexibility but don't want to have it involve sex or anything else in this section, that should not be a problem, including if that's a hard limit you set with a healthcare provider.

Lube, lube, lube, lube, lube: If you're using vaginal dilators or engaging in masturbation and genital sex with partners, lube gets even more essential than it was before. **Listen to me: you need lube.** When it came to things going inside the vagina or anus, you probably always would have benefitted from lube, even if you didn't wholly realize or accept it before, but you really will need it and benefit from it now. Because the tissues of the vagina, vulva, perineum, and anus become thinner and drier with the menopausal transition—especially once estrogen levels start declining—and postmenopause, they're less resilient. That makes them more prone to abrasions and fissures, as well as infections, including STIs. The supplementary lubrication that comes with the ovulatory phase of the menstrual/fertility cycle also will stop showing up once you're postmenopause.

For more on lubricants, when and how to use them, and a lube pep talk if you need it, see page 225 in the section on sex.

CHAPTER ELEVEN

BODIES, SKIN, AND LOOKS

"Your body is an heirloom. If we think about the purpose of an heirloom, it is a symbolic representation of resilience. We do not criticize an heirloom. We do not devalue it for its flaws and imperfections."

—*Sonalee Roshtawar*

Hungarian countess Erzebet Báthory was forty-nine years old when she was arrested in 1609. She may or may not have been a cannibal, sadistic torturer, and serial murderer who bathed in the blood of girls and young women in order to stay looking young. Given her power and wealth, how this all went down, and the tremendous lack of evidence, she was more likely the victim of a smear campaign that intentionally resulted in this reputation, as well as a slow death over three years of windowless isolation. That the men making this accusation did so as a power grab and a debt dodge seems far more realistic than the alternative. Yet everyone knows her as "the Blood Countess," not Erzebet, whom those sexist Protestant and Habsburg assholes robbed, smeared, and locked away until she died.

Are you surprised? I'm not, because patriarchy and misogyny. Also people clearly having no idea how hard it is to get bloodstains out of wood. The fact is, many of us have some strange ideas about bodies, looks, physical beauty, desirability, menopause and aging, and women.

It is appallingly easy to believe people, especially women and femmes, will do *anything* to avoid looking what's considered menopausal, middle-aged, or old, as well as fat or ugly. We easily believe that because both our overarching culture and many of our smaller cultures and communities have taught us that being any of those things, let alone *looking* those ways, is something to avoid at all costs. Cisgender women know how real pretty privilege and thin privilege are, so many who have had those earnestly fear life without them. If you think cisgender women live in terror of these standards, consider transgender women—and even more, transgender women of color—for whom standards of femininity are even more inflexible. Transmasculine folks are held, and more rigidly no less, to masculine ideals cisgender men made. The required presentation for those of us who are nonbinary, if we want to stand any chance of being recognized for who we are, is effectively looking like the secret love child of Peter Pan and Tinkerbell. That doesn't work with round middles, rivers of sweat, jowls, or babestaches.

It is easy to believe things like bloodbaths as spa treatments because some people *do* things like this to try and meet these standards. A "vampire facial" is an actual thing in 2020 that a Kardashian (who else?) made famous. It's your own blood, instead called "platelet-rich plasma," the "veal" of blood terminology, I guess. It's injected into your face or vagina, which I know is supposed to sound less gruesome than bathing in someone else's blood, and yet—it doesn't. The express reason to do it is all about how much younger it can apparently make you look.

The systems most of us grew up with, and live with the endless echoes of, make the actual or purported consequences of looking old, fat, unfeminine, not white enough, not sexy enough, or otherwise socially unacceptable in our world very

clear, all the time, almost everywhere we look. If we can lose power, value, benefits, privileges, protection, and even our ability to straight-up survive, well, who *wouldn't* go to great lengths to avoid that fate?

If we paid any attention to magazine ads and articles, to *Real Housewives*, to drugstore and department store shelves, to pharmaceutical ads, to the smooth faces of sixty-something actresses, it wouldn't be surprising if the thing we were most worried about with menopause, middle age, or both was how it might change our privilege and our appeal, mostly based on how our bodies and faces look. We're supposed to believe that. Fortunes literally depend on our believing that.

I can't tell you for certain what Erzebet Báthory did or didn't do. I doubt she bathed in other people's blood as an antiwrinkle treatment. It seems far more likely that Erzebet Báthory got screwed by the same systems and beliefs that are still royally screwing a whole lot of us right now.

THE WORLD DOES NOT, DESPITE UNDERstandable fears to the contrary, end when our bodies and the way they look change with menopause, aging, or both. If we had much to lose in the first place, we don't usually lose all of what we thought we might. Our appreciation of our bodies—and others' appreciation of them—doesn't *have* to end or diminish: that's our choice, not a predetermined destiny. We can even gain some things we may not have realized were in the cards for us, sometimes expressly *because* of losing some other things.

Just like every other part of all this, not everyone has the same changes or in the same ways or on the same timeline. Not everyone feels the same way about all this, and you get to have and feel your feelings about it, whatever they are. Per usual, I'm not going to tell you what to do, but if you insist, I might tell you to stop being such an asshole to yourself.

As Hanne Blank said, "If you are lucky enough to live long enough your body will change. Not 'might,' not 'could,' it *will* change. And it may change more than once. Thankfully, this is exactly what is supposed to happen. It's literally written in your DNA. There is no wrong way to have a body. Your body is what makes you possible, and as long as it's succeeding in that job, it is an excellent body."

THE BIGGEST "WHAT CAN YOU DO ABOUT it" for everything that follows in this chapter is this: **put energy into caring for yourself in ways that make you feel good, and nurture an adaptive acceptance of your body, like the rest of yourself, as a constant, always-changing work in progress.**

Changes with our body shape and size and other parts of our appearance are going to happen whether we like them or want them or not, and we're only going to be able to do so much about this arena of change. What happens here is mostly about our genetics and our past life history, which we can't change. It's less so about our present and future life circumstances, which we do have some control over, but how much and over what parts are variable as hell.

We're not going to be able to stop our bodies from aging or from responding to menopause. I propose that the Robert Wilson–esque idea that we can stay as we are premenopause forever with pills or cremes or even diet or exercise regimens is not just impossible but also sad, creepy bollocks. Most of us won't have much we can do to make giant changes to the shape or size of our bodies, to the way our skin looks, to how much hair we have. But I like to hope that most of us who have made it this far are—if we're not already there—ready to be more accepting of ourselves and our bodies, including how they look when they meet fewer and fewer beauty standards, as they will tend to in cultures like ours where beauty is set up as something you can age out of.

I'm still trying to wrap my head around the real possibility of living another forty or fifty years (and how on earth I'll afford it), and if I do, I don't want to spend the whole next half of my lifetime in a duel to the death with my body or appearance. I'm still traumatized and bruised from the first half's rounds, and mine weren't even that bad much of the time.

One more thing: things that get filed under looks—changes to our body shape and size, skin, hair, or nails—obviously aren't just about looks. They're part of our health, and some impact other systems of our bodies. They feel different ways physically, emotionally, and socially. Our bodies and their appearance are often part of our gender and sexual identities and other ways we experience and express some core parts of who we are. Weight or body-composition changes or changes to our skin can also feel unpleasant physically, even if we have no issue with them otherwise. For example, more weight in a given place can add a burden to an old injury, and hyperreactive skin can be a real PITA. I don't want you to get the idea I'm dismissing any of that. I have myself long possessed a frequently hurty, emotionally challenging, highly demanding body.

I'm not going to tell you to *love* your body, but I do encourage you to work toward accepting it. Sometimes our bodies are going to hurt us, limit us, cost us, or really piss us off. We are just not always going to love them. That's okay.

YOUR CHANGING BODY . . . YEP, *AGAIN*

Our body shape, size, and composition will often change to some degree during the course of a menopausal transition.

There are some typical ways those things can happen.

It's common for those who were more pear, hourglass, or straight-shaped to become more apple-shaped or to lean more in that direction than they did before, during, or after menopausal transition. If you didn't have a belly before, you might get one now. If you had a belly before, it might get bigger.

Some people gain weight during the menopausal transition or after sudden menopause. Others don't. Averages on this are all over the place, which would render them useless if they weren't pretty useless already by virtue of being about something we largely can't control anyhow. We're going to gain (or not) whatever we are, so unless you're concerned that it's happening because of something you might need treatment for (in which case you should check in with a healthcare provider), like a thyroid condition, it's just one of those things where you're going to see what happens and know what did when it's over.

Body composition also changes. Most often that change is increasing or increased fat mass and decreasing lean muscle mass, both changes that have been attributed in studies as clearly menopause related. The Study of Women's Health Across the Nation found an approximate doubling of fat mass at around two years prior to the final menstrual period and continued fat gains until about two years after, when fat and lean mass plateau. These composition changes are why some people don't see a change, or much change, in their weight: muscle weighs more than fat, so increased fat but decreased muscle mass can change body composition without noticeable weight changes.

There's an array of experience with how body changes with menopause interact with, impact, or reflect gender identities. Depending on how your body was before this and how it becomes, as well as your own gender (or lack thereof), these changes can affirm, have little to no impact on, or feel in conflict with an identity. There's a cultural narrative and sometimes a personal experience that looking older or going through menopause or midlife is universally masculinizing, or gender-neutralizing, but we don't all have that experience by any stretch.

WHY DO THESE CHANGES HAPPEN?

Surprise! A lot of this is hormonal. Fluctuating hormone levels and balances (between estrogen, progesterone, and also testosterone) in perimenopause often create changes in body size and weight. Changes in estrogen levels, especially once estrogen starts to decrease, can create changes in fat distribution, in how we process sugars and starches, and in our metabolisms on the whole. Increased follicle-stimulating hormone levels, which we see in late perimenopause and usually ever after, may be another player,

and increased cortisol levels, when they're in the mix, also likely play a part.

The body may also be trying to do something **protective** for our bones with fat redistribution and gain, particularly for once estrogen levels get and remain low. Our bodies, in their infinite wisdom, may be trying to do what they can to help ease us through this transition, period.

When we get to the part of perimenopause where estradiol starts going lower (or with sudden menopause from the jump), our bodies aren't getting the help from estradiol they're used to with regulating and supporting all the things estrogens help with, including our metabolism, but also other very important things.

Fat (aka adipose) tissue, especially around our middles, creates an extra source of estrogen, estrone. It is entirely possible that, especially once our estrogen levels start to drop, our bodies are trying to supplement it to help make our transition to lower levels and different sources easier on us. Research supports that postmenopause weight may help protect our **bones**. As eating disorders specialist and clinical psychiatrist Dr. Margo Maine says, "Your belly fat is not your spare tire, it is your life preserver."

SOME OF THIS INVOLVES OTHER MENOpause impacts or issues. Our metabolisms are greatly affected by sleep (or the lack of it) and by stress, for example. If we're fatigued, not only will we have less energy for movement but our digestion will struggle. Bloating can add water weight. Some of this is just about the aging process and where we're at in it. It's normal for metabolism to slow down as we age, and it's usually already been doing that for a while by the time we're in perimenopause.

The ways your body shape, size, and composition may change in this may be new to you or not feel like you, but it's all usually still just your body being your body, just in different ways than you've experienced so far. It also is often not itself a health or other problem. Most of us can and will get bigger or smaller, rounder or not, harder or softer without anything being the matter with us. It's normal for our bodies to change through our lifetimes in all kinds of ways.

IF YOU KNOW OR SUSPECT YOUR BODY IS changing in ways that are *not* good for your particular body and your well-being, I believe you, and I know that's real too. Weight or shape changes can be due to other conditions, like thyroid issues or polycystic ovary syndrome. If you have a weight change that feels very weird for you and your body as you know it, and you don't know why it's happening, by all means, check in with a trusted care provider.

Sometimes weight or shape changes can be a reflection of us not getting the amount of activity we need to keep up with mobility and feel good, not managing stress in ways that are best for us, or not getting the emotional support we need. By all means, if and when that's the case, do what you need to do to take care of yourself in this regard, as you would with any other system of your body or area of your health. I just want to remind you to take care of yourself and really center this in taking care of your whole self and how it makes you feel—as Rebecca Scritchfield puts it, try not to make your appearance your why for changes in this arena. Not only might your appearance not change when you do or adjust those things, but that just doesn't tend to be a motivator that helps with a positive mindset.

LOSE WEIGHT LOSS: DUMPING DIET CULTURE

If the way your body shape or size changes during any part of menopause involves gaining weight or looking bigger or fatter, you may think you need to try and lose weight. If you read menopause information or look for menopause supplements and other products, it's no wonder you think that, because it's ubiquitous. You may outright be told to lose weight by any number of people while within a fifty-year radius of menopause. I'd like to take a little time to explain why I think that is not good advice and why I think you should **not** try and do that, *especially* now, of all times.

I talk about fat and weight in a neutral way. That's because "fat" and "weight" are neutral, even though our world sure doesn't treat them that way. They aren't good or bad, noble or ignoble; they just **are**. They are part of us, like our noses, blood cells, or callouses, and are as much or as little as they are at any given time. They don't tell us or anyone else jack about our value as people, about the merit or success of our bodies or behaviors, or anything about our morality or lack of it.

If that approach is new to you, it might be refreshing. It might also be jarring, shame inducing, or even feel threatening. That's okay, and it's certainly understandable.

What diet culture and anti-fat bias has taught us and continues to enforce in us can be hard to shake, especially since it won't leave us alone for five goddamn minutes. It's hard, sometimes even painful—especially if we have sacrificed a lot to diet culture and are still holding out for a payoff—and it takes time to process, let go of, and recalibrate.

As Aubrey Gordon, author of *What We Don't Talk About When We Talk About Fat,* says in the July 2020 installment of her *Self* magazine column, "Having a Better Body Image Won't End Body-Based Oppression," "*none* of our bodies are received 'neutrally' by those around us. Countless data points show us, time and time again, that those of us whose bodies are marked by difference are treated differently in nearly every aspect of our lives. And simply changing our mindsets, feeling neutral about or loving our bodies won't address the bias marginalized people so regularly face.

"For those of us whose bodies lead to systemic adverse treatment, self-love isn't as simple as a mindset shift, a light switch to turn on. To be sure, self-love and body neutrality are powerful things. But they aren't so powerful that they can divert or erase others' harmful actions or make unjust systems more just. And body neutrality alone can't address our own learned biases, either. While working toward neutrality with our own bodies may make some limited shifts in how we see others', it won't do the work of uprooting our biases for us."

So. Wherever you're at with this, and whatever your body, be gentle with yourself, and please don't throw this book at anyone who isn't wearing safety goggles.

Weight and the having of it are often blamed for a host of menopausal ills, even though it's well known that things people consider to be overweight experiences during menopause, like hot flashes, bloating, and body shape changes or just having a crummy time, *also* happen to everyone else too.

Weight bias is so deeply internalized and entrenched that a lot of folks don't even see it to know they need to deal with it or make sure what they believe is even true. Many people, healthcare providers included, feel so confident in what they believe about fat, weight, and weight loss that they don't educate themselves to learn that what they believe was often *never* true or complete, and some of what was once thought to be sound has since been found to be otherwise.

The idea that "losing weight" is the answer to any and all menopausal misery is foolish for a thousand reasons. Don't worry, I'm not going to list them all; I know you don't have all day.

Losing weight can't fix cultural, interpersonal, and internalized sexism and ageism that can make *having* weight and fat in this world an awful experience. Losing weight isn't the answer to hot flashes, migraines, stress, dry skin, or other impacts of menopause. But most of all, telling someone to lose weight, suggesting they should, or even thinking they can is pretty ludicrous because **"losing weight"** is not an action we can actually even *do* in the first place.

Unless the weight is coming from a backpack, a kid attached to your leg, or your boots, you can't just "lose it." Weight loss is something that can *happen* to and in our bodies, sure, but losing weight is not an *action* any of us can actually *do*, like say, "increase your movement," "think of a cat," or, as you may have wanted to say to those who have told you to lose weight, "go fuck yourself."

What people *most* often do to *try* to lose weight, the actions people engage in in the pursuit of weight loss, is some kind of restrictive eating with rules, aka dieting. I'm talking about things like counting calories and trying to stay under a certain daily amount; focusing on, limiting, or avoiding particular foods or food groups; or focusing on, limiting, or avoiding food, period.

Dieting can do real, well-documented harm, is usually counter to health and well-being, and does some things that make menopausal impacts worse.

As many of us can attest, dieting is often a source of great frustration, self-loathing, and self-punishment. Dieting usually makes us feel worse about ourselves, not better. Dieting is a fickle and conditional frenemy to our self-esteem.

Dieting *causes* stress rather than helping us avoid or reduce it. Hunger makes it harder to fall and stay asleep. Restrictive eating can leave us too tired for movement, and if our main motivation for movement is weight loss instead of pleasure, we're less likely to want to move in the first place. Dieting messes with our cognition and makes it harder to focus, especially on anything that isn't food or body size. It can make our whole bodies drier inside and out, already an impact of lowering estrogen. It often impacts our digestion, our neurology, and our sexual lives in negative ways.

Rebecca Scritchfield puts it plainly: **dieting is a traumatic assault on the body**. She also noted that in reaction to, or as part and parcel of, dieting, we might also do things that *additionally* aren't supportive of our health, like smoking or overexercising.

Dieting requires us to be disappointed with our bodies—because it requires us to want to "improve" them. That can create or increase stress, depression, and anxiety and have a negative impact on our self-esteem, sexuality, and social relationships. Low self-esteem makes us more vulnerable to abusive, dysfunctional, or just crappy relationships. Leaning into disappointment in our bodies can make it harder to live and take care of ourselves with injuries, chronic pain and illness, or other disabilities we may have.

Dieting can get in the way of social support in menopause. Diet and weight talk often run rampant, unchecked, and enabled in menopause support groups and a lot of other peer social interactions. If we or others won't stop talking about dieting, we make relationships and spaces inaccessible for anyone for whom that talk is toxic, damaging, or dangerous.

The second-biggest risk group for eating disorders after adolescents is people in menopause.

People in a menopausal transition are very vulnerable to developing, continuing with, or relapsing into eating disorders. That has an awful lot to do with, as dietician and eating disorders specialist Erica Leon says, the fact that diet culture *preys* upon people in menopause. There's pressure to maintain a "youthful appearance" and not to look like you're in menopause. Menopause is also outside our control, so the desire to try and control what we can, like eating, can be strong.

Disordered eating—and much dieting would be considered such—presents a number of health risks. Some of those risks are already increased in perimenopause or postmenopause. Disordered eating can impact every system of the body, including the endocrine system. It increases already elevated risks of heart attack, stroke, and bone loss and can make us more likely to develop diabetes, thyroid disorders, and bacterial infections. Eating disorders don't play nice with other kinds of mental illness. The majority of death that occurs due to anorexia occurs to older, not younger, people.

Chronic dieting is associated with a host of ills, including some, like bone loss, stress, high blood pressure, or decreased insulin resistance, that menopause and aging already increase our risks of. People may, knowingly or unknowingly, give us positive affirmation for any visible weight loss that happens because of disordered eating, a particularly seductive reward if we're hungry for validation about our appearance as so many people are during and around menopause. They may congratulate us on our self-discipline or backside instead of expressing concern and offering help. It's all too easy to have an eating disorder in midlife in plain sight.

and, as Christy Harrison adds, "disproportionately harms women, femmes, trans folks, people in larger bodies, people of color, and people with disabilities, damaging both their mental and physical health." Dieting does everyone harm because it requires that we believe that one kind of body is superior—including *morally* superior—to another kind of body, a belief that is the basis of eugenics, racism, misogyny, and all manner of other horrible cultural ills and harms.

So far, it nets a $70 *billion* annual profit in the United States alone, and, as Rebecca Scritchfield points out, the level and intensity of belief many people have in it and all of its claims are near-religious.

"The body is not a wrong answer. The body is not a failed class. You are not failing."
—Sonya Renee Taylor

Accepting our bodies in menopause is vital to our well-being in and throughout this, but diet culture makes that really, really difficult.

Diet culture is the worst smoothie ever, made of religious asceticism (especially the Christian temperance movement), white supremacy, anti-fat bias, capitalism, manufacturing, the fashion industry, healthism and medicalization, economic class division, sexism, and exceptionalism. It makes being thinner and eating less, or eating "right," better and more virtuous,

Diet culture is why I've known how many calories are in a carrot or a Hostess Raspberry Zinger since I was eleven. It's why nearly all the living women in my family are perennially on a diet. Diet culture is why widely accepted systems of health evaluation have been based on things that aren't even **about** health, like the Metropolitan Life height and weight charts, insurance figures, and the body mass index, devised by mathematician Adolphe Quetlet and based on French and Scottish people so he could bolster his belief that people of color were criminals and show the "ideal" body to be a white European one.

When diet culture and menopause collide, it's easy to get the idea that thinness will equal a better menopause, that fatness will equal a harder one, and even that a shitty menopause is just what you get for being or getting fat.

THE THING IS, EVEN THOUGH IT SURE feels like it, institutions, doctors, celebrities, relatives, and other people don't determine the appropriate weight for us. Our own bodies mostly decide what our appropriate weight range is. **Our bodies know best.**

It's generally understood and accepted in weight-literate circles that we all have a weight set point our bodies can comfortably and healthfully maintain, usually ranging between about ten and twenty pounds. That set point is primarily determined by our genetics, our hypothalamus, and how the latter reads and interprets the conditions and environment of our body. *Health at Every Size* author, professor, and researcher Linda Bacon puts it like this:

Think of it as the preferred temperature on a fat thermostat. Like any thermostat, this one can be set at whatever point is most comfortable. The system then works tirelessly to do anything it can to bring your body into alignment with that point. It acts like a pull to get you back to the comfortable range. If you keep jiggling with the thermostat via diets, the mechanism breaks down. The result: Your body forces you to not only regain any weight you've lost, but you may even pay a penalty with extra weight gain—and a set point now set high to protect against future diets.

There's nothing wrong with gaining weight. But since the aim of dieting—and often at great cost to us and our bodies—is to lose weight, it's important to know that dieting only very rarely results in sustained weight loss, and that has likely nothing to do with anyone's dedication or lack thereof. Only between 3 and 10 percent of people who lose weight via restrictive dieting don't gain it back, and often more, within a few years. In other words, dieting doesn't even work to lose weight in the first place.

WHAT'S GOOD ADVICE ABOUT WEIGHT?

kiran nigam has some: "Don't focus on weight or fat. Focus on how you feel in your body. Experiment and explore, with curiosity, with love and care for yourself. Take notes, reflect, or journal to help you notice patterns. What shifts help you feel good in your body, and move you towards feeling nourished, well rested, clearheaded, steady energy, steady mood, less aches and pains? These are the shifts that will lead you to balance and optimal body system functioning."

Rebecca Scritchfield adds, "If you're noticing something is bothering you about your eating patterns, remember you're this whole integrated person, you're not just thoughts and feelings inside of a body. You're carrying with you all your life experiences, even ancestral experiences. If you're going to seek out some help or support with any of this, pick someone who does not recommend 'weight loss' or 'healthy weight management,' but who is instead focused on helping you with a positive well-being."

IF YOU WORK ON THE KINDS OF DEDI-cated care for yourself already mentioned in this section—like reducing and managing your stress, improving and increasing your sleep, getting real-deal emotional support and some movement in each day—you and your body are going to be on track to be in and stay in a good place with weight, whatever that place may be for your particular body. Our metabolisms work best when we're sleeping well, when we're not stressed to the max, when we're well hydrated, when we move in ways we enjoy, and when we pay attention to our digestion and how it feels instead of what a scale says.

If you pair those things with a good or better relationship with your body and food, one where you're kinder and more accepting of both of you and you eat to nourish yourself in all the ways, following your body's own guidance within your

ability, you'll be doing the things you actually *can* do to earnestly support your body, whatever shape and size it may be, and to take care of yourself at the same time rather than doing yourself harm.

There's no one right weight range for a given height, frame, gender, or age: there's just what our weight is for our unique bodies at any given time.

I know it's harder to believe during menopause, especially if you're not having a great one, but our bodies really do know what's best for them and best for us, most of the time.

Of course, even when we're accepting of our bodies and these kinds of changes, that doesn't automatically make change easy or without challenges. We might still have some hard or uncomfortable feelings, and the way a lot of people— friends, family, kids, healthcare providers, coworkers, street harassers—and institutions talk about and treat some of the kinds of changes we may be experiencing can be crummy, to say the least. We might also have some garden-variety practical struggles.

What can help with body shape and size changes?

❧ Tell diet culture to go to hell and keep it out of your life as much as you can. You might even be able to turn some of it on its head. When I was a kid and my young mother was fad dieting, she had these postcards of naked

Metabolic Syndrome

Metabolic syndrome sounds scary, probably because it combines two words we've learned to fear. The idea something may be syndrome-level wrong with our metabolism strikes at the heart of our anti-fat bias. That isn't to say, however, that what that term describes isn't serious or isn't something we shouldn't take seriously: it's both. The term is garbage, but what it describes is worth our attention.

What metabolic syndrome refers to is when someone has or is diagnosed with a combination of three or more of the following things known to increase risks of heart disease, stroke, and diabetes: a proportionally large waistline (or "apple" shape), a high triglyceride level, low HDL cholesterol, high blood pressure, and high fasting blood sugar. If some of those levels are normal but only because you're taking medication to control them, that still counts as having those things.

It's common to get a larger waistline in or with perimenopause or menopause (and it's also common for people to have that body shape, period), for blood pressure to elevate, and for blood sugar levels or insulin resistance to change. Some of these changes are common for many people with aging, all by itself, so it's not surprising the risk of metabolic syndrome is higher for menopausal people. Things we often struggle with during menopausal transition like fatigue can also play a part in some of the things that cause metabolic syndrome, like lower activity levels.

If you get this diagnosis, talk to your healthcare provider. They will most likely suggest what you'd expect to manage these issues, like dietary changes, medications, and reducing stress. They may also suggest you attempt weight loss. If your healthcare provider isn't weight-neutral and is suggesting any kind of weight loss attempts you don't want or you know to be unhealthy for you or in general, set a limit with them or, better still, see if you can switch to someone else.

fat women in sparkly makeup covered in cake on the fridge to ostensibly keep her from opening it and eating. But to queerbaby me, there were *gorgeous*, glamorous women in the kitchen who looked happy, sexy, and fun, and damn if that cake didn't also look good. You don't have to be seven to rewrite diet culture's scripts.

❧ Put a moratorium on negative body or diet talk with your friends, family, and anyone else. Aim (and ask everyone else to aim) to keep from body bashing or engaging in diet or weight loss talk. If and when someone does, you can ask them to save it for when you're not around or just excuse yourself.

❧ You can ask not to be weighed by healthcare providers unless it's essential, and it often isn't. You can bring a "Please don't weigh me" card with you to appointments and pull it out when you need it, or you can ask with words.

❧ I'm a superfan of putting ourselves in spaces and taking in media where we can soak in realistic body shapes, sizes, and other kinds of physical diversity. That can be anywhere from a bathhouse to the bus to queer porn, from the Y (yeah, I know what I said) to Instagram.

❧ Engage in things for your body that bring you pleasure and joy, that you feel good and whole in, and that give you some level of peace with your body: movement you're into, massage or other bodywork, body scans, masturbation, nonsexual pleasure-based self-touch, a trip to a spa, a daily stretching routine that's just about what feels good that day.

❧ If you have a habit of dieting or other kinds of restrictive eating, consider some help to change those habits. That might be books (see the resources section), a nutritionist and/or coach, or an eating disorders program. Many health insurance plans will cover at least some of these kinds of programs and healthcare, and public health like Medicare sometimes will too.

❧ Put things away that don't fit you right now. Who likes fighting with pants?

Bodies changing can be hard on our finances. The fact that changes in our bodies also often mean that clothes we like and already bought don't fit anymore—meaning we have to spend money on new clothes or tailoring old clothes—can make accepting body changes a lot harder, especially when we've gone up sizes, since that's not culturally celebrated like the other way around. Especially when no one is showing up at our door with thousands of dollars for new wardrobes.

If you can afford it, by all means, get yourself new clothes that fit and that you like and like yourself in. Just bear in mind that your size and shape may keep changing, especially before you're a couple years postmenopause.

If you're not in the money, a few helps and hacks:

❦ Clothing rental or subscription services: you can get or borrow a few new things each month that fit and that you're excited about. If your size keeps changing, you won't have bought things *again* that don't fit just a month later.

❦ Hit up a friend or two whose style you like and who are about your size. Ask if they can keep you on rotation for any hand-me-downs or long-term loaners.

❦ Find or start a clothing swap.

❦ When you buy new clothes, try and buy items that leave at least a size or two's worth of room for body changes. We may love super-tailored trousers, but right now, super-tailored trousers do not love us back.

❦ Check return policies and buy from folks with the generous ones when you can. Some shops or sellers allow for returns, changes, or swaps for up to a year, even when things have been worn and washed. Some even have a no-questions-asked policy.

❦ Buy secondhand from consignment shops or thrift stores. If you haven't been thrifting in a minute, or there aren't any shops nearby, you should know there are a handful of great secondhand clothing websites and apps now.

No matter how you do it, see if you can't treat getting new clothes as a form of self-care and self-expression. Even if you aren't yet comfortable with having to buy a new size or cut, that doesn't mean you still can't look for things you like that give you pleasure—that feel good on your skin, whose fabrics or lines thrill your aesthetic, or even just whose total lack of a waistband makes you feel better. Shopping can be extra stressful for a million reasons during menopause, so do what you can to make it a not-entirely-horrible experience. If you go out to shop, treat yourself to a nice long, solitary lunch somewhere you don't usually get to go. If you shop online at home, have some tea or a cocktail; maybe sit outside with a snack board and some music on or sucker a sweetie into giving you a foot rub.

SKIN, HAIR, AND NAILS

Because of the enormity of the antiaging market, or if you pay any attention at all to older people, you probably already know what can happen to your skin, hair, and nails. It's not that complicated or mysterious.

What happens?

❦ Skin becomes thinner: we can bruise or get scraped more easily, and wounds can take longer to heal.

❦ Skin becomes drier and less elastic: it can certainly feel drier and tighter; if we haven't already, we can develop wrinkles or more wrinkles; the texture

Focus on your best features

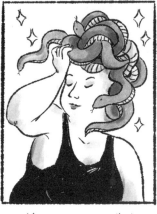

Dress in layers

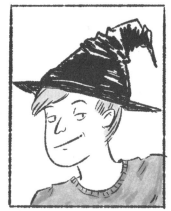

Accessorize!

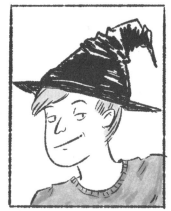

You can still be a sharp dresser

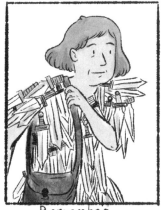

Wear natural fibers

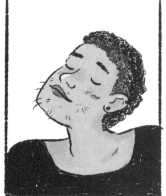

Express your feelings with fashion

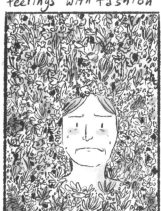

Remember clothes are a part of a woman's natural charm!

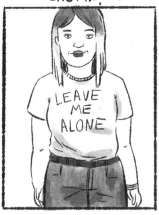

Stay out of the sun

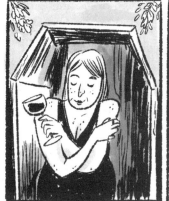

Experiment!

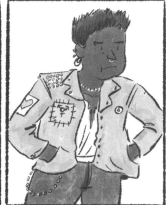

A Compendium of Menopausal Style Advice

of our skin can change (a lot of people describe one common change as skin looking "crepey"); it might look or get more ashy or flaky; and it may sit on our bones and over our muscles and fat differently than before.

- Skin can become more sensitive and more easily irritated.
- Skin can feel itchier, and skin issues like rashes, eczema, or rosacea may show up on the scene, or if you already have any of them, they may flare up more frequently or severely.
- Adult acne can develop or get worse, including cystic acne.
- Pore size increases, and skin may become oilier.
- Skin coloration changes, including the appearance of "age spots." (If you grew up hearing them called "liver spots" and worry they mean something is wrong with your liver, know that's a myth long debunked.) Our skin also becomes more susceptible to sun damage, which is why we see more of said spots.
- Hair thins, and there may be other hair loss (sometimes including pattern baldness), graying hair, or changes in hair texture.
- Facial hair increases, and there may be changes in body hair patterns: thicker in some places, thinner in others, and new growth perhaps in new places.
- Nails become less durable and thinner.

Why are these things happening?

- Estrogen and the moisture of our skin—and moisture in our bodies, period—have a *lot* to do with one another. Estrogen plays a role in sebum production and moisture retention, and our level of estrogen has a lot to do with the production of skin helpers like hyaluronic acid, elastin, and collagen. Less estrogen = less of all those things.
- Our skin is very reactive to systemic changes in our body, and big hormone fluctuations or changes freak it out—in a lot of ways, skin is the canary in the coal mine of our bodies. When something major is going on with our skin, it's usually because something major is going on in other systems.
- The balance of estrogen and testosterone is changing, a player in acne, dryness, and both hair loss and gain.
- Estrogen and progesterone play key roles in melanin production and synthesis.
- Plain old aging brings slower cell turnover, less collagen and elastin, and changes in circulation, all of which change skin, hair, and nails. Changes in our bones can also be responsible for some nail changes.

We don't usually look young, look young, look young and then wake up one day and BAM! We look old. Even when we don't see it, it's all happening and has already been happening gradually. What's great about that is that it lets us get used to those changes over time and learn to accept them, and if we need or want to do anything when it comes to them, that also lets us start doing those things any time (and also, with nonpermanent and reversible stuff, to stop anytime).

I said "want or need" because sometimes this stuff is a need. Some of these kinds of changes cause profound physical discomfort or pain, some can bring on or amp up gender dysphoria (including for cisgender femmes, who can experience some of these changes as feeling less feminine), and some are important for our health—like using sunscreen, for example, to try and avoid skin cancer. Some folks may have needs related to their survival—maybe the job you can't survive without right now requires you to at least look like you're *trying* to look a certain way. Again, we're all experiencing menopause and aging in the culture we live in, not in a vacuum.

Doing things about these changes is often about what we want. I hope I don't have to tell you this, but just in case, it's okay to do things when it comes to our bodies, skin, hair, and nails, their appearance, or both, and it's equally okay *not* to do things. It is also okay not to do them not just because you can't afford to or you worry about judgment but because you just do not want to. There is no universal requirement to keep skin moist, hair unfrizzy, and teeth white. There are people

all over the world doing just fine who let their appearance do what it wants and put their self-care or self-soothing energy, time, and money into other things instead. Likewise, no one is a betrayer of feminism, their gender identity, or their self-esteem by choosing to do things like getting into skin care, dyeing gray hair, or pursuing aesthetic treatments.

You know the drill by now: you get to feel however you feel about this stuff, and if you have any experiences of loss or grief about them, that is okay and doesn't suggest you're some kind of enemy to your own self-acceptance or body image. In fact, if you have those feelings, letting yourself have and feel them is probably the only way to get to or maintain acceptance of yourself and your body.

Author of *Unscrewed: Women, Sex, Power, and How to Stop Letting the System Screw Us All*, femme-nist royale, and my longtime friend Jaclyn Friedman said,

We have losses in life and we can grieve the passing of phases of life that are no longer accessible to us. There's nothing wrong with acknowledging there is some loss. I'm very attached to my hair as it is now. Who knows by the time it actually goes gray, but if it started happening right now, I would die. At first when I found that feeling, I was like, *How antifeminist of you. Why do you care? You should embrace it, blah blah blah.* But I've gotten to this place where it's like, you know what, my hair as it is makes me feel more me as I go through this transition. So fuck it, I'm going to do what I can and feels right to keep it as it is. These changes with perimenopause do mess with my idea of myself. Part of me is like, okay, here's an opportunity for you to learn that that's not where you derive your value from. You know, yet again, learn that lesson. But another part of me is just experiencing some of it as a loss, and thinking about how to mitigate it. I'm in both places about it right now.

You can and may be in two places at any given time too. Self-acceptance and self-love don't require that we have no hard feelings or nothing we don't like; they mostly just ask that however we feel about our bodies and ourselves, we're not a dick about it.

I know I've said it before, but there is a *lot* of anti-fat bias, misogyny, sexism, ableism, white supremacy, and transphobia, not to mention a host of other ills, when it comes to how appearance changes because of menopause, aging, or both are presented. In some resources or places where people are talking about it, it truly is a ***rough ride***.

It's also potentially going to be a rough ride if you're seeking out some arenas of healthcare or other kinds of help that are mired in normalized body and beauty toxicity during this. You may encounter assumptions about and assignments of what you want, are okay with, and believe: you might hear that *of course* you don't want to "look old," or *of course* you'd be willing to try a diet, or *of course* your body was "better" when you were younger, and *of course* you'd do just about anything—maybe even kill girls to bathe in their blood?—to get it back.

There's also a lot out there that says changes to our bodies and how we look around, with, and after menopause happen because we aren't doing all the things we should be doing. In other words, if, as we get old, we start looking old, it's our fault. If only we'd moisturized sooner, used sunscreen more, eaten "cleaner," and spent every cent and minute we had on our appearance, this wouldn't have happened to us.

JUST LIKE WITH SO MUCH WHEN IT COMES to aging and menopause, the things that happen in these arenas are more about genetics and the circumstances of our lives up until now; more about things outside our control, or not entirely within our control, than about things we did or didn't do that we could control.

Kimberly Dark said, "We don't handle bodily diversity well as a culture. There are women in their fifties who are extremely svelte, and their skin is taut, and this, somehow, is held up as the norm as opposed to the exception that it is. It gives us this sense that there's a right way to go through this and that we're doing it wrong. But if you end up with loose arm skin or with saggy breasts? It's often about what kind of skin you have far more than it is about what you did. And even when you do the 'right' things, you can still have saggy skin."

Just like with the rest of your body, this stuff also isn't about who is and isn't virtuous. The fact that your skin or hair looks a certain way has zip to do with your moral value or virtues, with how "good" a person you are or aren't.

What can you do for skin, hair, and nail changes?

• If all of these changes are only about appearance—they don't cause you any pain or discomfort or involve the loss of abilities you want or need—and you don't **want** to do anything, you can do nothing. I know I just said that, but I just don't want you to forget, especially since I know how rarely we all get that message.

• Accept yourself and your body. I know you know, but I'm saying it again.

• Yet again, Ya Basics: reduce and manage stress, improve sleep, move, get social support, quit smoking, and hydrate.

• More moisture and more things that retain moisture: whatever level you've been at with skin care, turn it up a notch or two. If you don't use any kind of moisturizer on your body or face, now's the time to add them. If you already do, look into moving up how hydrating what you use is and how much

it retains hydration. You might need to start adding something to lock in moisture for skin, hair, and nails on top of just adding moisture.

• Be gentler with yourself: when skin, hair, and nails become more delicate, we need to treat them that way. If you use an abrasive face scrub, harsh chemicals on nails, or superhot water when washing up, or haven't had to care much about what you wash your hair with, or use a lot of heat tools, you might need to make some changes and dial the intensity down.

• Be on the lookout for harmful ingredients. Look up "The Dirty 30" (which is not anywhere near as interesting as it sounds) for the most current list, but for our purposes with menopause, some you'll want to look out for because of negative impacts on the endocrine system specifically are bisphenol A, butylated hydroxytoluene, butylated hydroxyanisole, oxybenzone, parabens, phthalates, siloxanes, and triclosan.

• Keep up with or start using sunscreen: it's extra important to protect skin when it's getting drier and thinner.

• Try and add foods rich in the following, or, if you're deficient, supplement with biotin; niacin and other B vitamins; omega-3s; protein; vitamins A, C, and E; zinc; and iron—all skin, hair, and nail helpers.

• If you use makeup and don't like how what you've been doing is looking now, experiment—but there's no right way with this. There's a lot of "less is more" and "you can't be so sparkly" ageist advice with cosmetics and style, but you do you. If less or lighter is your way to go, cool, and if crayon-colored hair or MAWR SPARKLES feels like the thing, well, shine on, you crazy diamond.

- If you want to remove any of your body hair, by all means do. Just be aware that thinner and less resilient skin can mean more ouch or injury for most kinds of hair removal, so be careful. If you want to do things like style your new or more flowing body hair, go for it. Let me take a moment here to say that even if you identify as a woman, there is a long and storied tradition of mighty fine bearded ladies in the world. They'd be lucky to have you among their number.

- If things like haircuts, facials, or manicures are things you love and still want for yourself, but you now feel out of place or uncomfortable where you've been getting them from a menopause-and-gender-feelings place, you might try a barber shop or salon for men and see if that feels like a better fit. Queer and trans providers of these kinds of services might also be more comfortable for you, even if you're not yourself queer or trans.

- The evidence on what hormone therapy—specifically in this case, estrogen therapy—can do for the issues in this section is mixed. It has been found to help with skin-surface hydration and keeping skin thicker and more resilient, however, and estrogen-based therapies do help protect bones, which is a big deal, period, and can also help keep nails strong.

- Medical cosmetic procedures: a range of things from injections and lasers to surgeries are now available. But those things are so far outside my economic and social class, life, and personal and professional experience, I'd be as qualified to report on them as I'd be to report on life on Mars. If these things are something you want to look into, I can suggest that you use the same or similar tools from Chapter 5 to find qualified and quality providers of this kind of care.

- It's probably time to call in a pro (to contact a dermatologist or another kind of qualified provider) for help if something is changing that is causing you regular pain or ongoing discomfort (like eczema, cystic acne, or very dry skin) or may be a symptom of some kind of illness or condition and not just menopause (like big-time nail weirdness, rashes, or a lot of hair loss very suddenly).

PRETTY PRIVILEGE

Pretty privilege is privilege that comes with meeting cultural standards of beauty. That generally means things like being visibly able-bodied, being thin or the kind of curvy that's definitely not considered fat, being white or light skinned, having the kind of hair that meets white standards of beauty, having "good" teeth and skin, and otherwise meeting conventional cultural beauty standards, which also almost always include at least looking, if not being, young. All of those things don't translate into privilege for everyone or for everyone all the time in every place. But if the way you and your body have looked has meant things like getting a better job, having an easier time getting an apartment, receiving more of the kind of attention you wanted, or otherwise finding it easier to get things you needed to survive, and you feel afraid of changes that could make those things less likely or cause you to lose them altogether, pretty privilege has probably been at play for you. By all means, some other kinds of privilege may have been too—like white privilege or thin privilege—some of which you may also lose with changes from menopause; some of which you won't.

If you've had any of this kind of privilege, power, or protection, you certainly may feel fear and anxiety about your looks changing related to the potential or given loss of those benefits. Even if you think this kind of privilege is as gross, ableist, and sexist as it is, that still doesn't mean you'll feel great about losing it or that you're an asshole for not wanting to lose it. It's a rare person who wants to lose privileges, and the more marginalized you already are, the more devastating the loss of any more privilege can be. How we've learned to survive can be deeply linked to our privilege, and we truly might not know how to get by without it.

Losing privilege is anywhere from a bummer to outright terrifying and even dangerous. If we lived in a world where no longer getting one kind of privilege meant getting another equivalent kind of privilege, it would be easier. If we lived in a world where our social status *increased* with aging and we *gained* privilege with menopause and the changes it brings, that would obviously make this a lot easier. Alas.

HERE'S THE KIND-OF-GOOD NEWS: YOU really can't meet these standards anyway, not if you're just average-ish with average genetics and average income and average life circumstances like the rest of us or have even less in any or all of those departments. Even if you try. Not once you reach a certain stage of life, anyway. Not even if you're Helen Mirren or Angela Bassett. The loss of this kind of privilege, if we had it in the first place, comes for all of us eventually.

If you've never had these kinds of privilege, or you've only ever had very little, you might find freedom in entering this phase of life and your body you weren't expecting. Ageism sucks, and I'm not going to argue for enabling it, but a side benefit aging can bring is the acceptance that, at a certain point, no one will be pretty anymore, at least not in terms of conventional beauty standards, where one of the absolute requirements is youth. Reaching a time of life when no one expects you to meet those standards can be freeing. If you had pretty privilege that you had to work for, that made you feel unseen or unvalued as a whole person, or that seemed to cost you as much as it gave you, you might find benefits in what you've lost.

There's a bit in the movie *My Big Fat Greek Wedding* where Toula's father says to her, "You look so **old**." Toula is supposed to be thirty years old. Nia Vardolos, who wrote it and was playing her, was forty. Neither of them looks "old." But what, at that time, they do look like when he makes that comment is someone who isn't doing the things she is supposed to do to look pretty. She's wearing glasses, not contacts. She's not wearing makeup. She's dressed comfortably and plainly. She's not hyperfocused on what she looks like, period—in fact, he says that to her when she's asking for his support to go back to college, for chrissakes.

How refreshing to now or soon be able to *be* old enough to "look old" and have it just be a fact, not a put-down or a call to meet cultural beauty standards that most of us rarely met even when we were younger.

A LOT OF PEOPLE FEEL LIKE THESE KINDS of changes to the body are betrayals: that our body is supposed to look and behave the ways we want it to or to align with cultural standards and expectations, or both, and when it isn't, it is betraying us.

Our bodies are not betraying us by aging and going through processes of aging. Even when menopause isn't about aging—when it happens due to cancer treatments or nonelective surgeries—it *still* isn't betraying us. I get how it can feel like that. I've grappled with some of these feelings myself with chronic pain and other disability, with post-traumatic stress disorder, with unwanted pregnancies, and, yep, with menopause and looks too. I will undoubtedly grapple more in the years to come.

Our bodies are ultimately the result of our genetics, our lives to date, and whatever our current conditions are. They've all done some hard work to get us this far. All they're doing when it comes to menopause and aging is reacting and adapting and carrying on as best they can, which is, ultimately, their principal job description. We get to feel however we feel about all that, but none of this is about our failing or our bodies' betrayal: it's just about us being lucky enough to live long enough for our bodies to do this at all. They're not betraying us by changing. It's what they're supposed to do.

BODIES, SKIN, AND LOOKS

CHAPTER TWELVE
SEX AND SEXUALITY

"Sex is one of the few honest places inside us. It doesn't know how to lie, no matter if we change the narrative."
—*Susie Bright*

Of all the fears and worries people have about menopause, fears and worries about sex and sexuality seem to be some of the biggest and most common. Even as someone who really, *really* should know better, I've tangled with my own dread about genital and other body changes and my own share of concerns about what would or could change with my sexuality or sex life because of menopause. I have, myself, made some foolish assumptions.

If this is you, take a big breath. Let it all the way out.

From everything I can gather, people's sexual desires, interactions and relationships, sex lives, sexual selves, and sexual responses rarely get torpedoed *because* of menopause. And even when they do go kablooie in some way during or around this time, menopause more often seems a highly convenient scapegoat than the actual source of the problem.

For quite a few people, sparing temporary bumps in the road or new terrain they need to learn to traverse, things stay as good as they have been or get even better. Even when there *are* bumps in the road—including things like genital or desire changes, relationship or identity shifts, pain, depression, body image trouble, all things that can and do happen at other times of life too—studies and anecdata make clear that many older people are still having a good time, if not the best time. Not only is menopause itself unlikely to doom anyone's sex life, it can potentially be a bridge to the **best** sex lives some people have yet experienced.

A lot of people have also long had some wrong ideas about sex and sexuality that easily feed fears and worries about sex and menopause. For example, we know from broad study that for most people who really enjoy sex, sexual satisfaction is rarely about meeting beauty standards, perfecting techniques of sexual activities, being bendy, or getting someone to orgasm the fastest. Setting aside how bummerful the idea of getting to the *end* of pleasure *quickly* is, sustained sexual satisfaction just doesn't look like any of that stuff. Instead it's usually about things like acceptance of and knowledge about our own bodies and sexualities; being present, self-aware, and authentic; honest, open communication; emotional connection and sexual and erotic intimacy; and willingness to explore and keep learning what pleasure is for us—all things we usually continue to get *better* at over time. In the event we aren't already privileging or working toward all of that kind of stuff in our sexual lives, there's truly no time like the present.

Carol Queen and Shar Rednour put it perfectly in *The Sex and Pleasure Book: Good Vibrations Guide to Sex for Everyone*: "Pleasure is your birthright, and that fact doesn't have a sunset clause."

SEX AND SEXUALITY ARE WHOLE-PERSON, whole-body things. They're never just genital, even for people whose sexualities and sex lives are very centered in genitals. Without our brain and the rest of our central nervous system, we wouldn't even be able to feel our genitals, have sensory experiences, or orgasm. Without our life histories and personalities, the rest of our bodies, our thoughts, and our feelings, we wouldn't have sexualities.

As with the rest of bodies and life, every potential menopausal impact—from sleep problems to body-image issues, digestive troubles, hot flashes, stress, medications, depression or anxiety, dry skin, and every potential player in the mix—can also have a sexual impact. Some things that can happen for us through our experience of menopause, like identity shifts—gender, orientation, sexuality, embodiment, our sense of place in the world and our relationships, changing priorities—can affect sex and sexuality.

WHAT CAN CHANGE?

⬧ Levels or frequency of sexual desire or interest and the ways we experience sexual desire or interest—which can change in any direction, too, and not just once, like, for example, feeling increased sexual desire in early peri and a decrease in desire later in a menopausal transition

⬧ The experience of arousal, including the ability to become aroused, aroused in the way we're used to, or as intensely as it felt like we did before

⬧ The experience of orgasm, including ability to orgasm, the specific flavor of orgasm, or the ways you can and can't get yourself there

⬧ How we feel emotionally during and about sex and sexuality, including how

The current common worry about menopause and sex is that we won't want it enough or at all or won't be able to do (and, don't forget, provide) it: that menopause is the beginning of our sexual end. But not that long ago, the fear was we'd want it *too* much and be having *too* much of it.

Fear of the potentially insatiable, proliferous, *rabid* sexuality of menopausal and postmenopausal women and gender-diverse people, especially once the biological restriction and social controls of pregnancy and child-rearing are removed, has a long history in Western culture. This fear of people engaging in sex unharnessed from reproduction—seen as a convenient means to control sexuality and the people who have it, especially the people who have it who also have a uterus—has long been a primary feature in homophobia and transphobia as well as anti-contraception and anti-abortion sentiment.

The witch-hunting manual *Malleus maleficarum,* written in 1486 and used for centuries after, described witchcraft as born of the carnal lust of women who were insatiable by "normal" means (lesbian orgies featured large in what might apparently satiate a witch, though given the yawnfest colonial "normal" sex was, I suspect they'd have been more likely to satiate just about anyone). Sexual hunger is part of what makes a woman—or, more terrifying still, someone beyond the confines of gender entirely—a witch and part of why witches are so apparently terrifying: they're lusty, sometimes even letchy, and most of all, *old at the same time*. Horror! Louise Foxcroft reminds us that most of the women burned as witches in Salem were menopausal.

A few hundred years ago, our pal Edward Tilt of the poisonous douche said of his menopausal patients, "Many were driven to the verge of insanity by ovario-uterine *excitement*," providing not just this historical footnote, but perhaps the least sexy description of sexual desire ever.

Whatever the current cultural expectations are of us and our sexual desires and behaviors, be it purity or be it insatiability, it's unsurprising fears about what menopause might do to our sexualities are all about how we might not be able to meet (or be made to care about) those expectations anymore.

vulnerable or emotionally sensitive we feel

* Sexual sensation, including changes to what feels painful and what feels pleasurable, and other parts of our physical experience
* What we do and don't enjoy when it comes to sexual expression, how we enjoy those things, or how we feel about them
* Our conceptualization and experience of sex, our sexuality, and our bodies and/or ourselves as sexual
* Our interpersonal sexual dynamics
* Our patience

When impacts or changes happen *expressly* because of menopausal transition or postmenopause, they're usually because of the following:

* **Estrogen and other hormonal changes, fluctuations, or shifting balances:** Our pal patriarchy taught us that testosterone is a "male" hormone and that this purported dude-mone rules and dictates all things sex. Quelle surprise. Testosterone plays a part in sex and sexuality for most people, of all sexes and genders, but so do dopamine, vasopressin, oxytocin, and other hormones, including estrogen and progesterone. Fluctuations of the latter two can create changes in the production, balance, and uptake of all others, which can influence our sexual desire, sexual responsiveness, and sexual response, including arousal and orgasm.

Estrogen is the major player in genital changes and any breast or nipple changes. Changing balances and levels of estrogen and testosterone can also create changes to how we experience or enact sex or sexuality.

* **Genital changes:** Changes to vaginal and vulvar size, texture, elasticity, thickness, self-lubrication, and sensation can change our experience, framing, or ability with genital or other sex or the way we experience or conceptualize our sexualities. Changes with the bladder or urinary tract—like bladder control, urgency, or urinary tract infections—can also change or influence things here, including the ability to engage in some kinds of sex comfortably.
* **Fertility/menstrual cycle changes:** If sexuality or an understanding or concept of sex was connected to reproduction, being fertile, having menstrual or fertility cycles, or feelings in certain parts of those cycles, these can change sex and sexuality or how you experience them.
* **Other primary or secondary impacts of menopause:** This really can be anything or everything, and it's important to remember that a change or impact can be positive, negative, or neutral, and in this arena, it probably will be a combo of all three. These impacts can include thinning or more sensitive skin, feeling on fire (a friend recently told me she had the most amazing orgasm during a hot flash), sweating, fatigue,

body shape or size changes and the resulting physical and emotional effects, mood changes or mental health issues like depression, anxiety, body or gender dysphoria, pain or nervous system changes, your patience with other people (and their bullshit, which can actually lead to some helpful sexual boundary setting!), and all the extra stress we're usually dealing with.

Some things are also simply a part of aging:

- Changes in circulation, which can result in taking longer for blood flow to get to the genitals, a slower or longer path to arousal or orgasm, feeling less physically aroused or less sensitive, or needing more stimulation or a different kind
- Changes in the body's abilities or overall health, like the acquisition of health conditions like diabetes or an acquired disability like fibromyalgia, injury, or a loss of mobility
- A *desire* to deprioritize sex and sexuality or to experience sexuality or engage in sex in a more sensual or affectional than explicitly sexual way

The cultural, social, and interpersonal changes and issues—actual, feared, and sometimes feared-into-being—involved with the menopausal transition and aging can often play some of the biggest roles of all in impacts we experience in this arena. Tania Glyde says, "Menopause is a time when we may start to experience internalized ageism. Some people, especially feminine presenting ones, may start to feel invisible, where before they received too much unwanted attention. It can be confusing. We are so used to seeing altered images of unachievably young bodies that to turn from our computer screens to our own faces in the mirror may be a shock. It's worth checking in with these feelings and sharing them with others. They can be very isolating."

JOAN PRICE, SENIOR SEX ADVOCATE, educator, author, and all-around marvel was on the top of my list of people I wanted to talk to for this book. Joan is the author of four books about older-age sexuality, including *Naked at Our Age: Talking Out Loud About Senior Sex* and *Sex After Grief: Navigating Your Sexuality After Losing Your Beloved*. I want to be like Joan when I grow up. Joan says,

Most of us have *never* thought our bodies were right. If we never thought our bodies were right before, what's the big deal now? I've gotten wrinkly. I've gotten saggier. We own our bodies and our sexuality, and we can take joy in our bodies despite the sagginess of our skin, how low our breasts hang, or the puckers in our butts—or *because* of the changes of our bodies. We can say, "Hey, I'm a sexual being lifelong. I enjoy my sexuality. I own it. This is the body I'm living in. This is the body I am having sex in." Where did this notion come from that only a young, firm body and unwrinkled skin can be desirable? Our bodies have a capacity for giving us pleasure lifelong. There are so many reasons sex can be *better* as we age.

WHAT CAN YOU DO?

If you're someone who's already been having a satisfying sex life, you probably already do most of the things that are usually suggested when it comes to sex and menopause and that are connected with having or continuing to have a satisfying sexual life during and after perimenopause, like open and honest communication, making pleasure—very much including your own—a priority, healthy partnerships and wholly consensual interactions, and sexual exploration. If you're someone with disabilities, who has or has had sexual partners with disabilities, or who is otherwise already used to adjusting to physical, emotional, and other changes in sex and sexuality, in making and asking for accommodations as needed or wanted, same goes for you: you've probably already got most of this down.

If you *haven't* had a very satisfying sex life up until now, *and* your sexuality and sex life aren't already pretty adaptable when it comes to rolling with the physical and emotional changes and changing needs of yourself and your partners, I can almost guarantee that if you do many of

the things I'm going to suggest here, then you may well have menopause to **thank** for potentially radically improving how you feel about and in your own sexuality and your sexual life by the time it's over—and maybe even before that. No kidding.

First, there are a couple things that can help with most, if not all, of what's changed or changing.

IDENTIFY, ACKNOWLEDGE, AND DEAL WITH FEARS

Despite what erotic thrillers would have you believe, fear and anxiety don't usually make sex more fun. Especially when fear and anxiety are *about* sex.

Our sexual fears can easily become self-fulfilling prophecies. If we lean into fear that our bodies won't respond sexually anymore, that we won't orgasm, or that we'll feel pain, all of those outcomes become more likely. Just like with pain, fear can create a negative feedback loop our bodies and minds respond to.

A lot of these fears are based in the sexual frameworks and beliefs of our cultures, our relationships, or our own minds and sexualities that were *always* busted; they may just have been or seemed less impassable before than they might once things start shifting with menopause or once you know some of the change that's probably coming. So, in order to deal with some of our fears, we might first have to deal with some of—maybe even all of—our beliefs about them.

LIKE PATTI LABELLE, YOU MIGHT NEED TO GET YOURSELF A NEW ATTITUDE

The sex and sexuality frameworks many of us learned growing up are exceptionally limited, all the more so for the menopausal and postmenopausal. The limitations of those frameworks we might run up against the most, and find the most inflexible, are primarily about ableism, ageism, and heteronormativity. Developing an awareness of those limits and how they affect you and doing what you can to kick them to the curb or change them can help a lot. That might look like recognizing and letting go of the idea that desire has to be frequent or fervent or that being able to have sex means being able to have certain kinds of sex only certain ways or that there's one way sexy looks—and it doesn't look over forty.

Queering things up goes a long way, whatever your sexual orientation or identity. I mean centering sex on pleasure, joy, freedom, experimentation, and exploration, not reproduction, obligation, or rigid gender or sex roles. I mean sex that's about all kinds of pleasure and the whole of our bodies and selves, not just genitals, intercourse, or physical sex, and that cares about mutuality (when there's more than just you), intimacy, and connection.

With and after menopause, heteronormative sex and sexuality can become anything from boring or difficult to downright painful and oppressive. Those "rules" weren't really written with anyone but cisgender men in mind and doom *them* to substandard sex and relationships too.

You also might need to change how you think about and create your sex life through a disability lens. Even if you don't need to, you'll likely benefit from it.

In accessible sex and sexuality frameworks, ever-changing bodies and states of health, wants, needs, adjustments, accommodations, and even radical changes are a given and are just considered realities of being human. That's not the sexual praxis most of us learned, unfortunately. But if sex and our sexualities are to actually be about us, they *have to* allow for and be accepting of all of those things, because our bodies and our needs are always changing.

Even for those who meet and can continue to meet almost every other standard, you simply can't remain young: it's impossible. As a frequent side effect, you also won't remain able in all the ways you may have been when you were younger. You will age out of youth-based privilege if you haven't already, and your body will age with you, often bringing changes to your abilities.

Ageist beliefs about sex are not friends to our sexual lives or identities. If we believe that people postmenopause or in menopausal transition don't want sex, we are priming our pump to go that way (which might be helpful for you if that's a direction you want but counter to your wants if it's not). If we believe an orientation or other sexual shift can't be real or positive but must instead be some kind of meaningless midlife crisis, your belief may cause you to miss the boat on positive change. If we believe that no one who isn't young is sexually desirable . . . well, you see where this is going.

What else can help?

◆ Ya Basics—reducing and managing stress, improving your sleep, getting movement in, staying hydrated, quitting smoking, and getting social support—can all help with sex and sexuality.

◆ Estrogen therapy, particularly local estrogen, can usually help with genital issues, and testosterone therapy is often prescribed for desire/arousal issues, including if systemic estrogen therapy isn't helping with it, which it sometimes will.

◆ If genitourinary symptoms (like vulvovaginal dryness or pain or bladder issues) are going on and creating sexual issues, managing those (page 187) can help.

◆ Mental health and mood can have a big impact on sex and sexuality. For info on managing those, see page 129. Know it's always okay to take a break from sex and sexuality if and when you need to, whether that's about mental health or anything else: sometimes the thing that

helps your sex life most may be to put it on pause while you take care of other parts of yourself. If sex feels like an obligation in *any* way, changing that will absolutely help with your sex life and how you feel about it. I promise.

◆ You might look into sex therapy, counseling, and/or relationship counseling. Some sex workers also specialize in working with sexual life passages.

◆ Bodywork and other ways of experiencing touch that is nonsexual or not specifically sexual can help.

◆ You might try something new: that can be a new partner, adding partners, or a different kind of relationship, new toys or kinds of sex you haven't tried before, trying sex in new contexts, taking on different roles, or including different emotional dynamics in your sex life than you have before.

◆ If you're having vasomotor impacts and are just too darn hot to be physically close to someone else, but you still want to be sexual, mutual masturbation is one way to be sexual together without wanting to yell for the other person to get their painfully warm body away from you.

◆ If you're having sexual issues **and** don't even want to be engaging in sex (or a particular kind of it), rather than trying to change your body or make yourself adapt, this may be the perfect time to change your sexual life so you're only ever doing what you want to do and not doing what you don't. If you don't want to engage in any kind of sex at all, it is always okay to take sex out of your life, temporarily or permanently.

Plan sex and make real time for it: If there's something unsexy about planning, then I'm going to need someone to explain to me why I get so excited when I have a date. Any prep "in case of sex" *is* planning sex. So if you haven't been planning because you've got a negative mindset about it, try that on. It's just a date. Just give it a shot. That plan can be for masturbation or sex with partners, or you can make one standing date for each. Schedule what masturbation visionary and feminist educator Betty Dodson called "erotic recess" and treat it like recess, not like a community-service assignment.

If, when it's time for recess, you're not feeling it, that's always okay: do something else that's nice for yourself or your relationship with that time. One of the changes that seems common with aging is for the lines to get really blurry when it comes to pleasure, intimacy, and sex: whether or not something is expressly sexual matters less than if it—whatever it is—is enjoyable.

Lube, lube, lube, lube, lube, lube, lube: In the event you're not already a lube superfan, and shame has gotten in your way of using a slippery vat of lubey goodness, hear this: Lube is not a bummer or something to be embarrassed about. Lube is gravy on potatoes, pomade on a pompadour, or warm, melty syrup on pancakes, for crying out loud. Lube is a glorious thing that can make a potentially already good thing anywhere from a little better to downright magical. When George Harrison was posthumously inducted into the Rock & Roll Hall of Fame in 2004, Tom Petty, Jeff Lynne, Marc Mann, Steve Winwood, and George's son Dhani were already doing a gorgeous version of "My Guitar Gently Weeps." Then Prince slithered out and lit the whole thing up with a guitar solo a thousand times more delicious and amazing than you even expected it to be, and you already expected it to be pretty incredible, because Prince, okay? **Lube is that guitar solo.**

A lot of general information about sex and menopause recommends water-based lube. That was always what we suggested in the old days, because the alternatives were mostly oil-based, which doesn't work with condoms or other latex barriers. But we have more options now. Water-based still may be a kind you or your body parts like best or like to use for some activities. But even water-based lubes come with an array of potential extras they didn't used to, some of which can be extra helpful with menopause, like hyaluronic acid, aloe, tetrahydrocannabinol (THC), or cannabidiol (CBD).

The base of most lubricants is either water, oil, or silicone. Many lubes are hybrid and contain more than one of those elements.

There's no one right lube for every activity, no one lube everyone likes for a given thing. They don't all feel the same, last the same, or meet all the same needs, not to mention sensitivities, allergies, or other issues. If you don't already know what you like, or you don't know all of what's out there right now, you can often order samples or go into a shop and feel them for yourself.

When I talked with feminist sex toy shop and neighborhood sex education mecca Early to Bed owner Searah Deysach, she mentioned that one of the downsides to silicone-based lubes is that they remain inside the body longer than water-based lubes. That's a sound concern, especially if you're someone prone to infections or irritation. Glycerin, which is in many water-based lubes, *also* may or may not be a good fit for your genitals right now. If you are or have become more susceptible to yeast infections, you may want to take a pass on it. Try and steer clear of the yucky ingredients I

mentioned on page 212. Warming or cooling lubes and flavored lubes were never great for anyone's vagina, and that hasn't changed now.

Oil-based lubes are one good option: they provide some extra moisturizing that sinks in. It's sex *and* a spa! They can't be used with latex condoms or other barriers, but that's okay. Nonlatex condoms and barriers, just as effective when it comes to pathogens or sperm cells as their latex comrades, *can* be used with oils. Polyurethane condoms also drag less than latex ones and have a silkier texture, on top of conducting body heat better, all things that are nice, period, and all the more so in peri or postmenopause.

If you want to go DIY with lube and have only the contents of your kitchen and medicine cabinet at your disposal, be careful. Petroleum products (like petroleum jelly) are a no-no. Depending on how your body reacts to them, almond, olive, avocado, flax seed, and coconut oils can all be used as lubes, just again, not with latex. Aloe vera—the store-bought kind usually has additives, though, so read the label first—can work all by itself or mixed with one of those oils. Lubricating or moisturizing suppositories can also be used vaginally or anally (including CBD/THC types).

Expand your sexual horizons outside vaginal sex: What's presented as "foreplay" for straight people is often just other kinds of sex for the rest of us and for a lot of straight people too. Oral sex is sex. Manual sex is sex. A gazillion things that don't have "sex" on the end of them are also sex for a lot of people. Calling what's sex for a lot of us—for most of us, honestly—foreplay both systematically supports queer and trans invisibility and also helps keep a lot of people having sex in ways that aren't very satisfying.

Joan Price says, "Don't make sex one thing and everything else foreplay. Anything that arouses you sexually, that brings you sexual pleasure, that brings you to orgasm, all of those things are sex. Whether you do it yourself or with a partner with a toy, expand your notion of what great sex is to include all the different ways that you can enjoy sex." She also has some great advice if you need to learn how to explore sex differently with partners. "We can say to a partner, let's explore sex without vaginal intercourse for the next two weeks, and just see what else we do. See what else we like, try new things. The only rule is we've got to agree it's pleasurable. Let's just see what brings us pleasure, and then go forward."

Maybe for you that's adding massage or other whole-body touch, more talking, or more oral or manual sex (I mean the kind of sex you have with your hands, not having sex with a manual, though if it

floats your boat . . .). That could be anal sex, whether you're pegging or a receptive partner, bondage, sensation or temperature play (two words: "ice play"), role play, mutual masturbation, using toys or tools, cuddling, making out, sharing porn or erotica, phone sex or sexting, naked stretching or dance, or any other of a great number of things that you may or may not have experienced as sexual before.

A FEW WORDS ABOUT THE CLITORIS

Whether or not you or a partner wind up having vaginal impacts of menopause or postmenopause that also impact sex, there are a few basic things about the whole of the clitoris I think everyone benefits from knowing.

The clitoris is much, much bigger than it looks like from the outside. Externally,

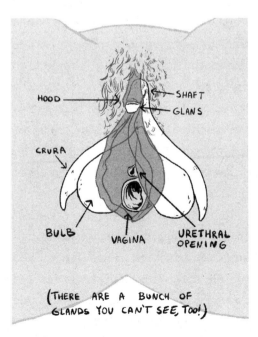

HOOD

SHAFT

GLANS

CRURA

BULB

VAGINA

URETHRAL OPENING

(THERE ARE A BUNCH OF GLANDS YOU CAN'T SEE, TOO!)

all we can see of it is the hood, glans, and some of the shaft. While the glans and shaft have the most concentrated sensory nerve endings by far (and there's a lot going on inside both of those we can't see), there are other parts of the clitoris inside the body, which we can't see at all, that are also part of what we feel with just about any kind of stimulation or sexual arousal that involves our genitals. Inside the body are the larger portions of the clitoris, the whole of which winds up being about the same size as the penis and also has analogous parts.

Surrounding the vaginal canal and the vulva are also the vestibular bulbs, the crura, and more of the shaft on the inside. The vaginal canal itself doesn't actually have that many sensory nerve endings past the first third of it: the internal clitoris is much of why vaginal stimulation can feel good and also why the vaginal canal tends to respond more to pressure than to fine touch. And when it *does* respond to fine touch, like with fingers strategically placed or a G-spotter toy, it's because that fine touch is stimulating tissue connected to—you guessed it—the clitoral body.

I'm telling (or reminding) you about this for a couple reasons.

In the event that you have vaginal changes or impacts that make some or all kinds of vaginal sex painful for you and you are not aware of this anatomy and these specifics, knowing might help you figure out some substitutions or new

things to explore. For instance, you might discover that rhythmic pressure to the whole of your vulva with a set of hands or on a thigh or toy mount creates some, or maybe even all, of the sensations you like with, say, intercourse, and with a partner positioned face-to-face, if that gives you an intimacy you enjoy, you can get it this way.

GHOSTS OF SEX LIFE PAST

Some things that worked for you in the past may stop working in peri- or postmenopause. Some or all of these things may never have worked for you, but maybe you got away with them before or were able to tolerate them. As a sex educator, I've seen the things that follow create sexual problems or barriers to good sex for people of all ages. I've also seen changes made with these things improve many people's sex lives.

Because humans, human sexuality, and human relationships are all so vast, what these things are is also vast. But I have seen some common threads in my travels, like people needing to change their tune on lubricants. What else won't work anymore, if it ever did to begin with?

Vaginal sex you aren't into, don't really want, or aren't excited about before you start (or while you're) doing it: With thinning and less flexible vaginal and vulvar tissue, the gradual smoothing of the rugae, and less lubrication from your own body, you're more likely to hurt yourself doing this, regardless of how it feels. This usually doesn't feel good earlier in life, but now it's even more likely to feel like shit in a host of ways. More than one person talking about trying to do this postmenopause has compared the feeling to a root canal. For anyone at all invested in your pleasure, you included, changing this shouldn't be a problem. You just need to get in the habit of doing more that turns you on first, whatever that is, be it other kinds of sex, winning at Scrabble, or both, and maybe for a longer period of time than you did before. And if you don't want to do it at all, you could stand to work on privileging your own wants and needs so that you can start only doing what you actually want and like sexually.

While we're talking sex and orifices, if your sexual life has been the kind where orifices of your body and what happens with them has mostly been about what feels good to your *partner*, now would be a great time to flip that. Author of *The Tragedy of Heterosexuality* Jane Ward puts this different paradigm well: "In queer space, what makes an orifice 'good' is not how it feels to the person going inside it . . . but how the orifice feels about *itself*: what it wants, what it can do, what it can enjoy."

A lack of sexual communication: If you do little to no talking before, during, or after sex with partners, it's going to be hard to get someone to pass the lube, to express what you can't do tonight because of a certain thing going on with your body or your mood, to help a partner learn to do in a new way something that y'all have been doing the same way for years, or to get aftercare you need because some part of menopause has shaken your sexual confidence. Hopefully you know this by now, but in case you don't, people who have great sex as a habit regularly communicate before, during, and after sex. It's not weird, disruptive, or unsexy, especially once everyone gets some practice.

If you've started or finished menopause and haven't started talking about your experiences, needs, feelings, and fears with it when it comes to sex and sexuality, that's a great place to start. That might feel daunting, but as Joan Price said, "What's the worst that can happen if you tell the truth? If you don't ask for understanding, you can't get understanding. Honesty is essential for successful aging, for aging with joy and with dignity, and with understanding and with intimacy."

Requiring body perfection: This was never a realistic or possible standard, but it may start to feel even more oppressive and depressing and can just plain FUCK YOU UP in perimenopause. Our bodies really couldn't be much more out of our control than they are now. It's almost like menopause had it up to here with our perfectionism and decided to burn it all down once and for all.

It's so hard to have a good time sexually when we are trying to be perfect or trying to hide that we're not. It's hard to give our attention to pleasure in this mindset. It's even hard to have a good time masturbating if your sexual image of yourself looks nothing like you, or is you, but twenty years ago. If menopause is making it harder for us to bring this and other kinds of perfectionism to our sexual selves and lives, it's doing us a favor.

Thinking sex is over with orgasm: Sometimes you're not going to come at all, even from things that got you there before, and sometimes that may be the case for your partner. You or a partner might not even feel like you want or need orgasm as much as you did before; pleasure or even comfort may become the priority. It might take you longer to get there than it used to, so it might be that your partner comes long before sex is over for you. Better now (and usually better, period) to figure that sex is over when anyone involved wants it to be over, whether that's about feeling done, feeling tired, or feeling like you'd actually rather have a bath or a cuddle, now that you think of it.

Quickies: Whether or not having sex in a hurry worked for you before, it is probably going to work for you even less as you progress through perimenopause and beyond. Even the way of thinking about sex that makes quickies work as a framework probably won't work for you in perimenopause, postmenopause, or both. Instead of thinking about sex as something that you need at least an hour for, you might even try thinking about it—and by "it" I don't mean intercourse, I mean all kinds of smaller sexual expressions and sensualities threaded together by intimacy and desire—as something you can, and perhaps should, stretch out over hours or even days. One of the bonuses of arousal and orgasm feeling more relaxed and less urgent or intense is that you can do that, making sex into a multicourse meal instead of a drive-through. And if you still want to do (or your schedule requires) short spurts, you might try treating those as appetizers or pieces of a whole rather than the whole thing all by themselves.

Things you liked before: Your favorite vibrator may become your least favorite (I hope there is a heaven for sex toys). Something that felt good with a partner before may stop feeling good. Your favorite body part or activity may change. Sex and sexuality are always fluid, but all the more so during times of major body, life, and identity change. If favorites stop being favorites, by all means, recognize and thank those babies Marie Kondo–style, but then do like Marie says and keep only what really sparks joy (and, in this case, nerve endings), clearing space for new favorites.

SEX AND DRUGS (AND MAYBE MIDNIGHT NACHOS, TOO?)

It would be silly for me to pretend that some of us do not mix sex and recreational substances. You may know plenty about that already.

Alcohol might not be playing nice with you in menopause, period, or with sex during peri- or postmenopause. It was never the best choice to mix with sex in the first place. It may make us feel more inclined to get down but makes our bodies *less* inclined to respond. If you're having issues with depression, mood regulation, or circulation, it might be a particularly lousy choice for you with sex. Oh, or if it gives you heartburn, which is never, ever fun during sexytimes.

If you want to try something else—even if alcohol is a thing you like and works for you—you might have a look at the list of adaptogens and other herbs on page 280. Those can help you relax or perk up in subtle, gentle ways. They also can be good choices for sober folks.

Cannabis is another option. Ashley Manta is especially keen on what topicals can offer in the menopausal space. She explained that "topicals like balms and lubricants decrease pain and help to nourish the tissue and also increase pleasurable sensations. They can make orgasm more accessible. Many people find that THC is better for sensation while CBD is better for inflammation. Ideally, you have a little bit of both." If you're just looking for one of those things, like something anti-inflammatory, you don't need to use both. But—and this is true for any form of either of these compounds—Ashley points out that THC and CBD work best together and that CBD in isolation is never going to be as effective as CBD in concert with THC.

If you're new to cannabis or other recreational substances, Ashley says to try them on your own first and explore them with masturbation. "Notice how it impacts your physical experience, your headspace and your sensory perception. Then you'll have a bunch of things you can tell a partner about before you get sexual together with this in the mix."

Both for consent and courtesy, Ashley advises, "negotiate before you medicate.

If you're going to be doing anything that causes a psychological state change, it's good to let your partner know." She suggests giving partners information like where you are presubstance, where you're trying to get with the substance, what you're using to try and get yourself there, and, if your partners don't already know, what it can look like if you're having a good time, if you're not, and what kind of care and help you want if the latter happens. Honestly, this kind of sexual communication is a boon, substance or no substance.

Ashley also mentioned a concept that's as helpful with sexual interactions or activity as it is with psychedelics: set (your mindset) and setting (your environment). Whether it's about using a substance with sex or exploring sex by itself with any of the changes or impacts menopause is having, having an awareness of both of these things and making adjustments to either or both as needed can help you out. For instance, if you come into a sexual experience or interactions in a bad mood, you won't be, as she puts it, setting yourself up for success. Doing what you can to come to any kind of sexual exploration in a good space in your head and to make sure your external environment meets your needs—like with privacy, time, aesthetics, and other sensory input you like, such as music or lights—is going to make your having a good time a lot more likely and can especially help if you're trying to

overcome some new challenges or learn new things.

TOYS!

Sex toys, tools, or whatever you like to call them are in a constant state of development. There are way more toys, including more accessible toys, out there now than in the past.

Be sure to avoid toys with toxic chemicals called phthalates. Phthalates also make toys more porous, so it's easier for bacteria to move into your toys and harder to clean them out. If a toy is very jelly-like, made of or contains PVC, labeled as a novelty, super cheap, or funky smelling when it's new, it probably has phthalates.

You or a partner might have the idea that if toys (or masturbation, for that matter) are involved, there's less intimacy. Yet, everything that people usually define as core to sexual intimacy is usually involved in using toys with or masturbating in front of partners: vulnerability, communication, collaboration, experimentation, and sharing pleasure. So, unless you or your partners are bringing less intimacy to sex that involves toys, that's just not likely to be the case.

A few additions to your toy/tool collection you might consider specifically with peri- or postmenopause in mind:

❧ An extra wand or other vibrator you can double up with. You might find two is better than one if you begin to need more stimulation (or stimulation to more places).

- Smaller and/or less textured dildos. Less is more can wind up being pertinent when it comes to vaginal sex, especially postmenopause. Having more options can help to make it no big deal if a size or shape that worked before doesn't feel good in the moment.

- If you wear a harness and that becomes uncomfortable, you can get soft silicone bumpers to slide between your genitals and the harness to reduce pressure.

- If you have penis-and-vagina intercourse and have pain, you might look into the Oh-Nut (it can also help when this kind of sex is painful with other conditions or situations, too, like endometriosis, prolapse, or after feminine bottom surgery). It's a soft, silky silicone helper that looks like a cross between a cock ring and a donut. It goes around the base of the penis and changes how deep, basically, a partner can go. If your partner straps on and there's pain, you can switch to a smaller dildo.

- Glass and stainless steel toys don't have the same kind of friction or drag as silicone or plastic. Stainless steel can also be made cooler or warmer by putting it in cold or hot water.

- If oral sex is an issue because of the kind of moisture involved or infections, you can try toys that simulate oral sex instead.

- There are wedges and other props made expressly for sex, but you can also use yoga bolsters or straps or pillows and

Some Risky Business

Perimenopause and menopause do not mean that sexually transmitted infections (STIs) are no longer a risk or less of one. In fact, because the process ultimately results in thinner, less resilient genital tissue, the risk of STIs increases. This, combined with other issues associated with aging, like less resistant immune systems and how many older people don't engage in safer-sex behaviors like barrier use and regular testing, is likely why the rate of STIs among middle-aged and older adults—people forty-five and up—has been exponentially increasing for years. Chlamydia cases in the United States nearly doubled for people between fifty-five and sixty-four between 2012 and 2016, for example.

Don't forget that if you're having or are going to have the kind of sex that can result in pregnancy, unless pregnancy isn't possible for you otherwise, until you are all the way on the other side of menopause, you may still be able to become pregnant in perimenopause. Whether that's something you want to prevent or make an end run for is your call.

rolled-up blankets. Adjusted positioning can help with things like joint pain, cramps, nervous system glitches, headaches, and other menopause-related impacts that can make sex less fun.

I have a few last big and **very important** memos to drop before we leave sexytown.

THIS IS NOT THE END (UNLESS YOU WANT IT TO BE)

You've probably experienced changes or shifts in sex or sexuality in the decades before now: changes in sexual frequency or opportunity, in your levels or intensity of desire or sexual response, in sexual orientation or other aspects of sexual identity, in how big or small a place sex and sexuality occupied in your self, your relationships, your life. Maybe you freaked out about them then too.

But I feel like people freak out far more about them in peri- or postmenopause—or even the possibility of them—and I'm pretty sure I know why. People seem to have the idea that any shifts or changes (they don't like or want) now are either forever or are the start of a downward spiral to the end. I don't know where everyone got that idea, but in case you have it, I want to relieve you of it. So long as you're still alive (and heck, for all I know, after you're dead too), sex and sexuality can, and probably will, keep shifting and changing. It's no more or less likely, for

example, that a decrease in frequency and desire is forever if it happens now as opposed to in one's twenties or thirties.

If something changes now that you don't like or that scares you, know that it is entirely possible that just like with so many changes and shifts before, these too may well be temporary.

Lastly, we can be so focused on what we might lose when it comes to sex and sexuality and menopause that we don't even consider changes that can create positive or wanted change—sometimes even liberation:

- Freedom from pregnancy and childbearing, as well as from the fear of unwanted pregnancy or childbearing
- Introduction of sex toys or lubricants to sexual interactions and relationships
- Improvements to sex and sexuality because of improved self-care
- Shifts in the focus of sex to other parts of the body besides genitals
- Discovery of new kinds of sexual attraction, interest, identity, or expression
- Greater confidence in asking for what we want and need and in setting limits and boundaries
- More enriching sexual relationships because of deeper and increased sexual communication
- Enjoyment of how sexual desire and sex feel without hormonal cycling
- Caring less about meeting beauty ideals as part of sexuality

- Potentially enjoying a wanted change in how urgent sexual desire feels—be it less or more
- Reduced expectation of sex or sexual behavior, particularly for asexual people
- Greater enjoyment of sex and sensuality because it takes longer to get to orgasm now
- Shiny radical sexual and physical self-acceptance from newfound IDGAF menopausal energy

We've known for a while that the popular idea that people "peak" sexually in their twenties or thirties may align perfectly with our culture's massive sexual ageism, but it doesn't square with the realities of people having satisfying sex lives throughout a lifetime. Even the idea that there's a "peak" at all is busted. So long as we're investing some measure of care, attention, and time in our sexualities and sexual lives, sex will usually keep getting *better* throughout life and be something we feel more and more satisfied with, not less.

Will it stay the same in every phase of life? Nope. When I talked to feminist sex editor, author, publisher, and firebrand Susie Bright—who has made it to the other side of menopause, by the way, and who remains as tremendous as you'd expect—about this, she talked about some postmenopausal sexual change and some of the ways those changes may lead us to a kind of sexual connection to ourselves we might not have had before or in a long time:

You may not feel the same kind of bulldozer sex drive that you're used to from your youth. You might feel relief at feeling less led by your clit. There's a certain satisfaction at being able to "take sex—or leave it." Instead of a heedless urgency, you may feel more relaxed and open, more curious. There's a new kind of "why not?" in menopause. Feeling good in your body isn't necessarily about feeling attractive, as you would define for a young person, or even loveable. It's not about being a catch. Ha! You become more aware of your body as you age, in part because of physical pain and loss, but also a shocking pleasure at what *endures*. The little things, and the persisting feelings, are the sweetest plums.

Does that mean there'll be no bumps in the road, no dry spells, no challenges, no bad lays? Of course not. This is still real life. Menopause or some impact of it might be one of those bumps. But by and large, satisfaction with sex and continuing to be alive tends to look not like a peak with valleys on either side but like a fairly steady upward trajectory throughout the whole of life.

YOUR EXPERIENCE OF MENOPAUSE OR ANY of its impacts may invite or even aggressively ask you to reevaluate your sexuality, your sexual life, and your sexual relationships, including your expectations of any or all of those things.

You might want something different from your sexual relationships and sex life than you have before, like more time and space to be sexual for and by yourself, a change in the model or dynamic of your relationship, a different kind of partner, more experimentation, or even some time for sex and sexuality to go on the back burner. There's no right or wrong here, just what's wanted and right for you. Separate from just being decent to ourselves and each other, there are also no rules.

We're all already outside the hegemonic cultural rules of sex and sexuality merely by being menopausal or postmenopausal people for whom no role is written. So if you haven't already, you can just lean into your sexual outlaw status and, as outlaws are wont to do, do what you want for a change.

CHAPTER THIRTEEN
OTHER PEOPLE

AT HOME, AT WORK, ON DATES, AND OTHER PLACES. HOW TO AVOID THEM WHEN YOU CAN AND HOW TO DEAL WITH THEM WHEN YOU CAN'T (OR DON'T WANT TO)

"I'm old enough and cranky enough now that if someone tried to tell me what to do, I'd tell them where to put it."
—*Dolly Parton*

Life goes on, as they say.

They neglect to mention that life goes on even if you space paying the bills, think it's Saturday for the first four hours of Tuesday, haven't slept for days, forget to turn off the burner, and leave the house without any pants. And when all of those things happen, it goes on without giving two shits that you're in menopause and barely holding it all together, with your phone service turned off, almost losing your job, and a reminder from your neighbor that it's October, you're no spring chicken besides, and also *Do you smell that—hey, is your kitchen on fire?*

And then, as if everything else we have to deal with weren't already much more than enough, there's **everyone else**: landlords, bosses, friends, partners, spouses, dates, parents, kids, the bus driver, coworkers, clients, chosen family, family you did *not* choose, doctors, your favorite ex, your shitty ex, *their* shitty ex, everyone in line at the grocery store, someone's terrible friend on Facebook, your upstairs neighbor, your crush, your nemesis.

Many of us are taking care of parents while also taking care of children, businesses, households, all the things. And yet, for all I hear about that, I rarely hear any empathy for us or anything to suggest that if we are doing all that mostly or even entirely on our own, that is **not okay**.

It can be daunting enough to figure out how to manage menopause. Now add the rest of our lives and everyone else in them into the mix. And if your life, as with so many of ours, has you at the center as a breathless octopus of service and care for everyone else? Well.

I cannot do all of this justice in a single chapter. This would make for an ideal encyclopedia series: *Menopause and Your Kids, Menopause and the Workplace, Menopause and Dating, Menopause and That Selfish Jagoff Driving Alone in the Carpool Lane*. I can't tackle all of this in great depth or detail, but I can get you started.

THE CONSISTENT SOCIAL MESSAGE HAS been that *we're* holy terrors during menopause. There's a 1950 ad for Premarin with a photo of a smug-looking, polo-shirt-wearing, standard-issue white husband and his sweetly smiling wife on a sailboat. The copy reads, "Husbands, too, like Premarin!" My fantasy is that she looks so happy because she's hatched a plan to throw the pills and his smug ass overboard and sail off into a beautiful life all her own.

I've seen this in menopause resources and advice, too, not just commercials from fifty years ago. So often social information we're given about menopause is about how *we* cannot make a mess of *other* people's lives and, most of all, the lives of *our poor, **poor** husbands*.

By all means, as in any other time of life, during any part of menopause, we should aim not to be total assholes to other people. Setting expectations and boundaries, and respecting them, is the name of this game all around, but that includes for and with us.

ENOUGH ABOUT EVERYONE ELSE. LET'S talk about us.

If there's such a thing as knowing how to do a thing too well, I know how to take care of and center other people *way* too well. The same may be said of you. This is not a chapter about how to keep taking care of everyone else and making everyone else happy while you hold on to your sanity and sense of self by a thread.

There are times when a given person's needs need to be prioritized and centered. This is one of those. If we still want to care for other people, be a superhero at work, home, or both, or save the whole world, we can get back to that when we're able and damn good and ready. But we might need or want to take a break from some or all of that during our menopausal transition; for others to lower their expectations of us (and we of ourselves) and step up for us more; and to ask for or make adjustments as we go through this. If you're like me, you tell other people they can and should do these things for themselves all the time: it's time to take our own advice.

Whatever the relationship, interaction, or environment, dealing with these arenas of life during menopause in ways that are best for you seems to come down to

◊ being honest about what's going on but also giving yourself whatever privacy and boundaries you want and need;

- accepting and leading with your needs and limits;
- saying enough with the self-sacrifice already;
- nurturing the part of your relationships that's about *you* being supported and cared for;
- asking for and accepting what you want and need, very much including any accommodations;
- dumping shitty, bad, or otherwise not-good-for-you relationships, interactions, or spaces—and when you can't, doing what you can to protect, distance, or emotionally disconnect yourself from them;
- getting practice bringing your post-menopausal IDGAF self to the table;
- making and insisting on the space—physical, emotional, social—you want or need for yourself.

FIRE ESCAPE

The essay "A Room of One's Own" centered Virginia Woolf's entirely reasonable supposition that a fixed income and the aforementioned room were essential for women to be able to write fiction.

She was forty-seven when she wrote it, by the way.

Woolf struggled with (and sadly succumbed to) suicidality and bipolar disorder, but if you ask this menopause-obsessed writer, she also gives a lot of clues that perimenopause was part of the struggle of her last fifteen years of life.

In her journals, she talks about feeling hot and cold, struggling with cognitive issues—her head "like an old cloth I don't know"—and "a curious throbbing."

I'm going to be wildly presumptuous and suggest that Virginia would have agreed with me that having a room of one's own is also essential for those in menopausal transition. The fixed income too, for sure, but let's be realistic.

I feel comfortable saying that a time will come in every person's menopause when everyone else's stuff gets tangled in their stuff, everyone else's body takes up space and air and makes the room or the bed or the car warmer and more can-of-sardines-like, and everyone else's dramas and crises and whatever the hell else loudly demands our attention and labor are Too. Damn. Much. A time when you need to get away from it **immediately**. Or else. You might need to get away for ten minutes, overnight, for days. (In some cases, "forever" may be how long you need. I support you, but that's a bigger matter; more on that later.)

If you don't want to do that, and you feel better surrounded by people asking a million things of you nonstop that they can all do themselves when you've only had three hours of sleep, that's cool, you adorable little masochist you. But for the rest of us, I suggest having some kind of physical and emotional escape hatch.

Ideally, that'd be your whole own place: a place you can do whatever it is you want to do (work, art, Zumba, MDMA, plotting revenge) and a place you can also try to sleep without the added complication of other people. One of my saving graces over the last year, especially once the pandemic hit, was having an office studio I could be alone in, with no one else's stuff in it, sometimes for days on end.

I need my own space to sleep sometimes (or to give up and stay up all night without having to worry about waking up other people), my own space to work, and my own space to feel however I'm feeling without having to deal with other people and their feelings and needs. It's been handy to have a space to feel free to cope with this stuff without having to care about things like wearing a top.

THERE ARE A BUNCH OF WAYS TO POTENtially make this happen. If you're lucky, you live somewhere with a guest room or space, a sunroom, or some other "extra" room. It's yours now. You claim this room for menopause. This is no time for hosting guests, anyway. If there's a room but not a door, you can make one, or at least make others understand there is an invisible one.

It may be your situation is such that a room of your own is just not an option, something far too many are far too familiar with in pandemic times. Maybe you can manage a nook of your own. A garage or back porch of your own. A corner of the living room behind a room divider of your own. A fire escape or balcony of your own. Hell, even a lounge chair of your own in a semi-quiet corner that everyone agrees to STAY THE HELL AWAY FROM when you're in it, and keep their stuff clear of, is way better than nothing.

A "room" can also be a different kind of dedicated space, like a day of the week or certain hours in the day where everyone agrees to leave the house so you can have it to yourself for a few hours or just plain leave you alone: no calls or texts, no *Hey, Mom, can you get me . . .* , no *Honey, did you see where I left my . . .*

There's also the kind of room that's about the larger space for yourself in menopause . . . we'll get to that later. Most of us need to limber up some more first.

THE INNER CIRCLE

You're most likely going to be in this major whole-body transition for a good period of time. No one in your life is going to be impacted by *your* menopause more than you. But people you're in relationships with, especially the people emotionally closest to you and in the greatest physical proximity, are going to be part of this. You get a choice about how much and which parts for the most part.

Your relationships should ideally be places of care and mutual support and benefit; it might even be that menopause provides avenues and motivations for more of that mutuality and support to happen than has before. Menopause might give you the gumption to ask for more of what you need from the people you're close to.

This can add some real richness to our relationships. It might be that as hard as having a kid in puberty while you're in menopause can be, it becomes a way to get closer and positively change one another's experiences of both (when the movie comes out, don't forget you saw it here first). This may be the thing that gets you to allow someone in your life to take more care of you than you've let people before, upping the intimacy and mutuality of your relationship. You might find an amazing friend or community in this.

But none of that can happen without a good foundation. It seems to me that foundation is all about support.

ACCOMMODATIONS AND ADJUSTMENTS

Because our bodies are changing and we're changing as people, our needs and limits are also changing. Just like we might need to ask for or make adjustments and accommodations with other things—work hours, pain medications, pants—so we might with or within our relationships.

That might look like

- changing what or how or when you eat in your household to better support what you need;
- switching around who gets which room or what space;
- creating household/community/relationship changes with things like body, age, or diet talk;
- doing things differently with sex or certain kinds of household labor that aren't working with your current abilities;
- changing schedules or reliance on you so that you have the ability to care for yourself.

DON'T MIND ME, I'M JUST A WALKING OPEN WOUND

During a lot of perimenopause, my hardest, most vulnerable feelings have lived

Abusive partners and trauma worsen menopause impacts, and during menopause—particularly if you have impacts or effects that an abusive partner doesn't like or finds disruptive (night sweats, vaginal dryness, fatigue)—abuse may also escalate. There's never a good time to be in an abusive relationship, but menopause seems like one of the toughest times. If you need help getting out or at least making a plan to leave, look up your local IPV/DV victims advocacy organization and seek out help and support. In the event it's you who has been or is becoming abusive, you can find helps for you via those channels, too.

full-time in my throat. My ability to contain or hide them is not what it was before. I try and beg strangers with my eyes to please, please not upset the delicate emotional balance I am barely (and sometimes not) maintaining by having the horrible audacity to ask me if I'm okay.

Ever been in that emotional space where, when someone does ask you that seemingly innocent question, you LOSE YOUR SHIT COMPLETELY? That space where, at best, you pour your whole heart out to some unfortunate kind fool who expected you to say that you were fine, because that's what you're supposed to say, not wipe snot on your sleeve in their break room for half the afternoon. I say at best, because at worst, the most broken part of you might decide to do its best Linda Blair *Exorcist* impression, sob-growling like a demon has your innards in its fist and telling them to go to hell while peeing on the floor.

I don't feel like *anyone* prepares you for how completely your emotional resilience can just bottom out in this and how vulnerable you can feel.

I'VE HAD TO START LEARNING TO DO some things differently. It's been hard, because it's in direct conflict with social and emotional armor I have been wearing for much of my life, but one of the things I've had to start teaching myself is to be honest with other people about how really, truly vulnerable I am. I have

been learning to say that out loud before talking about Big Things, when making plans, or when coworkers are asking for my participation or leadership. I'm getting better at accepting and owning my increased tenderness and fragility, even when I feel shame about it, as I often do. I've had to learn to better protect myself from people who aren't wise to be vulnerable around in the first place. There have been some people I had to stop seeing, talking to, or trying to maintain—read: fix—relationships with. I had to move some more intimate relationships to a more distanced place.

All of those things are net positives anyway. I've also recently been experiencing some of the most mutually open and tender relationships and interactions I've had in a long time, which seems unlikely to be a coincidence. It doesn't have to be a bad thing, this tenderness, so long as the appropriate TLC—be it from ourselves or others—or safe distance is involved.

KIDS. OH GOD. KIDS.

Dr. Lexx Brown-James, LMFT, CSE, CSES, is a licensed marriage and family therapist and sex educator in St. Louis and the author of *The Black Girls' Guide to Couple's Intimacy* and the children's book *These Are My Eyes, This Is My Nose, This Is My Vulva, These Are My Toes.* Dr. Lexx thinks menopause is not just a personal, individual event and issue but a family event, one that should involve kids as much as we'd involve them in anything else like this, such as pregnancy or menstruation, a divorce, or the loss of a job.

If what's said in support groups and books and what I overhear is any indication, going through menopause without a lot of—if any—communication with your immediate family about it is more common than not. People with kids, whatever their ages, in particular rarely seem to tell them what's going on, not even a kid version. Those of us with families that are more queer, more chosen, or both seem to fare better with this, but some of us might also just be talking a really good game.

LET ME PREFACE THIS BY REMINDING you that you get to have whatever boundaries you want and need. Keeping any part of this, even all of this, your own damn business is your prerogative.

Ultimately, talking to kids about this is mostly about making more room for yourself—if you're not hiding this, you don't have to sneak in self-care and other helps—letting them know what's happening so they're not scared and you can normalize it, keeping in relationship with them, and setting some expectations. There's nothing wrong with asking kids and other family members to step it up. Rather, that models for them how we all *should* care for each other.

Dr. Lexx and I agree: this is something you can talk to kids about as plainly as you can (even if you don't) talk to them about menstruation, toileting, having the flu, pregnancy, and other supernormal parts of life in these bodies we live in. In terms of how, here are a few basics.

Nothing bad is happening to you; your body is just changing: This isn't an illness, but it *is* a whole-body, whole-self event, and sometimes a long-term one. It's probably helpful to first tell them you're okay, just so that's clear, then explain this to them in an appropriate way for who they are and their development. If you're not sure what that is, figure out what stage of a pregnancy or menstruation talk they're at and how you'd deliver that, and tailor this one to suit. You can also tell them they'll go through this (if they will) or something like it (puberty) in life, too, and let them know about any other people they know on the other side of this, so they can know there is one.

Set expectations and boundaries: You can tell them it may have you feeling some kind of way, physically, emotionally, or both, and that you'll need them to cut you a break sometimes. You can let them know that if you behave in a way that's upsetting to *them*, they should talk about it with you, but also, so help them, if they start blaming everything you do that they don't like loudly on menopause, they're going to see what a real Italian Death Glare looks like and may never sleep soundly again.

Tell kids (and any other members of your household) you may want some of

their help while you go through this: You can let them know—maybe even make a list together—what kinds of things you might ask for, whether that's getting themselves dressed in the morning, being cool about food changes you need to make, switching rooms so you can sleep in the cooler one, not making body jokes, arranging more of their own rides instead of relying on you, or just trying to be a little more helpful and empathetic.

You have the opportunity to normalize menopause and other potentially uncomfortable or challenging life transitions for them, which is actually pretty damn cool, if you ask me. You're also showing them how partners and family members should support someone in menopause and other transitions. As Dr. Lexx said, "If your kids are going to go through this themselves and they see you making time and room for your own care, they will remember this. You've given *them* permission to take care of themselves in menopause. If your partner's supporting you, your kids get to see how a partner is supposed to act. If they're going to be the partner of someone going through this or something like it, they will get to be a good partner like from the beginning. Everybody wins. You get things. They get things."

I READ ALANIS MORISSETTE TALKING about how she's going through perimenopause *while* postpartum, and I don't

even know how to pick my jaw up off the ground to *try* and say something smart about that situation. I know she's not the only one in it, because having babies later in the life span has been becoming more common for a long time now. I open my mouth and all that comes out are seal-like sympathy grunts. You can't even *ask* babies to leave you alone. If this is you, and you're not asking for all the extra help from anyone and everyone in a ten-mile radius, I hope you know you get to. Hell, call me. Unless you've got your eye on martyrdom, call *someone*.

DATING IN MENOPAUSE

I'd have said a couple years back I may have a uniquely rosy perspective on this because I've had a pretty good experience. Then I started to hear what other people had to say about it, and it actually doesn't appear it's all that unique. Joan Price found someone she considers the great love of her life not just in, but literally because of, menopause. I think it's fair to say that seeking out and exploring new relationships, period, including platonic ones, might have been one of the things that saved my quote-unquote sanity during perimenopause. The fact that I wound up finding an astronomically fantastic partner who loves the shit out of me sure didn't hurt.

During menopause, as in any other time of life, you might experience a sexual orientation or other sexual identity shift you want to explore. If you're in an existing exclusive relationship, you might find yourself thinking about opening it up. If you haven't been dating for a long time, or even ever, you might like it better now when some of the pressures of dating as a younger person are gone. (For that matter, you might experience orientation or identity shifts that lead you away from dating: that's okay too!)

I think there's a reason it's fairly common for people to take new lovers or forge new platonic intimate relationships in or around menopause. We get to walk into something new **as we are** right now, in this moment, when we're perhaps inclined— even if for no other reason than sheer exhaustion—to just put ourselves all the way out there, ask for what we want, and have way less time for anyone else's bullshit. Making some adjustments is one thing, but it's a lot harder to fundamentally, radically change a preexisting relationship than it is to start something new, if you ask me.

In the event we forge lasting relationships while we're going through this, I feel like it's good practice for the extra mutual care and consideration we'll all want and need as we get older. Perimenopause is but the *start* of some level of endless indignity, not the end. This arena of our relationships now is the training wheels for what we may need from relationships in older age.

People with the kind of emotional maturity required to be generally safe for other people don't mind (and often even tend to appreciate) clearly stated limits and boundaries, are cool with folks who know what they want and don't want and aren't afraid to say it, and maybe, just maybe, are even into people who just keep it really real. I propose that when it comes to relationships during menopause—whether we're talking about dating and actual personals ads (I'm happy to write yours for you, by the way) or existing intimate relationships—it is absolutely okay, and perhaps even ideal, to lead with your clearly stated and honest wants, needs, and limits. I mean, who has time or patience for anything else at this point anyway?

I honestly think that, believe it or not, if you want to be dating, this may be one of the *better* times to do it. Since it's also one of the times in life when it becomes easier to say, "Oh, to hell with *this*," even when it's not, we still win.

MEN(O) AT WORK

It's fair to say a majority of workplaces are not particularly humane environments in the best of circumstances, and generally the lower the wage, benefits, security, and position, the lower the humanity. The amount of hours many have to work, what can be asked of our bodies, whether that's about being on our feet all day or having to sit, the minimal room often provided for our mental health and feelings, the minimal room often provided for being a woman or gender-diverse person at work, period—all of these things and more are terrible setups for self-care or respecting and adapting to limitations of our minds and bodies.

(Being your own boss or being *the* boss doesn't exempt you, by the by. I've been my own boss for the bulk of the last three decades. I've asked ask a lot of bullshit of myself—impossible workloads, crummy pay, hours I'd never ask anyone else to agree to—that I've often accepted as part and parcel of being self-employed, sometimes even when I *do* have flexibility to do things differently.)

What creates problems at work for people in menopause obviously depends on someone's experience of it, what kind of job they do, and what kind of power and agency they do or don't have there. For nearly everyone, whatever the job, if you're having fatigue, anxiety, issues with memory and concentration, or irritability, any or all of those can be everything from minor annoyances, to deeply disruptive and job risking, to outright dangerous. Some jobs will make it very difficult to manage things like menstrual flooding or vulvovaginal pain, and by all means, if what's expected of you at work doesn't make space for, say, visibly sweating your ass off in front of a team, class, company, or nation, then even something as common and benign as a hot flash can be a potential problem.

In the *Guardian*, Rose George wrote, "A study by Nuffield Health found that 72% of women felt unsupported at work when menopausal, and that 10% of women considered leaving their jobs as a result. A study by the University of Nottingham, released in 2011, reported that nearly half of women found it difficult to cope with the menopause at work. Nearly a fifth thought it affected how their colleagues and managers perceived their competence." A 2020 study of working women in Japan found, to the surprise of none of us having exactly this issue, that the greater the impacts of menopause someone was dealing with, the harder the time at work that person was having. It also found that when accommodations were made at work for menopausal people, the level of impact they were dealing with decreased.

We won't all have the same level of ability to create change for ourselves and others in our diverse workplaces or fields. And sometimes what we do will, all by itself, present challenges: driving a truck, doing sex work, or sitting at a desk all day with extreme vulvovaginal pain can be anywhere from horribly difficult to literally impossible. Doing surgeries or factory work with a big sleep deficit is not only very difficult but very dangerous for everyone involved.

Surveys have been done to learn what people in menopause want and need at work. It's all as reasonable and basic as you'd expect. In any given job, field, or workplace, you might not be able to get all of the things that can help, but you probably can at least get some. At the very least, you can likely ask, and potentially even ask as a group instead of all by your lonesome.

What's likely to help in most workplaces and what have people said they want to make it easier to be at work and in menopause?

ORGANIZATIONAL SUPPORT, SENSITIVITY, AND NORMALIZATION

In the United States alone, at least 20 percent of the workforce is likely in or recently has been in a menopausal transition or is experiencing or has experienced sudden menopause. When I've talked to friends about issues they're having at work with this, most said they don't or wouldn't even feel able to say anything about menopause, let alone ask for support or any kind of accommodations.

Workplaces and workplace management should be the ones mentioning menopause **first**, rather than putting that burden on their menopausal employees. It should be included in workplace policies and trainings, with informational flyers or memos from time to time. Workplaces can normalize and make room for menopause by treating it the same way they hopefully already treat pregnancy, disability, bereavement, and other common parts of the human life cycle.

A culture of comfort and respect should exist for people in menopause. At the very least, we need to feel safe and comfortable telling managers and other people we work with that we're in it if we're to find ways to make it work with work. A recent UK survey found that 59 percent of those experiencing menopausal symptoms said they had a negative impact on their work, and around half found it difficult to do their jobs. And "while nearly a third of women surveyed . . . said they had taken sick leave because of their symptoms, only a quarter of them felt able to tell their manager the real reason for their absence."

On her podcast, Michelle Obama said,

[Barack] didn't fall apart because he found out there were several women in his staff that were going through menopause. It was just like, "Well, turn the air conditioner on." A lot of the functions of day-to-day life when you're going through menopause just don't work. How we dress, wearing a suit . . . you can be drenched in sweat down to your core in the middle of a freezing-cold office and have to shower and change clothes and fix your hair all over again. There's a lot of stuff [we] need to talk about. Some of these cultural norms change, like how you dress, the temperature in the room. . . . The whole system of the workplace doesn't work for us in the right way.

If this kind of culture of comfort, respect, and adaptation isn't happening at your workplace, you can ask for it. If you have the desire and energy (and hopefully

247

some compensation), you can even offer to lead or help with the creation of those policies, including menopause education for employees and their coworkers, and other avenues of support and normalization.

Dr. Lexx talked about how most of us

can't show up for work like, "Look, I am in a puddle of sweat. I am barely breathing. And I'm very, very, very irritated. I do not need to meet with this client today." That whole suck-it-up-buttercup mentality we have taken on? Because we can't be seen as less-than in the workplace? Yeah, no. We have to lean on community. There is no suffering in silence. There is no suffering alone. Where is your community and specifically building that community so they can support you through this process? It's a process, a transformational process. Doing that alone sounds miserable and scary.

MORE FLEXIBLE HOURS, SHIFTS, BREAKS, AND SCHEDULES

Researchers estimate that absenteeism due to menopause can cost companies over $9.5 million annually. And that doesn't even account for what it costs *employees*.

Even though we know that some people seem to come out on the other side of menopause with superpowers—or, at least, things like better focus, improved depression, no more distractions or disruptions from menstrual cycles—that certainly benefit employers and workplaces, the collision of ageism, sexism, and ableism that even the suggestion of menopause brings seems to keep them from realizing that it's in their best interest to keep their menopausal employees around. Retaining employment and continuing to advance at work is a real struggle for many in peri- and postmenopause because of that -ism shit sandwich.

It obviously isn't better for employers to lose employees to sick time when they could, instead, allow an employee in menopause to get the work done if they just made some adjustments.

One adjustment with a potentially major impact is allowing for more flexibility with schedules, hours, and breaks. You might not *need* to call in sick if you were allowed to take more frequent breaks or longer breaks to grab a nap sometimes. Some of these kinds of adjustments can be made with letting more people work from home some or all of the time or organizing a system of pinch hitters for shift swapping as needed.

No pressure, but labor organizer Mary G. Harris Jones was a dressmaker in her fifties when she became "Mother Jones," considered one of the most dangerous women in America at the time for her organizing. Was she in menopause at the time? Maybe.

WHAT SHOULD BE BASICS ALREADY BUT OFTEN AREN'T

I'm talking about basic needs—like easy and always available access to water and toilets—and control over work environments and conditions like temperature control or windows and fans, access to extra uniforms or to uniforms made out of lighter materials or at least not sauna-inducing polyesters. Things like this might sound minor, but a lot of these "minor" things can add up to one majorly awful workplace.

What's making you or your menopause more miserable at work in basic ways like these? A delivery van without working A/C? A specific dress code? The fact that once you have to go, there's already not enough time to make it to the toilet because it's so far away? A lack of ventilation? You can ask for these things.

Strong anti-harassment and privacy policies should also be considered basics at any workplace. Sexual harassment remains a highly common experience for women and gender-diverse people at work. That doesn't magically vanish at midlife. Wouldn't that be nice. Not only is harassment at work unacceptable, but it also creates trauma and stress, both things we know are big players in making impacts of menopause more likely, frequent, or severe and making menopause more miserable, period. A menopause study on cardiovascular health found that "those who experienced sexual harassment at work had a twofold increased risk compared to women who hadn't of developing high blood pressure." High blood pressure is something we will have an elevated risk for postmenopause already, so this, obviously, is not a great start.

Ridicule is common with menopause. Every toxic joke or jab you've been the butt of or heard about periods or vaginas or breasts can find a new and equally awful home in menopause, uttered sometimes by coworkers or bosses. We've always needed our workplaces to have strong anti-harassment as well as privacy policies. We still do.

IF IT GETS REALLY BAD

Menopause isn't usually included in disability policies. That's sound in the sense that menopause isn't itself a disability. However, some of the *impacts* of menopause can certainly create disability or impact existing disability negatively. Severe depression can occur—sometimes for the first time—for some people with menopause transition and become debilitating. Rheumatoid arthritis often gets worse in perimenopause, so someone with this condition who was able to work with it before may find that peri changes that ability.

If you wind up having a menopause that creates disability or makes previously manageable disability unmanageable for you, you might look into filing for temporary disability if your field or workplace does not or cannot make adaptations you need in order to keep working.

Not everyone is going to be comfortable having some at work know that they're going through menopause, whether that's about a culture of sexual harassment, feeling unsafe as a transmasculine person, or something else. If you need or want to ask for changes or accommodations but you don't feel safe or comfortable saying it's about menopause, that's fine. The point is to get yourself the support and help you need, not to make you the Norma Rae of menopause (unless you want that, of course). Make it about whatever you need to try and get your needs met.

It also might get really bad because you work with nothing but overgrown frat boys or your manager is someone else's mean, racist grandpa or a believer, like my Irish Catholic great-grandmother, that the point of life—yours included—is to live, suffer, and die. Menopause-was-easy-for-me-what's-*your*-problem bosses and coworkers also exist, and boy, do *they* sound like assholes. Those situations might be the kind where you know, because you work there, you're better off saying nothing and just white-knuckling it at work and doing what you need to do *after* work for yourself.

A few things to help life go on even when we're losing our shit:

◊ If and when you can half-ass it, do: you can get back to being amazing at everything after menopause if you still want to.
◊ Use organizational tools like you are trying to solve a murder.
◊ Automate everything you can.
◊ Delegate, delegate, delegate.

◊ If you have savings, use some of them for yourself. This counts as an emergency.
◊ Replace some of the things you absolutely do not have to do with sleep.
◊ Pretend life right now is one of those competitive survival shows.
◊ Set limits. See also: boundaries.
◊ Get super into a weird, esoteric hobby to distract people from the parts of life you're lousing up.
◊ Lower your expectations of yourself. Lower your expectations, period.

GREAT BIG MENOPAUSAL LIFE 'SPLODY

It is not uncommon for some people in menopause to take a look at their whole lives or some big part of them and come to the conclusion that what it really needs is some gasoline and a match. There may come a time in this when our fucks *all* come home to roost, we size them up, and say, "Oh yeah? **Let's** *dance*."

This is often described as blowing up one's life or as a midlife crisis. There is no doubt a range of ways this goes, and

250

that certainly includes some people who had a good life they really liked and just decided to sabotage or abandon for whatever reason; for no reason. We're people: we sometimes do weird and reckless things, with or without menopause, including messing up a good thing. There are also those whose Ya-Ya Sisterhood careers to start something new, having passionate affairs, making big moves, delivering giant my-way-or-the-highway proclamations, forging communities, and reviving lost dreams, I rarely see what looks like some kind of big mistake. I see what more often looks like courage, wisdom, and self-trust.

> **"All I could think of when I got a look at the place from the outside was what fun it would be to stand out there and watch it burn down."**
> **—Shirley Jackson**

was not able to sustain them through something that got really rough for them in menopause—like suicidality or severe fatigue—and who just lost their basket. Sometimes "blowing up your life" is instead being unable to sustain your life, not getting the help you need, and drowning under the weight of it all.

But I want to make sure to mention those who I think might be the most representative of an exploded menopausal life, and that's the folks who torpedoed their lives or an aspect of them because they sucked, and they got the motivation, courage, or opportunity or just ran out of patience. I'm talking about people whose lives were already blown up, even if it wasn't obvious. They just finally walked out of the rubble.

WHEN I LOOK AT PEOPLE'S MENOPAUSAL or midlife stories of tossing away old

I've seen a lot of "don't make any major life decisions during this precarious time when you are clearly not in your right mind" advice tossed around in menopausal circles, often in reference to these kinds of major maybe-kabooms when people are thinking about them.

I disagree.

I WORKED AT AN ABORTION CLINIC FOR A couple years. My main job was to sit down with someone about to get an abortion and go over their forms, ensure that an abortion was what they wanted, tell them what the procedure and aftercare would involve, and check in about how they were feeling.

Sometimes, in that conversation, someone would tell me their whole story: what got them there and led to their decision. That conversation was one of my favorite parts of that job. (One of the others was quietly scaring the piss out of abusive boyfriends or family members, a delight I still can hardly believe I got paid for.)

As you might know, unplanned pregnancy is something that often forces a person experiencing it to quickly evaluate a great deal of their life, including their future. People I talked to in that spot not only had made a pregnancy decision but, as a result, had also often made other decisions and life plans as a by-product of that moment and decision-making process.

Sometimes they'd get there because their partners refused to cooperate with contraception or were outright reproductively coercive or otherwise abusive, and they'd decided to get out or plan to get out of those relationships as well as making their pregnancy decision. Sometimes, in trying to sort out what they wanted the next twenty years of their life to look like, they'd decided it didn't involve a child, period or yet, because they wanted to further their education, or start a business, or go somewhere first, or clean up the giant mess of their life so they could even start to figure out what they really wanted. Being at that kind of moment for ourselves is powerful.

I think that perimenopause and the menopausal transition can be that kind of moment too. This isn't to say that all or even any of this experience is A Shiny Empowerment Moment for everyone by any means. It might not be. It often isn't, and it's certainly not required. It also isn't to say that any big life 'splody that happens **must** be positive and empowering. Menopause—or is it everything else?—often has some impressively shit timing when it comes to the rest of our lives. Sometimes that timing is absolutely devastating. For example, Hillary Clinton's perimenopause was likely happening throughout the mid to late 1990s, just in case you weren't mad enough on her behalf already. Sometimes it's maddening bullshit. It does not usually feel empowerful to be racing between fires of our bodies and fires of our lives.

But I think even that *can* sometimes be positive and empowering in the long run.

Like Leela Sinha said, our tolerance for things we probably shouldn't have ever been so tolerant of in the first place can change now. We can find out we had too much on our plates. We can grieve things we have needed to grieve. If it's time for some big change, if you are just plain OVER whatever it is, and you are ready, willing, and able to walk away, 'splode it, or burn it all down? Here's my lighter.

CLOAK OF INVISIBILITY

At some point in your menopausal odyssey, you may start feeling less visible. As much as we might want other people to go away sometimes, we probably

> "The truth is, it's only when you stop worrying about becoming 'invisible' that you are able to see yourself. Then you are free. Free to decide what matters to you and what never will, whose opinions you value and whose you can disregard, and what exactly is worth your precious hours on this earth and what is a waste of damn time."
> —Benedetta Barzini

don't want to feel invisible to them either. The *fear* of invisibility alone can be debilitating.

Invisibility you experience may be sexual or romantic invisibility to men or butches some women feel around this time or other kinds of worries about erotic or romantic capital. You may feel your visibility waning in your work or community. You can feel it at home, in your own family. It can show up, or show up more than it already has, in daily life when you're trying to get an idea heard, order a drink, keep your place in line at the market, or just in asking for help, which was already hard enough to do, for fuck's sake.

Omisade Burney-Scott said,

I feel like as black folk are aging, there's already different levels of invisibility that we, like, contend with on a daily basis, like not being seen as human, not being seen as valuable, not being seen as lovable, not being seen as deserving of a good life. With aging, that gets exacerbated. How will—and *will*—I be seen or perceived at this stage of my life? Is it possible for my

authentic self to continue to become more fully actualized? Who are the folks who are going to hold that with me? How can I talk about what that feels like for me?

If you *already* felt invisible, if you're losing visibility with something or someone that mattered to you and your sense of yourself deeply, or if you're suffering in plain sight without anyone seeming to notice, it can be just awful.

There's little to say about that in brief that won't sound glib or dismissive, so the best I can do is to tell you to think of yourself like a boat in the fog and start by anchoring yourself. Find the people and places who see you and the ways you still see yourself and who will, like Omisade says, hold who you are with you. Maybe you stay holding on once the fog lifts; maybe you don't—that's up to you. But (if you even want it to in the first place) you can trust that fog will lift at least some if you can just wait it out.

There aren't only downsides, anger or sadness, to invisibility. Sometimes, it can be a literal cloak of invisibility, in the good ways.

OTHER PEOPLE

What can you do with your cloak of invisibility?

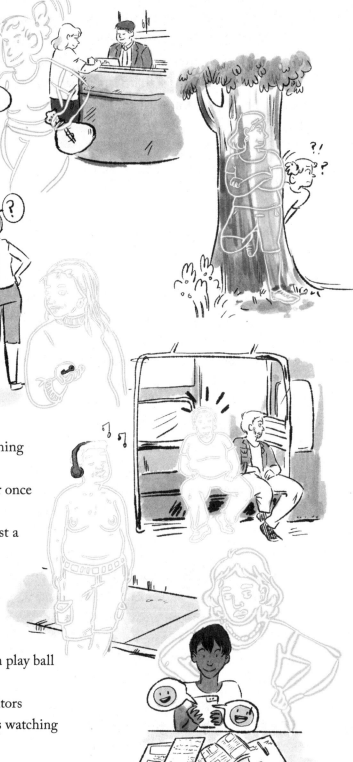

- Rob banks and never have to work another day in your life
- Win the *shit* out of hide-and-seek
- Use public transit for free
- Get into restaurants without reservations
- Move your nemesis's car keys every day
- Have the best time EVER on Halloween
- Sneak into work late without getting caught
- Never pay for a concert or game again
- Immediately vanish the way you long wished you could when you do something embarrassing
- Feel super safe on the train for once
- Garden in the nude
- Walk around town wearing just a pair of pants
- Swim in your neighbor's pool at night
- See if your kids are *really* doing their homework
- Make it look like your dog can play ball with ghosts
- Scare away door-to-door solicitors
- REALLY dance like no one is watching

I've heard people report a range of benefits from their newfound menopausal or middle-age invisibility: less catcalling and other street harassment, feeling safer or freer to do things in public, more freedom to experiment with gender expression or other kinds of presentation, a greater sense of privacy, being able to get away with things they'd get in trouble for if they were younger (yes, that is our weed you've been smelling in the park), feeling like less of a walking target. Having less care about what you look like to others; less care about how, or even if, others perceive you, period. Susie Bright told me Betty Dodson said one of her favorite parts of postmenopausal life was that she could leer at whoever she wanted to on the train without worrying anyone would notice.

The benefits, like everything else with this, aren't universal, of course. Some of us will get some that someone else doesn't, and we may be afforded some benefits only in specific places or circumstances.

In her son's documentary, *The Disappearance of My Mother*, Benedetta Barzini is working on carrying out her plans for a deeply wanted rest-of-life invisibility. She was very visible during some of her life, and in her seventies, what she wants is to leave her existing life behind and go to a new place, with nothing except herself. She's very clear: she doesn't want to go kill herself or die; she wants to vanish, to go somewhere else and live, but unseen.

She is working toward that: packing up all her things for her son, saying goodbye to friends, allowing him to do this film even though it's the last thing she wants for herself. She's actively working toward a dream that may or may not be realized, but she's all in, fully committed, focused on doing it in the ways she can as much as on the end goal. She's living in that end goal of invisibility all the time, even though she's technically not there yet.

By all means, if we're being taken for granted—which is what I think much of the most painful kind of invisibility is—in our personal relationships and other parts of our lives, and we want to try and repair them, we can. Sometimes, some people or systems just need a reminder, some hard limits, or both. Sometimes, with a poke people will see us and our needs and correct course. It's validating when that happens and, in some relationships, can be transformative. If we want to be seen, we get to yell, "See me!" Some people will see and hear us when we do.

Some other people won't. Continuing to try and get their attention, respect, or help when they refuse to give it is only going to make us feel like shit.

I propose that if you're not looking forward to it already, even if you're scared shitless, you try and reimagine invisibility like Benedetta has. What if we made grand plans for it instead of dreading and fearing it?

If we're invisible, fewer people are going to see, for instance, if our attempts at trying new things are successful or not, because they won't even notice us trying in the first place. We can potentially fall flat on our faces in front of everyone without it being humiliating because no one may even notice! You might have more confidence to do things that you didn't before. You might have the ability to just explore yourself and life more freely and find out who you even are and what you want in ways you couldn't with everyone watching.

There's a reason a cloak of invisibility sounds really cool to little kids (and to some of us very big kids, too): a cloak of invisibility can offer us freedom.

PART 3

YOU DON'T HAVE TO GO HOME, BUT YOU CAN'T STAY HERE

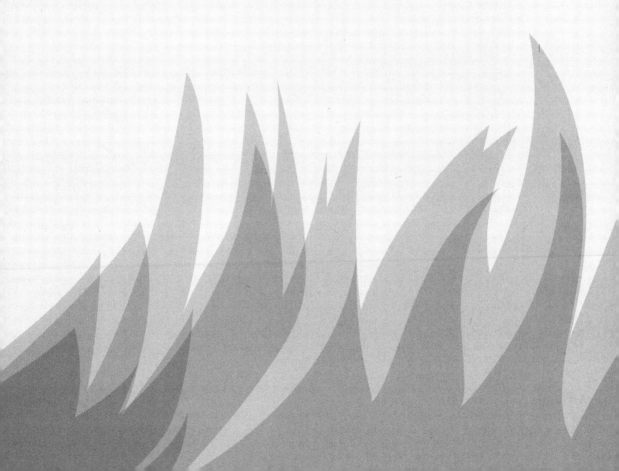

CHAPTER FOURTEEN
ARE WE THERE YET?

"Change never happens at the pace we think it should."
—*Judith Heumann*

As I write this, I am currently at 115 days without a period.

Before you get too excited for me, know this is not the first time I've gone this long without one in peri. Last year, I had a 162-day stretch without one that led me to foolishly believe I was, finally, in the final inning.

I was not.

When I walked out of the bathroom on day 163, after doing my best vocal impression of someone changing into a werewolf, my partner, standing on the other side of the door looking both sympathetic and scared, said, knowing the answer, "Your period?" There was a time I was over the moon to see my period, kissing the ground and anyone else. Even though it made me sick, pregnancy made me sicker and also made a giant mess of my already messy life besides. I was so grateful to see it then. Those halcyon days

are gone. Now when I get it, you'd think I found a dead rat in the toilet.

SOME PEOPLE AREN'T AWARE THEY'RE IN perimenopause, and so aren't trying to figure out if it's over or if it will, at least, be over some day before they die. For the rest of us, getting to the end of perimenopause, especially the longer and longer it goes on, can feel like a terrible reboot of Chutes and Ladders.

You keep making your way up, up, up the ladder, and then find yourself going down, down, down, sliding back to the maddening beginning all over again.

It's not really the beginning, of course: we remain as far along in this as we are, and having periods at any point in peri doesn't mean that we and our bodies go *all* the way back to where we were when we started peri. It sure feels like it though.

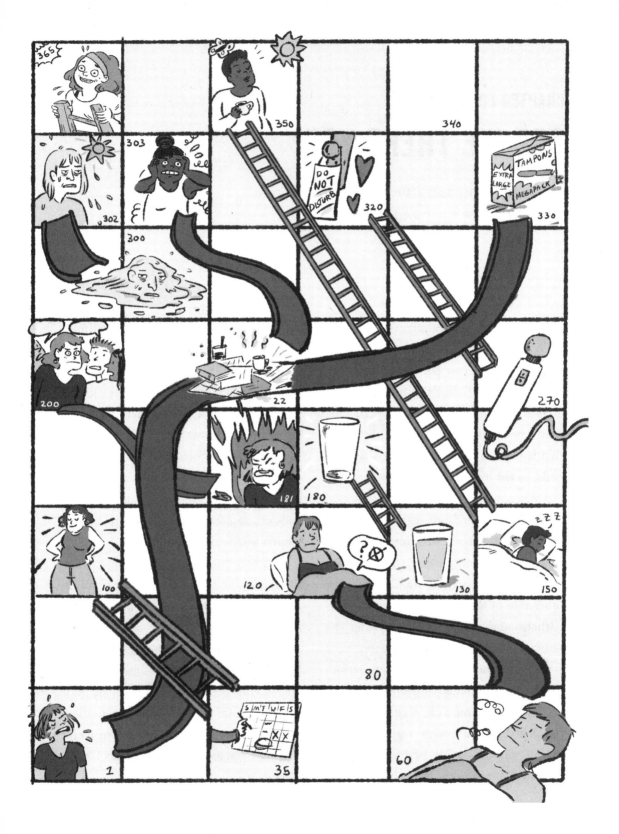

ONCE MORE WITH FEELING (AND, FOR some of us, with great desperation), perimenopause is considered over when it's been one year since what can then be referred to as the final menstrual period (FMP). Every time I type it, I imagine a metal anthem of the same name.

There's not any discernable signal when that FMP is going to happen, is happening, or has happened. For as much drama as often occurs with a first period, you won't usually even know you're having the last one.

Whenever this happens for you, whatever it is you feel you have earned in this—a badge, a trophy, sainthood, room to feel sad, a sex party, the most amazing sundae ever created—I psychically bestow it on you.

NOT KNOWING WHEN PERIMENOPAUSE will end isn't a big deal for everyone. Some won't feel like they're waiting at all. Some—ahem—will feel like the goddamn Frog Prince.

If you want, you can go to a healthcare provider and ask them to take your hormone levels. If you're at least close, you'll have the low estrogen and high follicle-stimulating hormone that's the hallmark of late perimenopause and postmenopause. Of course, even if you get those levels, you still could be years from the other side. Only you know what's useful for you and what is likely to make you even more frustrated.

If you haven't had regular periods for a long time, never did, or don't get periods because of something like a hormonal IUD, you may not find out when you're on the other side at all or for a long time. Again, if this is about a contraception method, Dr. Judith Hersh suggests you stop taking or remove the method around age fifty for six months and see what happens. (My editor, in her own painfully acquired wisdom, wants me to remind you to ask about any side effects you may have from coming off a method first, just so you're prepared. This is sage.) If you still don't get a period, it's likely because you're postmenopause, and you can verify that with hormone levels if you want. If you do get a period, you're not there yet and can either keep off that method or go back on and try again in another six months or more.

LOSS (OR NOT) AT THE ENDS

For the bulk of the time I've had them, my periods have, like Republican administrations, been painful and disruptive to my life and well-being. They've brought with them days of nausea, vomiting, and other decidedly unfun gastrointestinal adventures. They've usually included incredibly painful cramps for a couple days each time, the kind only helped by narcotics given to you by your friend who had oral surgery last month. My body reacts badly or not at all to many of the things that can help. My cycles have brought on migraines and icepick headaches when I don't have my periods, because, as everyone's mother has told us a million times, life isn't fair.

For thirty-some years, I did what I could to get used to and normalize a life, as many do, where for about 72 days out of 365 I felt like shit. I didn't get to do things I wanted to. I missed work I needed. I pushed through when I could and I had to. You might know how that goes. I don't remember anyone ever patronizingly asking me if I was on my period, probably because when I was, I was yelling invectives at them from across the street, so they already knew.

I never had a bad attitude about my periods, which is surprising, because they sure had bad attitudes themselves. Even with all the pain and disruption they caused, all for a reproductive system that wasn't even capable of finishing the things it started, I still liked them in a few ways. I liked the power the cultural fear of and disgust for menses gave me: it gave me ways to be scary when I wanted. There was a feralness to my menstrual experience—the pain of it but also the literal great bloody mess of it—that made me feel strong. I will certainly miss the delight of being the potential ruin of someone's fussy chair. Even though the end of mine brings great relief from pain and a ton of disruption, there are some parts of it I'll miss and have already been missing.

I DIDN'T ASK ANYONE I TALKED TO ABOUT these kinds of ends, but some brought them up on their own.

There's a sort of universally assumed hallelujah we're all supposed to say about our periods being over. For sure, some people are elated—Joan Price waxed poetic to me about the freedoms no longer menstruating gave her—and I obviously have my own brand of hooray. But I think the assumption that the end of periods will be nothing but relief, like the similar assumption that the end of reproduction will only bring feelings of loss, is just another resurgence of highly unuseful universalizing.

Jaclyn Friedman volunteered, "I really like my period. And—not everyone does or needs one to do this, obviously—but I associate it with being a woman. It's deeply bound in my experience of my own womanhood. I also loved having the rhythm of it in my life. My period hasn't been a burden."

Southerners on New Ground cofounder and LGBTQ activist and organizer Mandy Carter told me about how she first got hers while in foster care when she was twelve. She told me how traumatized she was for not knowing what it was. Her foster mother didn't tell her anything about it at all. No one ever really talked with her about it. Particularly since her periods were heavy and hard, that was something she held onto emotionally for years. Now that she doesn't have her period anymore, that means she doesn't have everything emotional she carried with it either.

Sometimes even the loss of something painful has its own weight or can leave an empty space behind. Mona Eltahawy said,

> One of the things that I struggle with the most is my period going. I am childfree by choice. I never wanted to have children. It's not like I feel that my fertility is gone. In that regard, thank you. All the different scares that I've had. **Thank you.** It's because I have had a period and I get a period every month, every month, within two or three days, which I've had since the age of eleven and a half. Outside of my parents and my brother, my period is the one thing in my life that I've had the most consistent relationship with.

With reproduction, the assumption made is usually the other way around: it's assumed we'll only feel loss. But again, being actual, whole people and not women in *Philip Roth* novels, it turns out we have a range of feelings.

I come from a long line of people, generally interconnected with ever longer, wider lines of people, for whom reproductive choice was often not an option or, when it was, was a deadly one. The end of the ability to reproduce has been solidly about freedom where I'm from, and for some people in my family, it's literally been lifesaving. I've also spent years of my life working with pregnant people who don't want to be pregnant and with people who want help avoiding pregnancy in the first place.

The end of my periods doesn't mean the end of my fertility or the end of my ability to have children. Setting aside what I did and didn't want when it came to kids, pregnancy and parenting (a whole book of its own), my body was never keen to remain pregnant when it became so, I had severe hyperemesis the few times I was pregnant, and I also never had the other life conditions (economic or social) that I specifically needed to support a pregnancy, me as a parent, or a child.

I made what little peace there was for me to make with all that way before now. But that's me, and I know that while I'm not alone in it, I am a bit unusual in that respect.

I know that for some, just having a body able to do this thing has felt like having a superpower. I read someone who said that the way soccer might feel like someone else's sport, pregnancy and birth felt like hers, so she's felt a kind of loss in how powerful it made her body, and she, as a person, feel.

The ability to continue a lineage is also loaded for a lot of people. Dr. Lexx said,

> I've seen people going through perimenopause or menopause depressed because of their loss of value from their loss of

reproductive power. I think it's entrenched from colonialism and white supremacy for Black women and women of color. How much am I worth now? Am I damaged? For Black, of-color, and indigenous women, you're made to feel it's your responsibility for perpetuating the race. So, if you haven't had children and perimenopause or menopause are happening, you've run out of time. What does this mean if I didn't further my family's lineage? I think even if we don't agree with this position, if we feel loss around it, we still get to grieve some of these losses.

I know menopause can happen after a long line of attempted, wanted pregnancies that never came to pass and that menopause can feel like a final failure. If it wasn't expected, it may be wholly heartbreaking. Or it can also feel like a massive reprieve and great relief.

I know it can feel like you're finally done, and even if you loved any or all of the parts of the ability or experience of pregnancy, you're happy to be done with it now. I also know you can wish you could keep on doing it and might grieve that you can't.

I know that for some, the end of the ability to become pregnant is the end of abuse: the end of being threatened, exploited, abused, or otherwise harmed because of it. Everyone with a uterus who's been living in most parts of the world, most certainly including the United States, gets to at least free themselves of the controlling yoke governments have on anyone who can procreate. Any and all of those things can obviously be incredibly liberating. But for some, even that is tempered by the known fact that anyone abusing them that way will find a new way to do it. Even liberation can feel unrewarding sometimes.

It can feel just exactly right. Or not at all.

It can feel like the end of a wonderful story or the end of a terrible one, and how anyone feels about either—or both—is as vast as the moon.

OF COURSE, AS MY MOTHER—WHO else?—felt it necessary to remind me, just getting to the other side doesn't mean it's all over. There's still a period—and potentially one as long as the one before menopause—of adjustment to the new chemical picture on *that* side too.

(My mother told me it took her about a decade in perimenopause and another decade on the other side to feel all the way through it. Knowing what I now know about patterns with menopause in families, it wasn't one of my better days.)

And then, of course, there's the matter that our bodies have always been changing and will continue to change so long as we're alive. The fairy tale in my mind—maybe in yours, too, but I don't want to be presumptuous—that after this I'd be done with all the big changes was always preposterous, and I should have known that all along.

FROM DAY 365 AFTER THAT LAST PERIOD on, the lowering estrogen and progesterone that got us there won't come to a complete stop. Their continued downward progression (for testosterone too) will be gradual over the rest of our lives. But we will usually start feeling more stable, because (1) there's no more hormonal cycling like there usually was from our first period on, and (2) there's also no more spikes or big fluctuations. Those hormones will all settle into a constant low level. It will usually—once we get used to it, anyway—leave us feeling more stable because we will be from a chemical standpoint. Learning this explained everything I never could figure out about how older women politicians deal with the behavior of many of their male colleagues so calmly.

As you've already found out, we might still have some menopausal impacts for a while, and that while could be as long on this side as it was on the other. There are some we won't have: we obviously won't be dealing with any menstrual issues, because that'll be all done. A lot of mood and mental health issues also improve or resolve. If we have felt a mental fog, and it hasn't let up at all yet, it might clear now. People who dealt with changes to sexual desire often express that those resolved for them too. But we might also still have vasomotor symptoms or new genital or bone issues, for example. And then, of course—and I say this because I am clearly my mother's child—there's everything that still awaits us in postmenopause and with plain old aging, both stages we will be in until we die.

There's no telling how long it'll take us, our bodies, and our psyches to get used to our new state of being to the degree that

All the things of life and health postmenopause are for another book entirely, one I am both entirely inexperienced and also much too tired to write. But some postmenopausal issues to keep on your radar since they're coming, and to take into account when you're making choices about managing perimenopause (such as with MHT, particularly as estrogen-based MHT can help protect against some of these risks), include

* osteoporosis and other bone-loss and related bone issues like fractures and oral health problems;
* increased risks of stroke, heart disease, and diabetes;
* more profound urogenital changes.

we feel like our menopausal transition is done. The same also obviously goes for what we make of it all emotionally. I'm trying not to let it scare me.

I'm trying to keep something Leela Sinha said in the front of my mind: "The key to having a body in this universe is adaptability and flexibility. The thing that makes you able to be okay with something like this and find what's good about it is when you trust yourself to be able to adapt."

How many times have I adapted even before this? *So* many times. This body has carried and helped me this far and, honestly, sometimes without any cooperation from me. Both it and I have already been through so much change and have dealt with so many kinds of garbage and hurt, but also with so much pleasure and joy and the ability to do so many things. I may feel like I can't do this some of the time, but both my body and I have actually done a helluva job, looking back, and even with some serious challenges.

It would be ridiculous, and certainly in bad faith, to assume my body—and I— won't keep on adapting.

CHAPTER FIFTEEN

THE MAYBE-GREAT BEYOND: POSTMENOPAUSAL PROJECTIONS

"Change, when it comes, cracks everything open."
—*Dorothy Allison*

When I drafted the outline for this book, this end chapter was tentatively titled "Who Am I Now?" I had the common idea that we lose ourselves in menopause and come out of it as less than we were or as someone else entirely.

I suppose that's still possible (if so, may I come out of it as a vengeance demon reincarnation of Sylvia Plath, please?), but that doesn't seem to be what happens for most everyone else, and it also feels unlikely for me.

That's the fear though, isn't it? We're absolutely given that message culturally: that come menopause, it'll be bye-bye us, especially the parts of us we're taught are the good parts. It can even feel like a threat, though the more I've thought about this and considered the usual sources of that threat, the more I suspect

it's a hope on the part of the threatener: they *want* us to go bye-bye with menopause. They're no less scared of us than their forebears were afraid of the menopausal of Salem they burnt, afraid of the old midwives and indigenous elders whose knowledge they criminalized, plagiarized, or erased, afraid of the powerful, purportedly guilty or hysterical women they slandered or locked up.

Unlike those with puberty or pregnancy, the changes with menopause are almost always painted as losses: loss of the ability to reproduce, power, privilege, allure, visibility, value—loss of ourselves. We certainly can experience loss of many kinds, but I feel like, on the whole, that picture of menopause *as loss* is a deeply demoralizing lie that sets us up to dread it—which then makes us more likely to have a tougher time of menopause, no less—and our lives and selves after it. The idea that we won't be our whole selves anymore is a particularly egregious lie.

In season two of the brilliant Phoebe Waller-Bridge's (I cannot wait to see what *she* does in menopause) show *Fleabag*, the title character encounters Belinda, played by Kristin Scott Thomas. Belinda is receiving one of those awards that's for "women in . . . " rather than, you know, people, and as Fleabag joins her at the bar, she explains why she thinks gendered awards are infantilizing bullshit. She then launches into this soliloquy:

"I've been longing to say this out loud—women are born with pain built in, it's our physical destiny—period pain, sore boobs, childbirth, you know. We carry it with ourselves throughout our lives. Men don't. They have to invent things like gods and demons. . . . They create wars so they can feel things and touch each other . . . and we have it all going on in here. Inside, we have pain on a cycle for years. Just when you feel you're making peace with it, what happens? The menopause comes, the fucking menopause comes, and it is the most wonderful fucking thing in the world. And yes, your entire pelvic floor crumbles and you get fucking hot and no one cares. But then you're free, no longer a slave, no longer a machine with parts, you're just a person, in business."

"I was told it was horrendous," Fleabag says.

Belinda replies, "It is horrendous, but then it's magnificent. Something to look forward to."

Setting aside some of what's not great in there (I swear, no one's entire pelvic floor "crumbles" just because of *menopause*, and, of course, the whole world doesn't just boil down to men and women, and just *oof* on the slave talk), this feels like the kind of talk about menopause we've been waiting for. Talk about the positive things it can bring, and not for everyone else—but for *us*. Talk about how we don't lose us but instead might just finally be able to really find and *have* us. Also, Kristin Scott Thomas apparently feels exactly about menopause as her character did, which is delightful.

Some of the problem is that these kinds of conversations and presentations are harder to find than they should be. But it's extra hard to find them if we're not looking for them in the first place. The invisibility so many complain about or fear is something most of us have been complicit in, and probably without even knowing it, because how do you know you're complicit in something you can't see in the first place?

By virtue of working on this book, I started to see more of who and what I hadn't seen before.

I began to discover the menopausal parts of people's lives I hadn't even considered looking for before or known might have been part of who I admired in them. Did you know Stevie Nicks had a horrible menopause? In an interview she said, "Rock and menopause do not mix. It is not good, it sucks, and every day I fight it to the death, or, at the very least, not let it take me over." But from what I can tell from the timing, she made *Trouble in Shangri-La*, arguably one of her best albums, fresh out of it. The Stevie Nicks I look up to isn't twenty-something Stevie—however great she was then too. She's postmenopausal Stevie, a much more interesting person. (Also, I now have acquired the skills to identify which albums I believe were a given artist's menopausal and postmenopausal works, perhaps one of my best parlor tricks ever.)

Learning about Stevie's menopause, Virginia Woolf's menopause, Michelle Obama's menopause, Susie Bright's menopause, Judy Norsigian's menopause, Patrick Califia's menopause, my neighbor's menopause, my mother's menopause, her mother's menopause, and the experiences of so many of the people I talked to and read about made so clear that I hadn't been told or shown a lot of things we all should. But I also hadn't known to start looking for them; nor did I have any idea what I'd find once I did.

LIKE OTHER CARD-CARRYING FEMINISTS of my generation, I've long loved *Thelma and Louise*. When it came out, I slapped a "Caution: Thelma and Louise on Board" bumper sticker on my Ford Tempo. I usually drove alone and enjoyed broadcasting what I felt was a message that I was two very angry women with nothing to lose all wrapped up in one person and so should not be messed with.

In the last half hour of the film, Thelma, after deciding not to go back to her old life, tells Louise something has just crossed over in her. She says, "I don't ever remember feeling this wide-awake." They're driving at night through dark canyons, without speaking, while Marianne Faithfull's "The Ballad of Lucy Jordan" (oh my god, the perfection of that choice) speaks instead. They're quiet, but who they are in those moments is so loud. They're contemplative, but it isn't soft; it's very intense: like a fire about to catch. It feels like a moment of two people not only having just figured out all of who they are but fully *being* all of who they are.

I know the ending isn't everyone's favorite. I suspect that as a suicidal person, it's more palatable to me, maybe even a little validating. But what feels like a bigger part of that ending to me than the suicide is the ownership of their choice. Their absolute, immutable agency, even in a moment where they seem so trapped. Their sureness, fearlessness. Their incredible acceptance of themselves but also of their lives and what the whole of them will be. The clarity that they've crossed over from being able to tolerate lives that they shouldn't have been tolerating in the first place, where they couldn't even know all of who they were.

That's what I think happens to a lot of us with menopause, whether that's about how it makes us feel physically or emotionally, what it takes or what it gives, what impact it has on our lives or just what's going on with the whole *rest* of our lives at the same time. If we can get there—which often involves taking better care of and better centering and prioritizing ourselves—something can cross over in us. We won't be a whole different person: we'll still be ourselves. We'll be ourselves who have broken through to a different place, potentially one where we are more able to be ourselves as *we* see us, more on our own terms. I don't mean to be dramatic, but a lot of us have *literally* walked through fire in this, okay? Just by virtue of getting through this, we'll have crossed over.

Who are we when we're driving across country in the solitary night, knowing our old lives are behind us, trying on freedom?

It might be how we managed menopause: there are a whole lot of seemingly minor everyday rebellions that could make a whole lot of difference in a lot of menopausal people's lives. It might be in how we think about menopause—even if there are losses that ache, we also may lose dead weight and crappy baggage.

It could be an adjustment in how you envision yourself in or after menopause:

What if you aren't lost or diminished but you've instead gone rogue? Just like *Thelma and Louise*, you get to decide what that looks like: that's the whole point. Maybe it looks like highway robbery or stranger sex, or maybe it looks like finally being able to stay in bed all day when you want to or saying no to people or saying yes to yourself.

HELLO FROM THE OTHER SIDE

I've got some good news for you this time. Are you sitting down? Of course you are. You're exhausted. Are you sitting up?

Nearly every postmenopausal person I talked to, whose writing I read, or whose voice I listened to said that life is *better* on the other side of this. Not just better than in *peri*menopause, because what isn't? A root canal can be better than this; listening to a man in his twenties talk about himself for an hour can even be better than this.

They sometimes even say life is better on the other side than it was for them *before* perimenopause.

When I first started talking to people about menopause, and I was talking to someone on the other side, I'd ask how it is in the same way that you'd ask someone how that supposedly edible fried bug tastes or how many days are left in electoral primary season. I'd steel myself for bad news. But I never got that dreaded answer. Joan Price said, "Menopause led me to make a change that determined the whole rest of my life. Menopause liberated me." She isn't at all alone in feeling that way. The more people I talked to about this, the more I'd get *excited*, instead of full of dread, when I realized I was talking to someone I could ask about postmenopause. I'd settle in, get cozy, and be all ears, like I was about to hear my favorite story.

It *is* my favorite story these days.

It is awesome knowing that life after menopause isn't the misery our culture so often indoctrinates us to believe it will be and that there's a veritable legion of people postmenopause who feel even *more* like themselves—even better, *more* at home in their bodies—and sometimes feel *so* good that even when menopause was miserable for them, they're expressing gratitude for it. It's an exhale, that whole thing.

Postmenopausal people express big feelings of freedom, self-acceptance, confidence, connection, and deeper intimacy, of being able to find a clarity about their wants and feelings and a greater ability to express them. This is legit. Margaret Freaking Mead talked about the power of this "postmenopausal zest."

Here are some other excellent surprises.

The risk of major depressive disorder goes way down postmenopause, and rates of depression are also considerably lower than they are for both peri- and premenopausal people. No one tells you that people having the best sex are more often *post*menopausal than premenopausal. It is potentially gender affirming for as many people as it may create gender conflicts for, and those for whom it creates conflicts may find they can resolve them by reimagining gender and identity in ways that feel more like home than the old ways ever did anyway. Most of the most disruptive physical and cultural parts of both pre- and perimenopause stop postmenopause: the often unpredictable disruption of hormonal cycling or menstrual pain and mood issues, hot flashes and night sweats (not for everyone, sorry to say, but for most, and they do get less intense, even if they continue), the anxiety, the worry, the fear, and (oddly often presented as a loss, like our loss of value to men who only value us for our biological offerings or vulnerabilities) the ways our world has exploited, oppressed, and limited us through them.

Almost everyone I talk to on the other side of all this tells me it's great. It speaks volumes that I keep being surprised by that and that almost everyone I tell that to keeps being surprised by it.

I should know by now that my own internalized ageism, ableism, sexism, and other emotional and cognitive sociomaladies are probably the primary sources of my ideas about what it's like after this. After all, my fears about this don't square with almost any of my experiences with people on the other side of menopause. When I run my fingers over my memory's rolodex of older women and gender-diverse people, I'm largely remembering people who are spirited, vibrant, beautiful, electric, and full of piss and vinegar. Everybody has their moments and their challenges, to be sure, but by and large, in my memory, everybody was usually doing pretty okay, and menopause certainly

Austrian royalty. We know she survived a concentration camp.

We know that Maude likes crashing funerals, stealing cars, making art (like the giant tactile vagina in the middle of her living room), inventing things, and engaging in small daily protest. She likes sunflowers and oatstraw tea; she thinks everyone should know how to play an instrument and that it's vital to always seek

> "I had more trouble in my life than anybody.
> But your first big trouble can be a bonanza if you live through it.
> Get through the first trouble, you'll probably make it through the next one."
> —Ruth Gordon

wasn't a thing putting everyone on a slow, crabby march toward death.

I FIRST SAW THE 1971 FILM *HAROLD AND MAUDE* when I was eleven. I deeply imprinted, perhaps becoming the only kid on earth who wanted to be a fictional octogenarian when I grew up.

I keep thinking about Maude not just because I always do but because we only see Maude at just shy of eighty in the film and learn little about who she was before. We know that Maude had a big love—who was in a penal colony, no less—and can tell from her face that the loss was horribly painful and never stopped being painful. We know that she loved growing up seeing posh

out new experiences. We know Maude takes a twenty-something lover, Harold, on the last few days of her life before she, as planned, takes herself out of life on her eightieth birthday.

We don't hear anything about Maude's menopause, but in order to get from Maude as a young girl in Austria to the Maude of the railroad car house with the hookah and the politely fuck-the-police Maude, she had to cross this particular bridge. Knowing all I know now about menopause, what it can ask of us, and how our experience of it can impact us, not only must menopause have happened to Maude, but Maude's menopause experience, and getting to the other side of it, was possibly part of how she would end up **exactly** as the eighty-year-old who had both eleven-year-old me and fifty-year-old me so starry-eyed.

How else was Maude so confident and comfortable in her body that she'd still model nude for her friend Glaucus? And take a young lover? Where else would she have learned to accept herself so ferociously and passionately but in menopause?

When it's learned that Harold has had sex with Maude, he's taken to several people for evaluation. Cultural norms being what they are, there's wide agreement in the movie that someone who wants to be sexual with an elderly woman who looks like an elderly woman must be pathological. A priest describes, each word dripping with disgust and disdain, the mere idea of Harold's young body with Maude's body: "[the image of] the withered flesh, sagging breasts and flabby buttocks makes me want to vomit."

Maude would have been very familiar with those attitudes. It's not like any of us are spared them, long before we get to be that age ourselves. It's also not like they can have zero impact: you can't just not feel strong, en masse cultural disdain for your body. I have to figure that if she got to the point where she was still down with her body and her sexuality at that stage of life, she *clearly* didn't get stuck in a body-hating rut or a desirability-insecurity

crisis in menopause. It seems obvious to me that she worked her way through those changes and then used those adaptive skills ever after.

Maude is a cloak of invisibility *ninja*. She even manages to steal cars while in polite conversation with police officers and priests by virtue of being assumed a sweet, unthreatening little old lady. She can walk through a funeral with a bright pink umbrella and still blend in. I get the impression she's even been overtly squatting in her amazing railroad car house for a good decade or more.

I firmly believe Maude learned the breath-of-fire technique she uses every morning to help manage hot flashes and menopausal stress. Desperate times, desperate learning of breathing techniques.

She, too, may have had a literal monster of a vaginal infection, an ex who emotionally abandoned her, fucking insensitive children/bosses/parents/lovers/cats, crummy health insurance, and a hideously long sexual dry spell in menopause, of all times; she, too, may have lost a home, thrown useless herbs across the room, cried for months, or experienced a strongly misanthropic phase with more than one highly detailed revenge fantasy. Even Maude's choices at the end of her life make clear she learned, somewhere in there, to be wholly self-possessed, without doing anything more than simply being, accepting, and celebrating herself. Maybe menopause was some of the most powerful stuff with which she created the Gospel of Maude: it would make perfect sense, wouldn't it?

WE *COULD* ACQUIRE SKILLS WE MIGHT pick up in menopause; adjust our mindsets or lives; change, end, or create the relationships we do; and learn whatever it is we learn about ourselves in other ways. Some of it, anyway.

In spite of myself and my deep resentment of some of my menopause experience, I have to acknowledge that it might even be, in some respects, the only way to learn some of the things we do in this. It is, truly, a unique and new experience.

The postmenopausal IDGAF is so often represented as *only* giving a fuck about yourself and giving none for other people. But Maude cares deeply about other people, about all people, but is still wholly IDGAF in about every way I can think of. Maude is Our Blessed Lady of IDGAF. Her brand of giving-no-fucks is based in freedom—everyone's freedom—not in lack of compassion or self-centeredness, even though she is certainly the center of all she is and does.

That menopause is perhaps a way to more power or sustained power or a new kind of power isn't what's most interesting, inspiring, or motivating for me personally. That it might be a way to finding more *freedom*? Now we're talking.

Mona Eltahawy finds a way—of course she does, because it's what she does—to merge power *and* freedom:

I cut my hair off because of the pandemic, but also for perimenopausal me, to make room for Mona that I am moving towards. Menopausal Mona. I'm moving towards this new era in my life. There's this beautiful line in Assata Shakur's poem *Love*: "Pregnant with freedom." I was like, *That's it! Pregnant with freedom*. I have wanted to give birth to myself, all the different times in my life where I am freeing myself from things. That's how I see this journey, to become pregnant with freedom, to give birth to myself, and to liberate myself using language that is usually a very patriarchal way of expressing what it wants women to be and what I've always rejected. I'm like, *No room in this womb for you! This womb is **mine!*** I feel this tremendous, incredible sense of power that I did not have before. If you talked to me about power two years ago and how I felt, I would do my feminist lip service to power, which I've always paid, but it would've, for me, sounded hollow. Now I am like, *Fuck everything. I will fucking destroy you.* I feel that no! I feel it! I feel such an incredible sense of power right now. I'm like, *Wow, if it's gonna get even more?* because I'm almost on the other side and I can't fucking wait.

Omisade Burney-Scott said that "by reimagining yourself constantly in this,

this aging thing, I feel like we're having so many conversations while we've been quarantining reimagining life, reimagining relationships, reimagining connection, reimagining intimacy, reimagining care."

Leah Lakshmi Piepzna-Samarasinha provided a gloriously dreamy-but-doable illustration of doing exactly that:

I want to change the street sign wherever we end up and call it Old Femme Road, like Lil' Nas X's *Old Town Road*, but different. Somewhere where you can't ride no more and nobody can tell me nothing. I want to envision a for-real future that's me as an old-ass femme, where I have pleasure and community and access, and where I don't have to be a skinny mountain climber who's able-bodied or else I might as well be dead or in a nursing home. I want to make a place where we can lie the fuck down and still have sensual, sexual, other forms of pleasure, but where I'm doing the prework to make it possible, which means the farm is all raised beds that are four feet, so if I become a wheelchair user, I can still be in my garden.

IN MY EARLY THIRTIES, I WAS IN EDINburgh for a friend's wedding, and the night before, a bunch of us headed out to a neighborhood pub. While we were there, two women came in. They looked to be in their fifties. One had slippers and pajama pants on; the other had actual pants on and half her hair in rollers. None of this was on my radar then, but looking back with what I know now, it's probably safe to say at least one of them—probably both—was menopausal in one way or another. The pants that probably fit slightly better last year or even last week, the rounder middles, the easy flush, the middle school awkwardness, the to-hell-with-it-all-I-surrender aroma.

They might well have started drinking before they got there, or maybe they were stone-cold sober—and Scottish—and just didn't give a damn. However they came to their very loud zeal, they soon fired up Billy Joel on the jukebox (really, Scotland?)—"Uptown Girl," even, of all things—started into some drinks, and almost immediately climbed onto the bar, trying to get the entire room to dance with them as they laughed and ah-ah-ah-ah-ah-ah-ahed for their own great delight and amusement.

Them. That's who I want to be—stay? be again?—when I'm their age. That's what I thought then (and probably also said very loudly and drunkenly, and hopefully they took it as I meant it), and that's what I still think now. Not the Billy Joel. *Obviously.* The point is I don't mean be them literally; I mean be them symbolically. Lord grant me the confidence—and if not the confidence, at least the bottomless proverbial scotch—of a menopausal woman at the pub in her rollers with her friend singing something completely horrible at the top of her lungs with boundless joy and not seeming to care about what any of her neighbors think. Let me bring that kind of flavor to my life at least with semi-regularity if I can't all the time (which I probably won't be able to, because who has the energy?).

Benedetta Barzini's dream speaks to me. Thelma and Louise's abandon. The clumsy, raucous, un-self-conscious joy of the Edinburgh broads. Leah's delicious community, Mona's power and hungry freedom, Omisade's ripe imagination. Maude's lyrical, quietly troublemaking, radical, beautiful, justice- and pleasure-centered life.

As much as my prickly, eye-rolling Gen X heart bristles at my saying so, I think the truth of the matter is that menopause—what it's asked of me, how it's felt, all this goddamn thing has put me through, reading about it, talking about it—creates some opportunities that

clarifying, courage inducing, fortifying. As tired as our menopausal transition can make us feel, it can also give us energy—energy from anger, from determination to get through this damn thing, from some of the neurochemicals hormonal shifts can fire up—and no small measure of chutzpah.

There can be opportunity and possibility even in some of our darker places. Feeling like we have lost any part of who we were, like we know ourselves less, or dealing with the loss of abilities, feelings, self-perceptions, or patterns that were integral parts of our identities can be massively disorienting and very painful. At the same time, that, and whatever grieving process we allow and make for ourselves, can clear the ground for some reconceptualization and some reinvention. We often learn to think about this as taking things away from us, and in some ways it does. But when we learn that, we rarely learn that in taking some

"Radical simply means 'grasping things at the root.'"
—Angela Davis

we could probably come by in other ways, and some people do, but gives us one way we might not have given ourselves otherwise.

The flux and limbo and chaos and uncertainty suck in a lot of ways, but they also offer us some things. They can be

things away, it might not limit us but instead make us more boundless.

Menopause isn't, and never was, *Change, The.*

I don't think the idea that it is has ever served anyone particularly well in this.

Even though menopause creates chemical and physical changes, some of them major, I don't think those changes, *in and of themselves, anyway,* are usually all that life changing.

I think if and when this experience feels like The Change, it's because it's been a catalyst or vehicle for bigger change. That may be change that happens because the world or people in it treat us differently. But it can, more powerfully, be a way to change how we see and experience ourselves and how we care for ourselves. Dr. Lexx said, "I think this can be when people who were born with a uterus start to get the empowerment of quitting the idea that self-sacrificing equals goodness."

In other words, this can be what change we make of it. And when it feels like *The Change* in a now-a-major-motion-picture kind of way, I'm pretty sure that's usually why, not because, or just because, babies can't be made anymore or estrogen levels are different. It's because any really big change is **us**, not hormones, not other people; not what happens *to* us, but what *we do with it.*

When people ask what they can do about some or all of their menopause, the answers are often very specific: this kind of hormone therapy or that plant medicine, this medication or that lubricant, this diet or that, this exercise or that sort of breathing. But I think it turns out that the big answer is simply (and

not so simply) this: **radical self-care and self-centering**. I'm talking about self-care and self-centering that shouldn't *seem* radical, especially since so much of it is what we all needed to be doing all along, what we long should have been supported in. (I'm also talking about centering ourselves in healthy ways, not about being a horrible, self-absorbed jerk to other people. I figure you know that, but the world being what it is, I'm saying it anyway.) And yet, here so many of us are, still just starting to consider that centering and caring for ourselves in real, sustained, dedicated ways may be the answer to this and so many of life's other burning questions.

We need to make more time and space for ourselves, however that looks for us, and, ideally, we need to be in relationships, workplaces, communities, and cultures that support us instead of, as is so often the case, standing in the way of or otherwise undermining us and our well-being.

There's no one medicine or herb or food or doctor or exercise that will universally make the experience of menopausal transition good or better for everyone: we're all just way too different. But I do think we can soundly say that radical self-care—and by that I really just mean that we always put our own oxygen mask on first, allowing ourselves what care we need for ourselves, uniquely, centering our needs—is a universally right approach for everyone's menopause. **Everyone's.**

277

When we start to make room for that way of living, managing even a tough menopause gets easier. Real-deal self-centering and self-care also make questions like why we still exist post-reproductively and what our purpose is appear to be the absolute garbage they are. We still exist because we do. Our purpose is all of what it has been and what we want it to be (including nothing at all but farting around, if that's what we wanted and still want). Radical self-care is what's going to get us through this kind of endlessly inane questioning of the validity of our existence, through menopause, and through all of the many other changes that are still yet to come.

THE WHOLE TIME I WAS WORKING ON this book, I had something Joan Didion wrote in 1979 written where I could see it:

A place belongs forever to whoever claims it hardest, remembers it most obsessively, wrenches it from itself, shapes it, renders it, loves it so radically that he remakes it in his own image.

I thought that was about this book, but as I look at it now, here, at the end of this book, in the endless middle of my menopause, this stage of my life, I realize it could just as easily be about myself, about ourselves, and even menopause, of all things.

We aren't lost in this, even if we experience and feel some loss in it. Even if we become, at times, so delirious from loss of sleep and overabundance of heat, stress, impatience, and hormones from hell that we *feel* lost. We aren't lost in this, even though the world most of us live in tells us that we are or will be. We're right here the whole time, and we're still right here on the other side. Who we are then depends on who we found ourselves to be in this and whom we bring to the other side.

A MENOPAUSAL (VERY) MINI-HERBAL

"For fast-acting relief, try slowing down."
 —*Lily Tomlin*

efore I say anything else: the standard-issue disclaimer! This is a list that includes a bunch of plant substances. **They are not safe merely by virtue of being plants or from plants.** Goji berries can be bad news for people using diabetes medications. Cocaine is an alkaloid of the coca plant. Hemlock is a plant. The poison ricin comes from plants. I love plants, but just like you and me, just because they're loveable doesn't mean they can't be dangerous. The following things may or may not have impacts you want or expect. Checking for possible interactions—either in general or at a certain dose—with existing medications, supplements, or other herbs you're using and any health conditions you may have is always a good idea, as is sticking with whatever recommended amount is suggested on the bottle or by a healthcare practitioner or herbalist. When at all possible, consult with a qualified care practitioner, and be sure and let any healthcare providers you're working with know if you're using any of these, especially if they're prescribing you anything else.

ADAPTOGENS, NOOTROPICS, AND OTHER KINDS OF PLANTS THAT MAY BE MORE HELPFUL THAN THESE DOUCHEY-SOUNDING NAMES FOR THEM SUGGEST

Adaptogens are plants—often known from Ayurvedic and traditional Chinese medicine (TCM), mostly herbs, roots, and mushrooms—or nutrients understood and found to provide a counterbalance to your cortisol levels. Adaptogens specifically aren't known to possess addiction, tolerance, and abuse potentials, and they also don't impair cognitive function. Many are also anti-inflammatory, which is a nice perk.

"Nootropic" is a term for substances that can potentially help with cognitive function. These can include pharmaceuticals like Adderall but also nutrients and plant substances. Like coffee, for instance, my own nootropic of choice since 1981. It's our ruby anniversary this year, apparently, an appropriate testament to the hot flash a cup of it always gives me now.

Unless you're very sensitive to any of these, the effects—any hot flashes notwithstanding—will be subtle. You're not likely to get blotto on gentian root or turn into Mozart with bacopa. Same goes for the few other kinds of plants mentioned here. They can be found in a range of forms, including teas, tinctures, and powders (which can easily be added to smoothies, juices, or other blended drinks, including warm ones, like lattes).

A FEW STRESS BALANCERS AND SLEEP HELPERS

Ashwagandha

B vitamins

Chamomile

Holy (or tulsi) basil (This one's a two-fer, potentially good for calm *and* cognition.)

Magnesium

Nettle (Like holy basil, it could fit in the list below too: it can help energize *and* de-stress.)

Raw cacao

Reishi and cordyceps mushrooms

Schisandra berry (This one, too, can calm and help with cognition.)

Turmeric root

Valerian root

A FEW ENERGIZERS AND COGNITIVE HELPERS

Amino acids L-theanine and creatine

Bacopa monnieri

Caffeine

Gentian root

Gingko biloba

Gotu Kola

He Shou Wu (Fo-Ti)

Licorice root

Omega-3s

Pine pollen

Rhodiola root

Shatavari

CANNABIS

Cannabis can potentially help with a range of menopause issues and impacts and has been suggested for this purpose in the Western canon alone for at least a hundred years. It may help with sleep, stress, mood, joint or genital pain, muscle tension, and sexual desire, among other things. It can sometimes help with focus and other times result in forgetting what you were supposed to be focusing on in the first place.

The two main compounds of cannabis are tetrahydrocannabinol (THC) and cannabidiol (CBD). As they explain simply at Leafly,

THC is defined by what cannabis makes you feel, while the effects of CBD can't be felt. The important distinction is that, unlike THC, CBD will not intoxicate you. It also addresses one of the most common reasons people choose to use CBD—pain management. CBD can also block some of the intoxicating effects of THC. By binding to cannabinoid receptors, it will keep THC from activating those receptors. This translates to a less intense psychoactive effect. . . . This does not mean that CBD, by itself, cannot offer an effect. High doses of CBD often produce a profoundly relaxing experience. Like stepping out of a hot tub, your body may feel tingly and relaxed, and your brain may be clear.

There are currently tons of different ways to use either or both: by smoking or vaping or through topicals, edibles, tinctures, patches, drinks, and suppositories (vaginal or rectal). You name it, there's a way to utilize cannabis in it right now. Menopausal folks might want to especially have an eye on CBD, THC, or CBD and THC lubricants and other genital topicals, which can help with pain or discomfort, as well as topicals for joint or muscle pain.

This really is something where, by and large, you're just going to have to experiment to find what works for you. You can also likely get pointed in your best directions by having a detailed discussion with a cannabis dispensary worker, a care provider, or a cannabis expert.

With CBD so much more accessible right now, and more often legal, as well

as something some people prefer or are only okay with, Ashley Manta pointed out something important: "CBD alone is most effective in very high doses, around 10 to 20 milligrams per kilogram of body weight. My colleague, Dr. Jordan Tishler, MD, often notes that doses of CBD much lower than that are likely placebo." Check those dosages when you're looking to buy CBD. You'll find that in a lot of CBD products being sold right now, many don't appear to have anywhere near the amount of CBD in them to actually do anything.

Don't forget that cannabis (even when it's CBD only), like everything else, can interact with some medications, so if possible, double-check with your healthcare provider, if you can, about cannabis use with whatever you are taking. If you can't, the internet can be a highly useful place for this kind of thing.

AND OTHER PLANTS

The following are some of the most common botanicals often suggested or used expressly for perimenopause and postmenopause, most often for vasomotor issues in particular. These aren't representative of anywhere near everything used or suggested in indigenous traditions or medicines: for those, you'll want to consult indigenous sources, providers, and educators. It's especially important to recognize that it's a distinctly Western approach to look for things to treat a "symptom," the way we do, an approach that won't work well or at all with some other modalities. For instance, herbal formulas in traditional Chinese medicine have been found effective for an array of perimenopausal impacts. But TCM involves taking all the systems of the body into account, so you are going to have much better luck getting a formula through a qualified practitioner than picking up something that works for a friend:

◊ Wild yam*
◊ Black cohosh*
◊ Evening primrose oil*
◊ Chaste berry (Vitex)
◊ Red clover*
◊ Maca
◊ Kudzu
◊ Motherwort
◊ Dong quai*
◊ Fenugreek
◊ Ginseng*

* Found as effective as or less effective than placebo in studies.

You'll run across reference to some herbs—like motherwort, black cohosh, He Shou Wu, and licorice root, for example—as *estrogenic*. The phytoestrogens discussed as follows can fall under that umbrella too. That means they may or do bind to estrogen receptors and may increase or act like estrogen. Studies on

this have been limited, inconclusive, and almost entirely only done on mice or cells in vitro, but a review of them suggests, as with phytoestrogens below, that in the event anyone needs to or is very concerned about avoiding estrogens, avoiding these may be wise for the time being since we just can't say for sure what the effects may be.

PHYTOESTROGENS

Phytoestrogens are some substances, namely isoflavones, that can bind, albeit very weakly, to estrogen receptors in the body. They're sometimes considered to have "estrogen-like" properties and often sold and recommended as alternatives to hormone therapy. Sometimes soy, which has phytoestrogens, is outright touted as what makes menopause easy for people who eat it often. You might hear about phytoSERMs or genistein, similarly, too.

Phytoestrogens are often believed or said to be superior to MHT because they're "natural" and believed to be safer as a result. They may be safer for many people, compared to some forms of MHT, but studies make very clear they are not likely to be even remotely as effective for menopausal impacts, if at all, as MHT.

Some studies and meta-analyses have found phytoestrogens or phytoSERMs effective for hot flashes, though usually no more effective than a placebo or a studied placebo group. Genistein has been found more effective with vasomotor impacts than other phytoestrogens, but again, nowhere near as effective as MHT.

From where I'm sitting, phytoestrogens mostly look like if they help, it's via a placebo effect. There have been many, many studies done on these at this point. It seems clear to me that if they were more effective than a placebo, we would have found out by now.

There also hasn't been long-term study on using these without an opposing progesterone. There could be, however slight, increased risks, when used unopposed, for people who still have a uterus. They may have effects on the endometrium we don't know about. Too, they might be antiestrogenic and block our bodies' estrogens, which obviously isn't what someone who wants to increase estrogen would want.

That all said, no amount of phytoestrogens at the level someone would get just by *eating* soy and other plants with phytoestrogens—rather than using supplements—would likely be unsafe for people, and soy and other plants can offer us other things, even if they don't do anything or much for our menopause impacts. If you can have it, soy offers a lot of known positive health benefits, including with cognition, heart disease, and osteoporosis. It just isn't the miracle cure for menopause it's sometimes touted as.

A MENOPAUSAL (VERY) MINI-HERBAL

APPENDIX

MENOPAUSE FOR THE REST OF US (AKA PEOPLE BORN WITH TESTICULAR SYSTEMS)

JOANNE MASON

Joanne Mason has retired from a lifetime in teaching and educational administration, a career she considers exceptionally rewarding and fulfilling. She has studied gender and sexual identity development extensively. She writes about nature and photography and has published numerous volumes of photography.

As a postsurgical trans woman in my seventies, a regular regimen of systemic estrogen has long been part of my life. I took estrogen and antiandrogens for years ahead of gender-affirming surgery, and I've continued with estrogen since. I've learned from experience that stopping or reducing my regular dose of estrogen brings about unmistakable manifestations of menopause. (Oh, joy! I can experience menopause on demand!)

At some point, those of us born with testicular systems may or may not experience our own versions of menopause. And we are not out of the woods if we're trans or otherwise gender-diverse and choose to medically transition.

As with any other kind of menopause, all of the menopause-like conditions we'll be looking at here have to do with hormones, which Heather has already discussed in Chapter 3.

I want to talk about testosterone first.

In general, the biochemistry of people born with a testicular system is more responsive to testosterone than that of people born with a utero-ovarian system, who are usually more sensitive to estrogen.

Testosterone levels diminish gradually with age for everyone, especially people born with testicular systems. The natural lowering of testosterone aside, depression, hypothyroidism, chronic alcoholism, and the use of medications, including corticosteroids, cimetidine, spironolactone (more on that in a moment), digoxin, opioids, antidepressants, and antifungal agents, can all affect testosterone levels, too.

For people born with testes, this condition of diminishing testosterone is called *hypogonadism* and is also referred to as *andropause*. This differs from what happens with menopause in a few ways: it doesn't mean the end of the ability to reproduce, its progression is more gradual, and its impacts are fewer. Testosterone levels are usually estimated to decline by about 1 percent each year after age thirty. About 30 percent of people will have noticeable impacts around age fifty. Many individuals may not experience any impacts from this until later, and some won't experience noticeable impacts period. Nevertheless, the consequences of a gradual testosterone decline are sometimes significant and can include the following:

- Loss of muscle mass
- Increased body fat
- Osteopenia (a condition involving the loss of bone mass, short of osteoporosis, and brittle bones from a loss of calcium)
- Cognitive impacts
- Irritability, depression, and other mood disorders
- Sleep disturbance

- Loss of motivation
- Sexual issues like difficulty with erection and decreased or absent sexual desire

Treatment for andropause can include testosterone supplementation. If you do this, it's essential to be screened initially and then monitored for conditions including adverse cardiovascular effects and prostate cancer. Some of the possible side effects of testosterone therapy can be partly mitigated by lifestyle changes like increasing exercise or quitting smoking.

THOSE OF US WHO ARE TRANSGENDER can elect to transition socially, medically, or both at any time of life. Purely social transition is not usually implicated in menopause-like conditions, although people born with testes who only transition socially will continue to be subject to hypogonadism or andropause described previously.

Trans women who have the desire, ability, and access can choose to transition medically, with hormone therapy, gender-affirming surgery, or both. Current surgical options include removal of the testes (orchiectomy) or more extensive gender-confirming surgery (orchiectomy plus vaginoplasty, the construction of a vagina). Some trans women pursue other surgeries—like breast enhancement, tracheal shave, and facial plastic feminization—but these have little or no effect in terms of menopause-like symptoms.

Most trans women also use hormone therapy—estrogen and possibly others—either in place of or in addition to surgery. Estrogen, in the form of estradiol, is also produced naturally in people born with testes, though not in the amount that the ovaries can produce. Even without any form of medical transition, this estrogen from the body helps with the maintenance of bone density and strength, brain function, and cardiovascular health. Unless indicated otherwise, when I talk about estrogen therapy, I'm talking about estradiol.

Most trans women having an orchiectomy will experience their own version of menopause almost immediately. That's because the usual requirements of that surgery demand that estrogen (and any other medications that can thin the blood) be halted for a period of time prior to surgery. Levels of estrogen in the blood will drop precipitously, bringing about an estrogen-withdrawal menopause. Estrogen intake can usually be resumed immediately following surgery (fortunately).

With or without surgery, the goals of estrogen therapy for trans people born with testes are twofold: to mitigate the effects of testosterone and to promote the development of physical changes usually associated with feminine secondary sex characteristics. (For more on how estrogen therapy can be administered, revisit Chapter 5.)

If the testes are not removed surgically, they continue to produce testosterone: this makes the progression of changes with estrogen therapy slow. Consequently, many trans women also take a testosterone blocker or antiandrogen, the most common of which is spironolactone. An antiandrogen is part of a typical regimen prior to surgery. Removal of the testes drastically reduces the amount of estrogen required, and an antiandrogen, if one has been taken, is then discontinued.

Sustained estrogen (before and after orchiectomy) usually leads to changes including

❦ decreased libido;
❦ slowing of scalp hair loss, where male pattern baldness progression stops but estrogen does not produce new hair growth;
❦ softer, less oily skin;
❦ breast development, with varying effects;
❦ redistribution of body fat;
❦ decreased muscle mass;
❦ decreased facial and body hair growth, though existing facial hair is usually not completely eliminated;
❦ improved mood.

These results are all gradual, with full development taking as much as three to seven years. The results become enhanced when estrogen therapy is accompanied by removal of the testes or by the use of antiandrogens in concert with estrogen.

For people with intact testes who take estrogen without an orchiectomy, additional results can be expected:

⬦ Decreased spontaneous erections
⬦ Decrease or cessation of semen production
⬦ Testicular and possibly penile atrophy

Hormone therapy in trans women leads to overall psychological improvement, an increase in feelings of well-being, and reduction of gender dysphoria. One systematic review of the research literature concluded that hormone therapy in trans women produced statistically significant psychological improvements, including reductions in depression, psychological distress, anxiety, hostility, and agoraphobia, and an improvement in interpersonal sensitivity. It isn't clear whether these psychological benefits are a biochemical response to the estrogen or the result of greater feelings of self-acceptance and happiness that follow gender-affirming changes. It's probably a combination of both, although estrogen does lead to an increase in serotonin, which may contribute to mood improvements. Notably, these improvements appear with hormone therapy alone, with or without surgery.

Progesterone is another option in hormone therapy for trans women. The metabolism of progesterone is complex. Progesterone acts in concert with estrogen, each reinforcing the effects of the other. Paired with estrogen, progesterone may add the following effects:

⬦ More rapid feminization
⬦ Decreased testosterone production
⬦ Increased breast development
⬦ Increased bone formation
⬦ Improved sleep and relief of vasomotor symptoms (see page 65)
⬦ Cardiovascular health benefits

As noted above, estrogen results in an increase in serotonin. Progesterone has the opposite effect, decreasing serotonin and possibly leading to depression. Dosages of progesterone for trans women that are too high create a risk of breast cancer. However, carefully monitored, progesterone in concert with estrogen can be a helpful part of hormone therapy.

Most of the changes above attributed to estrogen use by trans women are permanent; however, some are reversible. This is what leads to menopause-like conditions when estrogen is stopped or significantly reduced. While the degree of these effects can vary depending on such factors as the length of time on estrogen, dosages, individual estrogen levels, and other medications being taken, the following can occur in fairly short order:

Questionable Practices

There are two practices that, if not completely discredited, are in my view seriously misguided. One way to view hormone therapy in trans women is to view its objective as replicating the gonadal steroid level of hormones in people with intact ovaries. This view is fine so far as it goes. But some medical practitioners have inferred that since hormone levels in people with intact ovaries cycle according to the menstrual cycle, hormone levels in trans women should be induced to cycle as well. This is achieved by taking progesterone for seven to ten days while reducing or stopping estrogen during that period. This practice does not account for the well-being of the trans person. In the first place, actually duplicating the menstrual cycle is next to impossible. In the second place, varying hormone levels in this manner is likely to lead to emotional impacts like mood swings or depression. This practice still has advocates today.

The other approach I question is based on the belief that since people born with ovaries experience a significant reduction in hormone levels at menopause, then trans women should reduce or stop estrogen at middle age, around forty-five, to replicate the phenomenology of ovarian people. This practice, which amounts to inducing menopause in trans women, is just cruel in my view. Fortunately, this practice is rarely advocated today, but it is still encountered.

- Hot flashes (Wow, I can personally attest to this condition.)
- Sleep disturbance (Yes, that too.)
- In some instances, resumption of scalp hair loss
- Increase in oily skin
- Mood variations and instability, irritableness, and occasionally depression

There are other options for gender affirmation or transition for people born with testes, for nonbinary or otherwise gender-diverse people, or for trans women who don't want to use the more common approaches. These include no changes or transition at all, a purely social transition, or limited hormonal treatment through microdosing. Just as nonbinary or transmasculine people can do with testosterone, microdosing in this case can consist of taking an antiandrogen or androgen blocker such as spironolactone and/or small doses of estradiol. This approach tends to generate a subtler degree of feminization or just a gentle push away from undesired physical characteristics or

As for menopause, there is little or no convincing evidence about whether herbal, soy, nutritional, or other treatments can produce the same outcomes hormone therapy can in the first place, and transgender support sites seem to acknowledge this.

feelings. Our medical knowledge of microdosing is new and limited; so is our knowledge of what happens when someone goes off a low dose or microdose of hormones.

Trans persons sometimes consider stopping or reducing estrogen—and so, experiencing this kind of menopause—for a number of reasons including cost and other common barriers to access. Additionally, some trans people choose to detransition, stop transitioning, or otherwise stop taking estrogen simply because they don't feel they want or need it any longer.

OBTAINING GOOD HEALTH AND MEDICAL care is of great importance to trans women. In general, it's important for trans people on hormones or following surgery to have their health monitored.

In seeking medical care, a helpful internist or family doctor can be a godsend, but unfortunately not all are educated about trans health or even try to be helpful to trans people. A good endocrinologist is usually more knowledgeable about the hormonal aspects of trans care, but I have found that not all endocrinologists are equally committed to sensitive and supportive care for trans people.

Transgender people have existed forever, but it's only recently that older trans people have begun to be such a large and visible critical mass. Cultures around the world have been changing, and acceptance of trans people has never been greater.

Estimates of the number of transgender people vary greatly, mainly due to the lack of clear criteria and methods for counting a population with so many varieties of identification. According to a 2011 report by the National Gay and Lesbian Task Force, 37 percent of trans women are age forty-five or older, and 21 percent of trans women were fifty-five or older when they transitioned. As the population ages, these numbers will surely increase. Although lots of attention is being paid today (and rightly so) to trans youth, for those of us who are aging (rapidly it often seems), our health needs, lives, and experiences are a real concern. Unfortunately, much of the current focus and research on trans healthcare is on younger trans people just beginning hormone therapy. Far less information and research exist for older trans people who are beginning to deal with issues of aging.

Aging affects trans women much as it does menopausal or postmenopausal people born with utero-ovarian systems. The biology of trans women postsurgery and after many years of hormone therapy sure seems more or less the same as that of people born with ovaries postmenopause, but the fact is we just don't yet know. What *is* clear is that the endocrinological profiles are nearly the same. Surgery and years of hormone therapy succeed in driving our testosterone levels to near zero while raising estrogen levels to nearly the same as those in people born with utero-ovarian systems. There's also research to suggest that the neuroanatomy of older trans women is closer to that of those born with utero-ovarian systems than to those born with testicular systems prior to transition. Our health and medical needs also tend to converge. With only a few exceptions, the health concerns of trans women and cis women as we all age become pretty much the same.

Thus, many of the treatments that are appropriate for menopausal or postmenopausal people born with a utero-ovarian system will also be appropriate for trans women. Similarly, treatments and approaches for managing menopause for people with utero-ovarian systems will probably also often be helpful in managing corresponding impacts for those of us born with testicular systems. The most successful approach to managing healthcare has been, for me, a good gynecologist who is aware of trans concerns.

A POSITIVE DEVELOPMENT IN RECENT years has been the increasing number of good trans care clinics available. These combine the practice of multiple disciplines and practitioners knowledgeable about and trained in providing healthcare for trans people.

Healthcare for older trans people should be about more than just hormones and biochemistry. All the rest of our health concerns are important too. This certainly includes our psychological needs as well.

While challenges continue to confront us, helpful resources exist. Numerous organizations, churches, and community groups are building welcoming communities. SAGE: Advocacy and Services for LGBT Elders (www.sageusa.org) is one such organization and a powerful resource we should all be familiar with.

If a sympathetic and caring practitioner is found, I find the best approach is to say upfront that you are trans and to ask directly if the practitioner is (1) knowledgeable about trans healthcare, and (2) supportive of trans people. If so, provide your complete medical history. Let the practitioner know if you are not out so they will be sure to provide appropriate confidentiality. Inform them about your preferred pronouns. (See more in Chapter 5 about how to find good healthcare providers.)

Even with a supportive and friendly practitioner, it is still often necessary for us to educate healthcare providers. Trans elders are at significantly greater risk for poor general health, disability, depression, and stress in comparison with people of the same age who aren't trans. Both trans people and healthcare practitioners should be familiar with the information and guidelines in the *Standards of Care for the Health of Transsexual, Transgender, and Gender Nonconforming People* of the World Professional Association for Transgender Health.

I AM FINDING BEING AN OLDER TRANS woman to be a freeing experience.

No longer am I preoccupied with old uncertainties and self-doubts. *Am I feminine enough? Am I too feminine? Do I pass? Is passing an issue? What do my friends really think of me? Family? Is my job, career, affected by my transition?* Rather, I am free to simply be who I am.

There is no one right way to be a trans woman. In my younger years, I was always focused on my feminine presentation. I dressed well and very femme: I always wore makeup and lots of jewelry. Now, I'm more relaxed. I live in jeans. I don't worry about how my presentation is being perceived or if I'm being seen as a trans person. I'm just me, and my presentation is determined simply by what's comfortable for me and appropriate for whatever I'm doing.

Most interesting to me is discovering that my gender identity is becoming more fluid. I still identify as a trans woman, but one who now gravitates more toward nonbinary. (I have always been uncomfortable, intellectually as well as emotionally, with a binary gender paradigm.) This is apparently a thing. I've heard it said by more than a few people (trans as well as cis) that aging is sometimes experienced as a process of "degendering." Or perhaps "regendering." There is even research to support this idea, suggesting that in later life, gender identities become altered in ways that diminish gender differences and clear-cut gender representations.

ACKNOWLEDGMENTS

"Excuse my dust."
  —*Dorothy Parker's suggestion for her epitaph*

I LOVE ATTRIBUTION. ON AN AVERAGE day, I could happily say thank you until my lips fell off, and this is no average day. This is the day I've somehow managed to finish editing this book, of all books, in these conditions, of all conditions. (This is also the last day of the Trump administration, Dolly Parton's seventy-fifth birthday, *and* the day I found my Red Bull stash.) Here I thought that I was being ambitious and more than a little masochistic by just trying to write a perimenopause book from the belly of *that* particular beast. Little did I know everything else that would happen over the course of the last yearish: to me, to all of us.

It's not a complete mystery to me how I pulled this off. I'm absolutely bonkers, for one, obviously. The lesser-known factor is the incredible help and support that I received in this, even while so many of the people who gave me that help and support were themselves in their own various circles of hell; perimenopause included for some, no less.

I have, per usual, surpassed my word count, so they're going to make me keep this brief, a horrible torment when you're the Fozzie Bear of the piece, but I see the tomatoes poised midair, so I will do my best in limited space. Some of you belong in more than one of these lists, but I had to pick but one: please place yourself in all the lists you belong in and know I see you across them. There is no doubt that to my great horror, I will certainly manage to forget someone. Please know it is a measure of my exhaustion and my overextended mind if I do, not of my affection or gratitude. I will write your name in your copy with my blood and tears if that makes you feel any better.

EVERYONE I INTERVIEWED FOR THIS book was part of it, whether their words **293** made it directly onto the pages or not. There's not a single person I spoke with who didn't spark something new in my head or my heart. I'm so grateful for the time all of you gave me, and for the greater depth and breadth of voice, perspectives, and experiences you gave me and this book. Y'all were the freaking dream team. I couldn't be more grateful for the genius and generosity of S. Bear Bergman, Hanne Blank, Jennifer Block, Susie Bright, Dr. Lexx Brown-James, Omisade Burney-Scott, Mandy Carter, Soraya Chemaly, Ronete Cohen, Nina Coslov, Kimberly Dark, Searah Deysach, Mona Eltahawy, Tasha Fierce, Jaclyn Friedman, Tania Glyde, Dr. Judith Hersh, Sharon Lamb, Aida Manduley, Ashley Manta, Emily Nagoski, kiran nigam, Judy Norsigian, Leah Lakshmi Piepzna-Samarasinha, Joan Price, Therese Schecter, Rebecca Scritchfield, Dawn Serra, Leela Sinha, and s.e. smith.

I had some much-needed and deeply appreciated help with some of the research, fact-checking, tactical, editorial, and other logistical bits of all this. Bless your hearts and your fantastic minds: Staśa Morgan-Appel, Michelle Demole, Amanda Friese, Riley Johnson, Laura Jones, Lesley Kinzel, and Jenn Price.

Joanne Mason: thank you for daring to do something no one has done before with me for this book, and for your dedication to the arduous process of getting it right.

Archie Bongiovanni: I just couldn't have asked for a better illustration partner for this. When I already had some ideas, your take on them was always so damn perfect, and when I just threw things out there for improvisation, you always delivered something super amazing. Thank you! Natural fibers forever!

The team at Hachette Go! involved in the production of this here book is just freaking fantastic. All of the icepacks, edibles, and accolades to you, Michelle Aielli, Michael Barrs, Michael Clark, Alison Dalafave, Amanda Kain (*THAT COVER!*), Jennifer Kelland, Mary Ann Naples, Amy Quinn, and Lauren Rosenthal. Bless.

Catherine Buni, Marisa McAdoo, Michell Campbell Hayford, Melanie Davis, and Karen Rayne: thank you for your reads and feedback.

Ann Whidden: I don't even know what to say about your help and just . . . you, save that I adore you. Thank you for everything.

Anna Sproul-Latimer, there couldn't have been a perfecter thing for us to join forces for. I'm so happy you're on my team.

Thanks to my team at Scarleteen, as always, particularly Sam Wall and Rachel Ronquillo Gray for helping hold down the fort so I didn't have to drown in both menopause *and* adolescence 24/7.

Thanks so much to everyone who filled out my survey and to the gang over at the All Gender Peri/Menopause Group who've kept me motivated to finish this thing, made me feel less alone, and lent me support in my own perimenopause and its various maddening mysteries.

To some other members of my chosen friend/fam, thanks for your support (be it with the book or with things that might have otherwise sabotaged my ability to do the book), company, input, ideas, or mere existence in the world: Cath Airola, Veronica Arreola, Emily Burns, Trina Grieshaber, Kate Harding, Ricky Hill, Briana Holtorf, Carson Jones, Janine Jones, Becca Nelson, Daryl Lynn Johnson, Pam Keesey, Jenny Lobasz, Zoe Mendelson, Jacob Mirzaian, Jennifer Peepas, Mark Price, Danya Ruttenberg, Christian Ruzich, CJ Turett, Jess White, Elizabeth Wood, everyone who fights all the good fights at Women and Children First Bookstore, and Deanna Zandt. To my dog, Troublepants, and to Fiona the hippo and her all-too-often-unacknowledged mother, Bibi, who I know can't read, but to whom I express gratitude for here all the same.

To my amazing therapist, Brandy Parris, who has helped me get myself through so much during perimenopause, including this book and everything along with it. My gratitude to Dr. Prema Sanne for her care as well.

Dad, I'm so glad you hung in there. I know it wasn't and still isn't easy: I love you. Maria, I love you, too. Listen: you're going to need this—don't wait to read it until later, trust. It's also okay to call and ask for help (but maybe send a bottle of vodka over first?).

Mom. Who'da thunk that this would be the time of life, of all times, we'd finally be able to start building a decent relationship? It's certainly been one of the better and more unexpected parts of this entire perimenopausal misadventure. Thank you for your help, your support, your openness, your acceptance, and your love. I love you.

Anwar Fucking Khuri: Bless your sweet innocent heart for being so excited when I got the contract for this book even when I told you that you had no idea what perpetual torment the process involved. I've never had a partner so supportive and invested in my work on a book, and even while our world kept falling down and catching on fire around us, no less. Of course, there's never been someone like you in a million ways, and this is but one. I know you won't be so thrilled the next time: that's okay. I'm just hoping you'll still be around, because I love you so much and can't imagine life without you. I just thought you oughta know.

Finally, my beloved Renée Sedliar. Who else could I have done this with? I mean, who else would I want to do this or *any* book with? You are and remain the great love of my editorial life, pal. I'm so happy you found me way back when, so grateful you continue to champion my work, and so sorry when you have to co-suffer for my art. If I believed in marriage, I'd have proposed by now; if I could make you babies (or, more aligned to your wants, kittens), I'd have done that for you. Since neither is the case, I offer you my ideas, my books, and my book-related freakouts, which seems like a raw deal, but (a) you know they mean the most to me, and (b) at least you don't have to pay for the vet or college. Every author should be so lucky as to have an editor like you, but since they're not, I'm glad that at least I get to be. Thank you for *everything*, my clammy comrade. xoxo

RESOURCES (AKA DELIRIUM HOME COMPANION)

HERE ARE A FEW PLACES TO GET STARTED in some key areas with things that I've long or recently liked, loved, or appreciated most. What we love or hate, feel or don't in the menopause space is so personal, a thing reviews of menopause books (ouch!) make painfully clear. These are just some of my own faves. Find me—it's easy—and feel free to ask if you want more specific suggestions or help finding faves better suited to you.

Most of these aren't about menopause specifically; there is a lot of other stuff out there, but unfortunately almost none of it is inclusive in a few ways. A lot of menopausal literature and other resources are also full of fat shaming, ableism, assumptions about healthcare access or economic ability, and other painful or toxic land mines, access barriers, and tone deafness.

When it comes to websites and apps, a lot of *that* is also for profit. You can perhaps understand why I don't want to make or give you a list that includes a bunch of that stuff.

Instead, I've kept the specific-to-menopause content to some of my favorite things I found in my travels, most of which aren't current (so shouldn't be considered accurate as far as things like current medical info goes), and most of which also are not inclusive in ways I wish they were. I do believe, however, they still have considerable merit otherwise, and the same is the case for books listed in the other sections of this list that aren't wholly inclusive. I greatly look forward to a second edition of this book where I'll hopefully have a lot more to choose from that is inclusive of a lot more of us.

MENOPAUSE
BOOKS, ARTICLES, AND HISTORY

1100s: *The Trotula of Salerno*
1800s: Lydia Pinkham and her vegetable compound
~1934–1978: the unsung (mostly) feminist mass media of Maxine Davis

1973: *Menopause: A Positive Approach*, Rosetta Reitz

1975: *Menstruation and Menopause: The Physiology and Psychology, the Myth and the Reality*, Paula Weideger

2003: *Age Ain't Nothing but a Number: Black Women Explore Midlife*, edited by Carleen Bryce

2003: *The Black Woman's Guide to Menopause*, Carolyn Scott Brown

2006: *Our Bodies, Ourselves: Menopause*, Boston Women's Health Collective

2010: *Hot Flushes, Cold Science: A History of the Modern Menopause*, Louise Foxcroft

2015: *The Madwoman in the Volvo*, Sandra Tsing Loh

2015: "Pause," Mary Ruefle, *Granta*

2020: *Menopause (a Comic Treatment)*, edited by MK Czerwiec

2021: "How can therapists and other healthcare practitioners best support and validate their queer menopausal clients?," Tania Glyde, *Sexual and Relationship Therapy*

WEBSITES, FILMS, SHOWS, AND PODCASTS

British Menopause Society (thebms.org.uk)

National Institute for Health and Care Excellence menopause guidelines (https://www.nice.org.uk/guidance/ng23)

North American Menopause Society (menopause.org)

Women Living Better (womenlivingbetter.org) and the great fantastic that is Nina Coslov

2016–current: *Better Things*, television series, Pamela Adlon

2018: *Pause* (*Pafsi*), film, Tonia Mishiali

2019–current: *Black Girls Guide to Menopause*, podcast, Omisade Burney-Scott

2021: *Barb and Star Go to Vista Del Mar* is not about and doesn't even mention menopause, yet is still somehow a menopausal Muppet movie except people are the muppets. I don't know how they did it, but they did.

For more links, including online support groups, playlists, Lydia Pinkham cocktail recipes, and more of my random but specifically menopause-themed mania, see heathercorinna.com/isonfuckingfire

EVERYTHING ELSE
A PATRIARCHY SURVIVAL KIT

1973: *The Portable Dorothy Parker*

1984: *Sister Outsider*, Audre Lorde

1993: *Stone Butch Blues*, Leslie Feinberg

2006: *Gender Trouble: Feminism and the Subversion of Identity*, Judith Butler

2007: *Whipping Girl*, Julia Serano

2015: *This Bridge Called My Back: Writing by Radical Women of Color* (third edition), edited by Cherríe L. Moraga and Gloria E. Anzaldúa

2015: *Trauma and Recovery: The Aftermath of Violence—from Domestic Abuse to Political Terror*, Judith Lewis Herman, MD

2016: *We Were Feminists Once: From Riot Grrrl to CoverGirl®, the Buying and Selling of a Political Movement*, Andi Zeisler

2017: *Living a Feminist Life*, Sara Ahmed

2019: *Rage Becomes Her: The Power of Women's Anger*, Soraya Chemaly

2019: *Down Girl*, Kate Manne

2019: *The Seven Necessary Sins for Women and Girls*, Mona Eltahawy

2020: *Life Isn't Binary*, Alex Iantaffi and Meg-John Barker

BALMS FOR DIET CULTURE, BODY IMAGE, MOVEMENT, SEX, AND SEXUALITY

2000: *Still Doing It*, Joani Blank

2011: *Naked at Our Age: Talking Out Loud About Senior Sex*, Joan Price

2013: *Feminist, Queer, Crip*, Alison Kafer

2014: *Body Respect*, Lindo Bacon, PhD, and Lucy Aphromor, PhD, RD

2015: *Come as You Are (the Surprising New Science That Will Transform Your Sex Life)*, Emily Nagoski, PhD

2016: *Body Kindness*, Rebecca Scritchfield, RDN

2017: *Every Body Yoga*, Jessamyn Stanley

2017: *How to Understand Your Gender: A Practical Guide for Exploring Who You Are*, Alex Iantaffi and Meg-John Barker

2017: *Unscrewed: Women, Sex, Power and How to Stop Letting the System Screw Us All*, Jaclyn Friedman

2018: *Hunger*, Roxane Gay

2018: *Queer Sex: A Trans and Non-binary Guide to Intimacy, Pleasure and Relationships*, Juno Roche

2019: *Fearing the Black Body*, Sabrina Strings

2019: *Fat, Pretty and Soon to Be Old: A Makeover for Self and Society*, Kimberly Dark

2019: *Pleasure Activism: The Politics of Feeling Good*, written and gathered by adrienne maree brown

2020: *A Quick and Easy Guide to Sex and Disability*, A. Andrews

2020: *Fitness for Everyone: 50 Exercises for Every Type of Body*, Louise Green

2020: *Magnificent Sex: Lessons from Extraordinary Lovers*, Peggy Kleinplatz, PhD, and A. Dana Ménard, PhD

2020: *Restorative Yoga for Ethnic and Race-Based Stress and Trauma*, Gail Parker

2020: *What We Don't Talk About When We Talk About Fat*, Aubrey Gordon

2021: *Hell Yeah Self-Care!*, Meg-John Barker and Alex Iantaffi

2021: *Pussypedia: A Comprehensive Guide*, Zoe Mendelson and Maria Conejo

2021: *The Body Is Not an Apology: The Power of Radical Self-Love*, second edition, Sonya Renee Taylor

HOW TO GANG UP WITH EACH OTHER

1969–present: *Our Bodies, Ourselves*, Boston Women's Health Collective

1987 (book) and 1991 (film): *Fried Green Tomatoes at the Whistle Stop Café*, Fannie Flagg

1995: *The Story of Jane*, Laura Kaplan

1999: *All About Love: New Visions*, bell hooks

2014: *Trans Bodies, Trans Selves*, edited by Laura Erickson-Schroth

2018: *Care Work: Dreaming Disability Justice*, Leah Lakshmi Piepzna-Samarasinha

2018: *Rewriting the Rules: An Anti Self-Help Guide to Love, Sex and Relationships*, Meg John Barker

2019: *I Hope We Choose Love: A Trans Girl's Notes from the End of the World*, Kai Cheng Thom

2019: *Turn This World Inside Out: The Emergence of Nurturance Culture*, Nora Samaran

2020: *How We Show Up*, Mia Birdsong

2020: *Mutual Aid: Building Solidarity During This Crisis (and the Next)*, Dean Spade

2020: *Disability Visibility: First-Person Stories from the Twenty-First Century*, Alice Wong

2020: *You Belong: A Call for Connection*, Sebene Selassie

IN CASE OF LIFE 'SPLODY

1969: *I Know Why the Caged Bird Sings*, Maya Angelou

1974: *Pilgrim at Tinker Creek*, Annie Dillard

2007: *The Year of Magical Thinking*, Joan Didion

2013: *Wild*, Cheryl Strayed

2016: *When Things Fall Apart: Heart Advice for Difficult Times*, Pema Chödrön

2017: *Emergent Strategy: Shaping Change, Changing Worlds*, adrienne maree brown

2017: *Trainwreck: The Women We Love to Hate, Mock and Fear…and Why*, Jude Ellison Sady Doyle

2017: *Unfuck Your Brain: Getting over Anxiety, Depression, Anger, Freak-outs, and Triggers with Science*, Faith Harper, PhD, LPC-S, ACS, ACN

2019: *Burnout: The Secret to Unlocking the Stress Cycle*, Emily Nagoski, PhD, and Amelia Nagoski, PDA

2020: *From Shitshow to Afterglow: Putting Life Back Together When It All Falls Apart*, Ariel Meadow Stallings

2020: *Too Happy to Be Sad Girl*, Angel Aviles

NOTES

CHAPTER ONE

8   "As author of *Care Work: Dreaming Disability Justice . . .*" Leah Lakshmi Piepzna-Samarasinha, telephone interview, 06/04/20.*

11   "As disability activist, writer, and my genius friend s.e. smith pointed out when we talked about this . . ." Zoom interview, 04/03/2020.*

12   "'Our bodies are complex, with lots of things going on inside them. And they are wise . . .'" Information from consultations by email and phone with kiran nigam, 05/19/20, 6/28/20, 7/16/20, 8/13/20, and 1/12/21.*

17   "As Black southern feminist mother, leader, and organizer Omisade Burney-Scott . . ." Zoom interview, 5/29/20.*

17   "Writer, storyteller, and author of *Fat, Pretty and Soon to Be Old: A Makeover for Self and Society* Kimberly Dark told me . . ." Zoom interview, 07/21/20.*

CHAPTER TWO

24   "Paula Weideger said in the 1970s . . ." Paula Weideger, *Menstruation and Menopause: The Physiology and Psychology, the Myth and the Reality* (New York: Knopf, 1973), 143.

25   "Giovanni Marinello and Jean Liébault chronicled . . ." Susan Mattern, *Slow Moon Climbs: The Science, History, and Meaning of Menopause* (Princeton, NJ: Princeton University Press, 2021), 270; Barbara Seaman and Laura Eldridge, *The No-Nonsense Guide to Menopause* (New York: Simon & Schuster, 2008), 17.

25   "English physician Thomas Sydenham . . ." Thomas Sydenham and John Pechey, *The Whole Works of That Excellent Practical Physician, Dr. Thomas Sydenham . . . the Fourth Edition, Corrected from the Original Latin, by John Pechey* (United Kingdom: R. Wellington, 1705).

25   "In 1774, John Fothergill published . . ." John Eliot and John Fothergill, *A Complete Collection of the Medical and Philosophical Works of John Fothergill* (United Kingdom: John Walker, 1781); Michael Stolberg, "A Woman's Hell? Medical Perceptions of Menopause in Preindustrial Europe," *Bulletin of the History of Medicine* 73, no. 3 (1999): 404–428, www.jstor.org/stable/44445288.

26   "John Lizars's answer . . ." Louise Foxcroft, *Hot Flushes, Cold Science: A History of the Modern Menopause* (London: Granta Publications, 2011).

26   "Mortality rates were as high as 86 percent with some surgeons who performed the practice . . ." Herbert R. Spencer, "The History of Ovariotomy," *Proceedings of the Royal Society of Medicine* 27, no. 11 (1934): 1437–1444. doi: 10.1177/003591573402701101.

26   "Isaac Baker Brown was Lawson Tait's rival . . ." Helen King, professor emerita, "The Rise and Fall of FGM in Victorian London," *The Conversation*, October 7, 2020, https://theconversation.com/the-rise-and-fall-of-fgm-in-victorian-london-38327.

26   "This, apparently, was a bridge too far . . ." John Studd, "A Comparison of 19th Century and Current Attitudes to Female Sexuality," *Gynecological Endocrinology* 23, no. 12 (2007): 673–681. doi: 10.1080/09513590701708860.

27   "Tilt's treatments for menopause . . ." Daisy Butcher, "Menopause: The Female

Mummy's Curse," *S Y N A P S I S*, October 18, 2017, https://medicalhealth humanities.com/2017/10/17/menopause-the -female-mummys-curse.

27 "You can find him describing those in prior postmenopause as . . . " Edward John Tilt, *The Change of Life in Health and Disease: A Practical Treatise on the Nervous and Other Affections Incidental to Women at the Decline of Life* (United Kingdom: J. Churchill, 1857).

27 "W. W. Bliss held the ovaries . . . " Louise Foxcroft, *Hot Flushes, Cold Science: A History of the Modern Menopause* (London: Granta Publications, 2011), 137.

30 "Estrogen produced from human placenta . . . " J. A. Houck, "How to Treat a Menopausal Woman: A History, 1900 to 2000," *Current Women's Health Reports* 2, no. 5 (October 2002): 349–355. PMID: 12215307.

30 "In the early 1940s, synthetic production began . . . " "The History of Estrogen," University of Rochester Medical Center, February 2016, www.urmc.rochester.edu /ob-gyn/ur-medicine-menopause-and -womens-health/menopause-blog/february -2016/the-history-of-estrogen.aspx.

31 "How could such a serious deficiency disease as menopause seem 'normal' to her?" (and the rest of the Wilsonian garbage that follows) . . . Robert A. Wilson, *Feminine Forever* (M. Evans and Co., 1966).

32 "In 1963, Wilson and his wife, Thelma . . . " Judith A. Houck, "'What Do These Women Want?': Feminist Responses to Feminine Forever, 1963–1980," *Bulletin of the History of Medicine* 77, no. 1 (2003): 103–132, www .jstor.org/stable/44447695.

33 "Ann Neumann writes . . . " "The Future Is Menopausal: Ann Neumann," *The Baffler*, November 18, 2019, https://thebaffler.com /salvos/the-future-is-menopausal-neumann.

34 "According to their son, Ron Wilson, she died . . . " Louise Foxcroft, *Hot Flushes, Cold Science: A History of the Modern Menopause* (London: Granta Publications, 2011).

34 "Ron Wilson has also exposed . . . " Margaret McCartney, "Women Have Been Oversold HRT for Decades," *Guardian*, February 19, 2015, www.theguardian.com /commentisfree/2015/feb/19/misinforma tion-menopausal-women-drugs-companies -hrt.

34 "Ron is still working today . . . " Ron Wilson, "Premarin Regrets," *Tuesday's Horse*, February 10, 2010, https://tuesdays horse.wordpress.com/2010/02/10/premarin -regrets.

34 "In 1969, in his book *Everything You Always Wanted to Know About Sex but Were Afraid to Ask*, psychiatrist David Reuben . . . " Frances B. McCrea, "The Politics of Menopause: The 'Discovery' of a Deficiency Disease," *Social Problems* 31, no. 1 (1983): 111–123. doi: 10.2307/800413.

34 "In 1973, in *Feminist Studies*, Carroll Smith-Rosenberg dissected . . . " Carroll Smith-Rosenberg, "Puberty to Menopause: The Cycle of Femininity in Nineteenth-Century America," *Feminist Studies* 1, no. 3/4 (1973): 58–72, www.jstor.org /stable/1566480.

CHAPTER THREE

37 "It's currently estimated that by 2025, there will be somewhere in the neighborhood of one billion people . . . " Reenita Das, "Menopause Unveils Itself as the Next Big Opportunity in Femtech," *Forbes* magazine, July 24, 2019, https://www.forbes.com/sites/reenitadas /2019/07/24/menopause-unveils-itself-as -the-next-big-opportunity-in-femtech /?sh=46a8e18b6535.

40 "Dr. Nanette Santoro and Dr. Jerilynn Prior . . . " Nanette Santoro, "Perimenopause: From Research to Practice," *Journal of Women's Health* 25, no. 4 (April 1, 2016): 332–339. doi: 10.1089/jwh.2015.5556; N. Santoro, J. R. Brown, T. Adel, and J. H. Skurnick, "Characterization of Reproductive Hormonal Dynamics in the Perimenopause," *Journal of Clinical Endocrinology &*

Metabolism 81, no. 4 (April 1, 1996): 1495–1501. doi: 10.1210/jcem.81.4.8636357; Jerilynn C. Prior, "Perimenopause: The Complex Endocrinology of the Menopausal Transition," *Endocrine Reviews* 19, no. 4 (August 1, 1998): 397–428. doi: 10.1210/edrv.19.4.0341.

40 "'misunderstood, confusing and long'": Maryse Zeidler, "This UBC Researcher Wants to Demystify Perimenopause," *CBC News*, September 13, 2020, www.cbc.ca/news/canada/british-columbia/perimeno pause-jerilynn-prior-ubc-1.5721781.

41 "By the time most of us start to transition into menopause, our stockpile of oocytes . . ." "Hormones and the Menopause Transition," *Obstetrics and Gynecology Clinics of North America* 38, no. 3 (September 2011): 455–466. doi: 10.1016/j.ogc.2011.05.004.

42 "Author, menopause researcher, and Women Living Better cofounder Nina Coslov always wants to be sure people know that . . ." Zoom and email interviews, 04/07/20, 04/08/20, 06/23/20, 12/15/20. *

42 "Dr. Prior says . . ." "Perimenopause: The Ovary's Frustrating Grand Finale," The Centre for Menstrual Cycle and Ovulation Research, August 19, 2019, www.cemcor .ubc.ca/resources/perimenopause-ovary %E2%80%99s-frustrating-grand-finale.

45 "Why Are Estrogen and Progesterone Causing Such a Ruckus, Anyway?": D. C. Deecher and K. Dorries, "Understanding the Pathophysiology of Vasomotor Symptoms (Hot Flushes and Night Sweats) That Occur in Perimenopause, Menopause, and Postmenopause Life Stages," *Archives of Women's Mental Health* 10, no. 6 (2007): 247–257. doi: 10.1007/s00737-007-0209-5; Nanette Santoro and John F. Randolph, "Reproductive Hormones and the Menopause Transition," *Obstetrics and Gynecology Clinics of North America* 38, no. 3 (September 2011): 455–466. doi: 10.1016/j .ogc.2011.05.004; Hannah Nichols, "Estrogen: Functions, Uses, and Imbalances," *Medical News Today*, updated on March 12, 2020, www.medicalnewstoday.com/articles /277177; "Progesterone and Progestins," Hormone Health Network, www.hormone .org/your-health-and-hormones/glands -and-hormones-a-to-z/hormones/progester one; "What Is Estrogen?," Hormone Health Network, www.hormone.org/your-health -and-hormones/glands-and-hormones-a -to-z/hormones/estrogen; Harvard Women's Health Watch, "When Thoughts Become Obsessions," Harvard Health Publishing, January 2006, www.health.harvard .edu/newsletter_article/When_thoughts _become_obsessions; "Understanding the Reproductive System," Women Living Better, December 31, 2019, https://women livingbetter.org/reproductive-system.

50 "Dr. Judith Hersh, an OB/GYN, NAMS-certified menopause practitioner . . ." Zoom interview, 06/01/20.*

53 "'Premature' Menopause or Primary Ovarian Insufficiency . . ." Boston Women's Health Collective, *Our Bodies, Ourselves: Menopause* (New York: Simon & Schuster, 2006), 61.

53 "POI is menopause that happens . . ." "Primary Ovarian Insufficiency in Adolescents and Young Women," American College of Obstetricians and Gynecologists, July 2014, www.acog.org/clinical/clinical -guidance/committee-opinion/articles /2014/07/primary-ovarian-insufficiency -in-adolescents-and-young-women.

54 "Sinéad O'Connor recently talked about . . ." Geoff Edgers, "Sinéad O'Connor on Religion, Dealing with Pain and the Right to Be Forgotten," *Independent*, March 23, 2020, www.independent.co.uk/arts -entertainment/music/sinead-oconnor -tour-dates-where-songs-a9412336.html.

55 "As you may recall, modern American gynecology . . ." Brynn Holland, "The 'Father of Modern Gynecology' Performed Shocking Experiments on Slaves," History.com, August 29, 2017, www.history.com/news /the-father-of-modern-gynecology-per formed-shocking-experiments-on-slaves.

NOTES

55 "This kind of abuse continues today in disproportionate use of hysterectomy . . . " Beata Mostafavi, "Understanding Racial Disparities for Women with Uterine Fibroids," University of Michigan, August 12, 2020, https://labblog.uofmhealth.org /rounds/understanding-racial-disparities -for-women-uterine-fibroids.

GENERAL HYSTERECTOMY INFORMATION:

OBOS Common Medical Conditions Contributors, "When Is a Hysterectomy Needed?," Our Bodies Ourselves, October 15, 2011, www.ourbodiesourselves.org /book-excerpts/health-article/when-is-a -hysterectomy-needed.

"Hysterectomy," National Women's Health Network, updated 2019, https://nwhn.org /hysterectomy.

"Why It's Necessary: Hysterectomy," NHS, last reviewed February 1, 2019, www.nhs.uk /conditions/hysterectomy/why-its-done.

56 "the further away from that time someone is . . . " Boston Women's Health Collective, *Our Bodies, Ourselves: Menopause* (New York: Simon & Schuster, 2006).

CHAPTER FOUR

60 "But since they're all associated with better health outcomes . . . " Jennifer Wolff, "What Doctors Don't Know About Menopause," *AARP The Magazine*, August/ September 2018, www.aarp.org/health /conditions-treatments/info-2018/meno pause-symptoms-doctors-relief-treatment .html.

61 "can amplify . . . some of the long-term health risks . . . like bone loss, insulin resistance, and cardiovascular risks . . . " Nancy F. Woods et al., "Increased Urinary Cortisol Levels During the Menopause Transition," *Menopause* 13, no. 2 (2006): 212–221. doi: 10.1097/01.gme.0000198490.57242.2e.

63 "Nutritional support for stress . . . " Information from consultations by email and phone with kiran nigam, 05/19/20, 6/28/20, 7/16/20, 8/13/20, and 1/12/21.*

64 "Emily Nagoski, PhD, and Amelia Nagoski, DMA's . . . " Emily Nagoski and Amelia Nagoski, *Burnout: The Secret to Unlocking the Stress Cycle* (New York: Ballantine Books, 2020), 3–22.

65 "Studies of menopausal sleep . . . " "Data Briefs—Number 286—September 2017," Centers for Disease Control and Prevention, September 7, 2017, www.cdc.gov/nchs /products/databriefs/db286.htm; Howard M. Kravitz and Hadine Joffe, "Sleep During the Perimenopause: A SWAN Story," *Obstetrics and Gynecology Clinics of North America* 38, no. 3 (2011): 567–586. doi: 10.1016/j .ogc.2011.06.002.

67 "If you can't manage it with bedtime . . . " Audrey Noble, "Plot Twist: The Key to Better Sleep Is Not a Bedtime—It's a Wake-Up Time," Pocket, https://getpocket.com /explore/item/plot-twist-the-key-to-better -sleep-is-not-a-bedtime-it-s-a-wake-up -time.

68 "Cannabis and sexuality educator and *The CBD Solution: Sex* author Ashley Manta . . . " Zoom interview, 4/16/20.*

71 "Headspace says . . . " "Sleep Hygiene Tips," Headspace, www.headspace.com /sleep/sleep-hygiene.

77 "I asked professor, body acceptance activist, author of *Fat* . . . " Hanne Blank, email interview, 4/27/20.*

78 "Health at Every Size dietician, *Body Kindness* author, and angel of diet-culture mercy Rebecca Scritchfield says . . . " Zoom interview, 6/16/20.*

80 "smoking is associated with hot flashes . . . " Boston Women's Health Collective, *Our Bodies, Ourselves: Menopause* (New York: Simon & Schuster, 2006), 76.

80 "smokers usually have lower estrogen levels . . . " Shannon Perry, "Quit Smoking for Your Estrogen's Sake," Gennev, last updated July 30, 2020, https://gennev.com /education/smoking-menopause.

80 "Smokers also tend to start perimenopause . . . " "Penn Medicine Study Reveals Genetics Impact Risk of Early Menopause

Among Some Female Smokers," Penn Medicine News, February 5, 2014, www.pennmedicine.org/news/news-releases/2014/february/penn-medicine-study-reveals-ge.

83 "'The biggest lie that we're told . . .'" Aida Manduley, Zoom interview, 5/30/20.*

CHAPTER FIVE

97 "Rose George wrote for the *Guardian* . . ." Rose George, "What Science Doesn't Know About the Menopause: What It's for and How to Treat It," *Guardian*, December 15, 2015, www.theguardian.com/society/2015/dec/15/what-science-doesnt-know-about-the-menopause-what-its-for-how-to-treat-it.

98 "Prescriptions for hormone therapy . . ." Angelo Cagnacci and Martina Venier, "The Controversial History of Hormone Replacement Therapy," *Medicina* (Kaunas, Lithuania) 55, no. 9 (September 2019): 602. doi: 10.3390/medicina55090602.

98 "The WHI was also primarily about white women . . ." Adam Ostrzenski and Katarzyna M. Ostrzenska, "WHI Clinical Trial Revisit: Imprecise Scientific Methodology Disqualifies the Study's Outcomes," *American Journal of Obstetrics and Gynecology* 193, no. 5 (2005): 1599–1604. doi: 10.1016/j.ajog.2005.07.085.

98 "In fact, later results from the WHI and other studies show a *beneficial* risk-to-benefit ratio . . ." Roger A. Lobo, "Where Are We 10 Years After the Women's Health Initiative?," *Journal of Clinical Endocrinology & Metabolism* 98, no. 5 (2013): 1771–1780. doi: 10.1210/jc.2012-4070.

99 "According to one principal investigator for the study . . ." Lauren Vogel, "Landmark Trial Overstated HRT Risk for Younger Women," *CMAJ News*, April 12, 2017, https://cmajnews.com/2017/04/12/landmark-trial-overstated-hrt-risk-for-younger-women-109-5421.

99 "In an NPR interview in 2013 . . ." Nancy Shute, "The Last Word on Hormone Therapy from the Women's Health Initiative," NPR, October 4, 2013, www.npr.org/sections/health-shots/2013/10/04/229171477/the-last-word-on-hormone-therapy-from-the-womens-health-initiative.

100 "NAMS makes clear custom-compounded . . ." "Hormone Therapy & Menopause FAQs," North American Menopause Society, www.menopause.org/for-women/expert-answers-to-frequently-asked-questions-about-menopause/hormone-therapy-menopause-faqs.

103 "Personalization alone has radically improved . . ." Santiago Palacios et al., "Hormone Therapy for First-Line Management of Menopausal Symptoms: Practical Recommendations," *Women's Health* 15 (2019). doi: 10.1177/1745506519864009.

103 "Some forms of MHT can reduce some major health risks . . ." "Hormone Therapy Risks / Benefits," Cleveland Clinic, https://my.clevelandclinic.org/health/treatments/15245-hormone-therapy/risks--benefits.

104 Hella Basic MHT Literacy: general background for this section: Frances B. McCrea and Gerald E. Markle, "The Estrogen Replacement Controversy in the USA and UK: Different Answers to the Same Question?," *Social Studies of Science* 14, no. 1 (1984): 1–26, www.jstor.org/stable/284699.

104 "At the time of this writing . . ." Nicole K. Banks, "What Are the UK National Institute for Health and Care Excellence (NICE) Guidelines on Menopausal Hormone Replacement Therapy (HRT)?," Medscape, September 24, 2019, www.medscape.com/answers/276104-193557/what-are-the-uk-national-institute-for-health-and-care-excellence-nice-guidelines-on-menopausal-hormone-replacement-therapy-hrt.

105 "Primary possible effects . . ." Tara Allmen, *Menopause Confidential: A Doctor Reveals the Secrets to Thriving Through Midlife* (New York: HarperOne, 2016), 173.

106 "When used for less than one year . . . " "Risks: Hormone Replacement Therapy (HRT)," NHS, www.nhs.uk/conditions /hormone-replacement-therapy-hrt/risks.

106 "estrogen-only MHT may even help *prevent* breast cancer for some . . . " G. L. Anderson et al., "Effects of Conjugated Equine Estrogen in Postmenopausal Women with Hysterectomy: The Women's Health Initiative Randomized Controlled Trial," *JAMA* 291, no. 14 (2004): 1701–1712.

106 "The North American Menopause Society explains that SERMs . . . " SERMs factsheet, North American Menopause Society, www.menopause.org/docs/default-source /for-women/serms-faqs.pdf.

107 "A SERM-estrogen combination can also sometimes be used . . . " "Hormone Therapy & Menopause FAQs," North American Menopause Society, www.menopause.org /for-women/expert-answers-to-frequently -asked-questions-about-menopause /hormone-therapy-menopause-faqs.

107 "Some synthetic progester*ones*, specifically, are . . . " Santiago Palacios et al., "Hormone Therapy for First-Line Management of Menopausal Symptoms: Practical Recommendations," *Women's Health* 15 (2019). doi: 10.1177/1745506519864009.

108 "Testosterone does a lot of different things . . . " "Testosterone Replacement in Menopause," British Menopause Society, April 6, 2020, https://thebms. org.uk/publications/tools-for-clinicians /testosterone-replacement-in-menopause.

109 "Possible risks:" World Professional Association for Transgender Health (WPATH), *Standards of Care for the Health of Transsexual, Transgender, and Gender Nonconforming People*, 7th version, WPATH, www.wpath .org/media/cms/Documents/SOC%20v7 /Standards%20of%20Care%20V7%20 -%202011%20WPATH.pdf.

113 "Dr. Luana Colloca found that . . . " Luana Colloca et al., "Overt Versus Covert Treatment for Pain, Anxiety, and Parkinson's Disease," *The Lancet: Neurology* 3, no. 11 (November 2004): 679–684. doi: 10.1016/ S1474-4422(04)00908-1.

CHAPTER SIX

122 "While at least 25 percent of people . . . " "Menopause FAQs: Hot Flashes," North American Menopause Society, www .menopause.org/for-women/menopause -faqs-hot-flashes.

122 "They're more common when we're stressed . . . " Boston Women's Health Collective, *Our Bodies, Ourselves: Menopause* (New York: Simon & Schuster, 2006), 76.

122 "What we know about **hot flashes** . . . " "How the Body Regulates Heat," Rush, August 18, 2014, www.rush.edu/health -wellness/discover-health/how-body -regulates-heat.

122 "'transient sensations of heat, sweating . . . '" Ramandeep Bansal and Neelam Aggarwal, "Menopausal Hot Flashes: A Concise Review," *Journal of Mid-life Health* 10, no. 1 (2019): 6. doi: 10.4103/jmh.jmh_7_19.

123 "What Is Their Deal?" D. C. Deecher and K. Dorries, "Understanding the Pathophysiology of Vasomotor Symptoms (Hot Flushes and Night Sweats) That Occur in Perimenopause, Menopause, and Postmenopause Life Stages," *Archives of Women's Mental Health* 10, no. 6 (2007): 247–257. doi: 10.1007/s00737-007 -0209-5.

124 "Nina Coslov explains . . . " "Night Sweats and Hot Flashes," Women Living Better, November 2, 2020, https://womenliving better.org/night-sweats-hot-flashes.

126 "If you feel ashamed . . . " Martha A. Sánchez-Rodríguez et al., "Association Between Hot Flashes Severity and Oxidative Stress Among Mexican Postmenopausal Women: A Cross-sectional Study," *PLOS ONE* 14, no. 9 (2019). doi: 10.1371/journal .pone.0214264.

126 "Instead, it and other kinds of therapy *can* . . . " "Cognitive Behaviour Therapy (CBT) for Menopausal Symptoms," British Menopause Society, April 9, 2020, https://

thebms.org.uk/publications/tools-for
-clinicians/cognitive-behaviour-therapy
-cbt-menopausal-symptoms.

127 "recent studies have found that ongoing acupuncture . . . " Carolyn Ee et al., "Acupuncture for Menopausal Hot Flashes," *Menopause* 24, no. 8 (2017): 980–987. doi: 10.1097/gme.0000000000000850.

127 "The median duration of vasomotor impacts . . . " Nancy E. Avis et al., "Duration of Menopausal Vasomotor Symptoms over the Menopause Transition," *JAMA Internal Medicine* 175, no. 4 (2015): 531. doi: 10.1001/jamainternmed.2014.8063.

CHAPTER SEVEN

131 "In a piece by Rhitu Chatterjee for NPR . . . " Rhitu Chatterjee, "As Menopause Nears, Be Aware It Can Trigger Depression and Anxiety, Too," NPR, January 16, 2020, www.npr.org/sections/health -shots/2020/01/16/796682276/for-some -women-nearing-menopause-depression -and-anxiety-can-spike.

131 "Recent studies on mental health and menopause . . . " Wulf Rössler et al., "Does Menopausal Transition Really Influence Mental Health? Findings from the Prospective Long-Term Zurich Study," *World Psychiatry* 15, no. 2 (2016): 146–154. doi: 10.1002/wps.20319.

132 "Those entering a menopausal transition . . . " Barbara L. Parry, "Perimenopausal Depression," *American Journal of Psychiatry* 165, no. 1 (2008): 23–27. doi: 10.1176/appi.ajp.2007.07071152.

136 "In some studies, those with schizophrenia . . . " Martha Sajatovic et al., "Menopause Knowledge and Subjective Experience Among Peri- and Postmenopausal Women with Bipolar Disorder, Schizophrenia and Major Depression," *Journal of Nervous and Mental Disease* 194, no. 3 (2006): 173–178. doi: 10.1097/01. nmd.0000202479.00623.86.

136 "A recent study found a link between higher dietary fiber . . . " Yunsun Kim,

Minseok Hong, Seonah Kim, Woo-young Shin, Jung-ha Kim, "Inverse Association Between Dietary Fiber Intake and Depression in Premenopausal Women," *Menopause*, December 21, 2020. doi: 10.1097/ GME.0000000000001711.

139 "Leela Sinha described as . . . " Zoom interview, 4/24/20.*

140 "As *Rage Becomes Her* author Soraya Chemaly said . . . " Zoom interview, 06/24/20.*

140 "If menopause makes it harder . . . " "Ep. 2: Women and Anger with Soraya Chemaly," *Empowered Health*, November 20, 2019, https://empoweredhealthshow.com /women-anger-soraya-chemaly.

143 "'Perimenopause during this particular time . . .'" Mona Eltahawy, Zoom interview, 05/31/20.*

145 "Aida Manduley says, 'When you ignore feelings . . .'" "How to Feel Your Feelings and Why You Should Try," Aida Manduley, November 14, 2019, http://aidamanduley .com/2019/11/14/how-to-feel-your-feelings -and-why-you-should-try.

147 "Studies show that trauma and its effects . . . " Becky Upham, "Past Trauma Linked to Hot Flashes and Other Menopause Symptoms," *Everyday Health*, last updated November 19, 2018, www .everydayhealth.com/menopause/menpausal -symptoms-worsen-with-ptsd-abuse; Rebecca C. Thurston et al., "Childhood Abuse or Neglect Is Associated with Increased Vasomotor Symptom Reporting Among Midlife Women," *Menopause* 15, no. 1 (January 2008): 16–22. doi: 10.1097/gme.0b013e 31805fea75; Elizabeth Hlavinka, "Trauma May Up Risk for Menopause Symptoms in Older Women," *MedPage Today*, November 19, 2018, www.medpagetoday.com/obgyn /domesticviolence/76441.

147 "A recent cross-sectional analysis . . . " Carolyn J. Gibson et al., "Associations of Intimate Partner Violence, Sexual Assault, and Posttraumatic Stress Disorder with Menopause Symptoms Among Midlife and Older Women," *JAMA Internal*

Medicine 179, no. 1 (2019): 80. doi: 10.1001/jamainternmed.2018.5233.

148 "Hypervigilance or hyperarousal . . . " Judith Lewis Herman, *Trauma and Recovery* (London: Pandora, 2015), 40.

CHAPTER EIGHT

158 "Higher levels of stress during perimenopause . . . " Gail A. Greendale, Carol A. Derby, and Pauline M. Maki, "Perimenopause and Cognition," *Obstetrics and Gynecology Clinics of North America* 38, no. 3 (2011): 519–535. doi: 10.1016/j.ogc.2011.05.007.

162 "The Seattle Women's Midlife Study . . . and the Study of Women's Health Across the Nation . . . " Nancy Fugate Woods and Ellen Sullivan Mitchell, "The Seattle Midlife Women's Health Study: A Longitudinal Prospective Study of Women During the Menopausal Transition and Early Postmenopause," *Women's Midlife Health* 2, no. 1 (2016). doi: 10.1186/s40695-016-0019-x; Pauline M. Maki and Victor W. Henderson, "Cognition and the Menopause Transition," *Menopause* 23, no. 7 (2016): 803–805. doi: 10.1097/gme.0000000000000681.

162 "When I talked with professor, author, psychologist, and feminist human-development whiz Sharon Lamb . . . " Zoom interview, 04/24/20.

CHAPTER NINE

165 "twice as likely to experience chronic pain . . . " Carolyn J. Gibson et al., "Menopause Symptoms and Chronic Pain in a National Sample of Midlife Women Veterans," *Menopause* 26, no. 7 (2019): 708–713. doi: 10.1097/gme.0000000000001312.

166 "Autistic people, those with ADD/ADHD, or both, may experience an amplification of their experiences . . . " R. L. Moseley, T. Druce, and J. M. Turner-Cobb, "'When My Autism Broke': A Qualitative Study Spotlighting Autistic Voices on Menopause," *Autism*, January 31, 2020. doi: 10.1177/1362361319901184.

CHAPTER TEN

171 "The Trotula . . . " Monica H. Green, *The Trotula: A Medieval Compendium of Women's Medicine* (Philadelphia: University of Pennsylvania, 2001).

172 "new irritable bowel syndrome (IBS) or IBS made worse . . . " Margaret M. Heitkemper and Lin Chang, "Do Fluctuations in Ovarian Hormones Affect Gastrointestinal Symptoms in Women with Irritable Bowel Syndrome?," *Gender Medicine* 6 (2009): 152–167. doi: 10.1016/j.genm.2009.03.004.

172 "The reduction of moisture in our bodies . . . " Xin Yang et al., "Estrogen and Estrogen Receptors in the Modulation of Gastrointestinal Epithelial Secretion," *Oncotarget* 8, no. 57 (2017): 97683–97692. doi: 10.18632/oncotarget.18313.

172 "Dr. Siri Carpenter explained . . . " Dr. Siri Carpenter, "That Gut Feeling," American Psychological Association, September 2012, www.apa.org/monitor/2012/09/gut-feeling.

175 "As Claire Maldarelli wrote in *Popular Science* . . . " Claire Maldarelli, "What Happens if You Eat Too Many Tums?," *Popular Science*, May 28, 2018, www.popsci.com/too-many-tums.

184 "genitourinary impacts . . . " "Changes in the Vagina and Vulva," North American Menopause Society, www.menopause.org/for-women/sexual-health-menopause-online/changes-at-midlife/changes-in-the-vagina-and-vulva.

185 "vaginal pH changes from . . . " Ananya Das et al., "Vaginal pH: A Marker for Menopause," *Journal of Mid-life Health* 5, no. 1 (2014): 34. doi: 10.4103/0976-7800.127789.

CHAPTER ELEVEN

197 "Research supports that postmenopause weight . . . " Mohammad Reza Salamat, Amir Hossein Salamat, and Mohsen Janghorbani, "Association Between Obesity and Bone Mineral Density by Gender and Menopausal Status," *Endocrinology and Metabolism* 31, no. 4 (2016): 547. doi: 10.3803/enm.2016.31.4.547; Blandine Laferrère

et al., "Race, Menopause, Health-Related Quality of Life, and Psychological Well-being in Obese Women," *Obesity Research* 10, no. 12 (2002): 1270–1275. doi: 10.1038/oby.2002.172; Ellen W. Freeman et al., "Obesity and Reproductive Hormone Levels in the Transition to Menopause," *Menopause* 17, no. 4 (July 2010): 718–726, 1. doi: 10.1097/gme.0b013e3181cec85d.

201 "The second-biggest risk group for eating disorders . . ." Barbara Mangweth-Matzek et al., "The Menopausal Transition—a Possible Window of Vulnerability for Eating Pathology," Wiley Online Library, July 11, 2013, https://onlinelibrary.wiley.com/doi/full/10.1002/eat.22157; Harvard Women's Health Watch, "Disordered Eating in Midlife and Beyond," Harvard Health Publishing, February 2012, www.health.harvard.edu/womens-health/disordered-eating-in-midlife-and-beyond.

201 "Erica Leon says . . ." "#240: "Aging, Diet Culture, and Body Changes Around Menopause with Erica Leon," *Food Psych*, podcast with Cristy Harrison, May 18, 2020, https://christyharrison.com/foodpsych/7/aging-diet-culture-and-body-changes-around-menopause-with-erica-leon?fbclid=IwAR3DuaU3cKPDaZz40mug-GJQiYQ7z1oFPCNH4LR2BvOEnWj1MpnNy5ds9ek.

202 "Diet culture is the worst smoothie ever . . ." Sabrina Strings, *Fearing the Black Body* (New York: New York University Press, 2019), 122.

202 "as Christy Harrison adds . . ." Christy Harrison, "What Is Diet Culture?," ChristyHarrison.com, August 10, 2018, https://christyharrison.com/blog/what-is-diet-culture.

203 "*Health at Every Size* author, professor, and researcher . . ." Linda Bacon, *Health at Every Size: The Surprising Truth About Your Weight* (Dallas, TX: Benbella Books, 2010).

203 "Only between 3 and 10 percent of people . . ." Harriet Brown, "Planning to Go on a Diet? One Word of Advice: Don't," *Slate*, March 24, 2015, https://slate.com/technology/2015/03/diets-do-not-work-the-thin-evidence-that-losing-weight-makes-you-healthier.html.

210 "my longtime friend Jaclyn Friedman said . . ." Zoom interview, 04/14/20.

CHAPTER TWELVE

217 "Even when there *are* bumps in the road . . ." P. J. Kleinplatz, "Sexuality and Older People," *BMJ* 337 (2008): a239. doi: 10.1136/bmj.a239; Peggy J. Kleinplatz and Ménard A. Dana, *Magnificent Sex: Lessons from Extraordinary Lovers* (New York: Routledge, 2020); Joani Blank, *Still Doing It: Women and Men over Sixty Write About Their Sexuality* (San Francisco: Down There Press, 2000).

218 "Instead it's usually about things like . . ." Peggy J. Kleinplatz and A. Dana Ménard, "Building Blocks Toward Optimal Sexuality: Constructing a Conceptual Model," *Family Journal* 15, no. 1 (2007): 72–78. doi: 10.1177/1066480706294126.

219 "Louise Foxcroft reminds us . . ." Louise Foxcroft, *Hot Flushes, Cold Science: A History of the Modern Menopause* (London: Granta Publications, 2011), 184.

221 "Tania Glyde says . . ." Email, 9/14/20.

221 "Joan Price, senior sex advocate . . ." Zoom interview, 05/15/20.

226 "When I talked with feminist sex toy shop and neighborhood sex education mecca Early to Bed owner Searah Deysach . . ." In-person interview, 06/20/20.*

CHAPTER THIRTEEN

242 "Dr. Lexx thinks . . ." Zoom interview, 06/29/20.*

246 "In the *Guardian*, Rose George . . ." Rose George, "What Science Doesn't Know About the Menopause: What It's for and How to Treat It," *Guardian*, December 15, 2015, www.theguardian.com/society/2015/dec/15/what-science-doesnt-know-about-the-menopause-what-its-for-how-to-treat-it.

246 "A 2020 study of working women in Japan . . ." North American Menopause Society, "New Study Links Number of Menopause Symptoms with Job Performance," *EurekAlert!*, December 1, 2020, www.eurekalert.org/pub_releases/2020-12 /tnam-nsl120120.php.

247 "'while nearly a third . . .'" Megan Reitz, Marina Bolton, and Kira Emslie, "Is Menopause a Taboo in Your Organization?," *Harvard Business Review*, February 4, 2020, https://hbr.org/2020/02/is-menopause -a-taboo-in-your-organization.

247 "On her podcast, Michelle Obama said . . ." "What Your Mother Never Told You About Health with Dr. Sharon Malone," *Michelle Obama Podcast*, Spotify, August 12, 2020, https://open.spotify.com/episode/6ro JUCIX5Gqs8j4QkDHEWT?si=R GLkzG6vQqaykMPtUXhfSg.

249 "A menopause study on cardiovascular health . . ." Mara Gordon, "Sexual Assault and Harassment May Have Lasting Health Repercussions for Women," NPR, October 3, 2018, www.npr.org/sections /health-shots/2018/10/03/653797374 /sexual-assault-and-harassment-may-have -lasting-health-repercussions-for-women.

CHAPTER FOURTEEN

262 "Southerners on New Ground cofounder and LGBTQ activist and organizer Mandy Carter . . ." Zoom interview, 05/19/20.

A MENOPAUSAL (VERY) MINI-HERBAL

279 "Adaptogens specifically aren't known to possess addiction . . ." A. Panossian and G. Wikman, "Effects of Adaptogens on the Central Nervous System and the Molecular Mechanisms Associated with Their Stress-Protective Activity," *Pharmaceuticals* 3, no. 1 (2010): 188–224. doi:10.3390/ph3010188.

279 "Nootropic" is a term for . . ." Markham Heid, "Nootropics, or 'Smart Drugs,' Are Gaining Popularity. Should You Take Them?," *Time*, January 23, 2019, https:// time.com/5509993/nootropics-smart -drugs-brain.

280 "A Few Stress Balancers . . ." and "A Few Energizers . . ." Agatha Noveille, *The Complete Guide to Adaptogens: From Ashwagandha to Rhodiola, Medicinal Herbs That Transform and Heal* (New York: Adams Media, 2018); "The Ultimate Guide to Using Over 21 Adaptogens (Bookmark Me, Baby)," *The Chalkboard*, February 28, 2019, https://thechalkboardmag.com/how-to -use-adaptogenic-powders-guide; Stephanie McClain, "Your Ultimate Guide to Adaptogens: What Are They and Do They Work," *The Beet*, April 7, 2020, https:// thebeet.com/what-are-adaptogens-herbs -and-plants-that-can-help-reduce-stress -and-anxiety.

280 "As they explain simply at Leafly . . ." Leafly Staff, "CBD vs. THC: What's the Difference?," Leafly, August 17, 2020, www .leafly.com/news/cbd/cbd-vs-thc.

282 "Studies on this have been limited, inconclusive . . ." Karen M. Prestwood, "The Search for Alternative Therapies for Menopausal Women: Estrogenic Effects of Herbs," *Journal of Clinical Endocrinology & Metabolism* 88, no. 9 (September 1, 2003): 4075–4076. doi: 10.1210/jc.2003-031277; Brian J. Doyle, Jonna Frasor, Lauren E. Bellows, Tracie D. Locklear, Alice Perez, Jorge Gomez-Laurito, and Gail B. Mahady, "Estrogenic Effects of Herbal Medicines from Costa Rica Used for the Management of Menopausal Symptoms," *Menopause* 16, no. 4 (July–August 2009): 748–755. doi: 10.1097/gme.0b013e3181a4c76a; D. Dixon-Shanies and N. Shaikh, "Growth Inhibition of Human Breast Cancer Cells by Herbs and Phytoestrogens," *Oncology Reports* 6, no. 6 (1999): 1383–1390, https://doi .org/10.3892/or.6.6.1383.

282 "They're sometimes considered to have . . ." M-n. Chen, C-c. Lin, and C-f. Liu, "Efficacy of Phytoestrogens for Menopausal Symptoms: A Meta-analysis and Systematic Review, *Climacteric* 18, no. 2 (2015): 260–269. doi: 10.3109/13697137.2014.966241.

282 "Some studies and meta-analyses have found . . ." Alice L. Murkies, Gisela

Wilcox, and Susan R. Davis, "Phytoestro-gens," *Journal of Clinical Endocrinology & Metabolism* 83, no. 2 (February 1, 1998): 297–303. doi: 10.1210/jcem.83.2.4577; A. E. Lethaby, J. Brown, J. Marjoribanks, F. Kronenberg, H. Roberts, and J. Eden, "Phytoestrogens for Vasomotor Menopausal Symptoms," *Cochrane Database of Systematic Reviews* 4 (October 17, 2007): CD001395. doi: 10.1002/14651858.CD001395.pub3.

APPENDIX

286 "... significant and can include the following": J. Bain, "Andro-pause: Testosterone Replacement Therapy for Aging Men," National Li-brary of Medicine, National Institutes of Health, 2001, www.ncbi.nlm.nih.gov /pmc/articles/PMC2014707/#; Brian Krans, "Male Menopause: Overview, Symptoms, and Treatment," *Healthline*, September 16, 2018, www.healthline.com /health/menopause/male; Sean Iwamoto, Justine Defreyne, Micol S. Rothman, Ju-dith Van Schuylenbergh, Laurens Van de Bruaene, Joz Motmans, and Guy T'Sjoen, "Health Considerations for Transgender Women and Remaining Unknowns: A Nar-rative Review," *Therapeutic Advances in En-docrinology and Metabolism* 10 (August 30, 2019), www.ncbi.nlm.nih.gov/pmc/articles /PMC6719479.

286 "Treatment for andropause can include..." P. Singh, "Andropause: Current Con-cepts," US National Library of Medicine, National Institutes of Health, December 2013, www.ncbi.nlm.nih.gov/pmc/articles /PMC4046605.

287 "improved mood": Eva Moore, Amy Wisniewski, and Adrian Dobs, "Endocrine Treatment of Transsexual People: A Review of Treatment Regimens, Outcomes, and Adverse Effects," *Journal of Clinical Endo-crinology & Metabolism* 88, no. 8 (August 2003): 3467–3473.

288 "antiandrogens in concert with estro-gen": "Feminizing Hormone Therapy," Mayo Clinic, www.mayoclinic.org/tests -procedures/feminizing-hormone-therapy /about/pac-20385096.

288 "For people with intact testes who take estrogen ... " "Feminizing Hormone Therapy," Mayo Clinic, www.mayoclinic .org/tests-procedures/feminizing-hormone -therapy/about/pac-20385096.

288 "Notably, these improvements appear..." Jaclyn M. White Hughto and Sari L. Reisner, "A Systematic Review of the Ef-fects of Hormone Therapy on Psycho-logical Functioning and Quality of Life in Transgender Individuals," *Transgender Health* 1, no. 1 (January 2016). doi: 10.1089 /trgh.2015.0008; Hillary Nguyen, Alexis M. Chavez, Emily Lipner, Liisa Hantsoo, Sara L. Kornfield, Robert D. Davies, and C. Neill Epperson, "Gender-Affirming Hormone Use in Transgender Individuals: Impact on Behavioral Health and Cogni-tion," *Current Psychiatry Reports* 20, no. 12 (October 11, 2018): 110.

288 "However, carefully monitored, progester-one ... " Jerilynn Prior, "Progesterone Is Important for Transgender Women's Ther-apy," *Journal of Clinical Endocrinology & Me-tabolism* 104, no. 4 (April 2019): 1181–1186; E. Simpson, "Sources of Estrogen and Their Importance," *Journal of Steroid Biochemistry and Molecular Biology* 86, no. 3–5 (Septem-ber 2003): 225–230.

290 "As for menopause, there is little or no con-vincing evidence ... " Lassey, "Herbal Hor-mones for the Transsexual," Transgender Support Site, 2015, http://heartcorps.com /journeys/hormones/herbal.htm; Cecilie Unger, "Hormone Therapy for Transgender Patients," *Translational Andrology and Urol-ogy* 5, no. 6 (December 2016): 877–884.

291 "become pretty much the same ... ": J. A. Wanta, "Review of the Transgender Lit-erature: Where Do We Go from Here?," *Transgender Health* 2, no. 1 (July 1, 2017): 119–128; Sean Iwamoto, Justine De-freyne, Micol S. Rothman, Judith Van Schuylenbergh, Laurens Van de Bruaene, Joz Motmans, and Guy T'Sjoen, "Health Considerations for Transgender Women

and Remaining Unknowns: A Narrative Review," *Therapeutic Advances in Endocrinology and Metabolism* 10 (August 30, 2019), www.ncbi.nlm.nih.gov/pmc/articles/PMC6719479; Jaime M. Grant, Lisa Mottet, Justin Edward Tanis, Jack Harrison, Jody Herman, and Mara Keisling, *Injustice at Every Turn: A Report of the National Transgender Discrimination Survey* (Washington, DC: National Center for Transgender Equality; National Gay and Lesbian Task Force, 2011).

291   "These combine the practice of multiple disciplines . . ." Amy Bournes, *Guidelines for Gender-Affirming Primary Care with Trans and Non-binary Patients* (Rainbow Health Ontario, 2019); M. B. Deutsch, ed., *Guidelines for the Primary and Gender-Affirming Care of Transgender and Gender Nonbinary People*, University of California San Francisco Medical Center, 2016, https://transcare.ucsf.edu/guidelines.

292   "World Professional Association for Transgender Health": World Professional Association for Transgender Health (WPATH), *Standards of Care for the Health of Transsexual, Transgender, and Gender Nonconforming People* (Minneapolis: WPATH, 2012).

292   "appropriate for whatever I'm doing . . ." Meredith Talusan, "On Being a Trans Woman, and Giving Up Makeup," *New York Times*, May 26, 2020.

292   "There is even research to support this idea . . ." Sarah Karlan, "Here's What Older Trans and Nonbinary People Want You to Know," *BuzzFeed News*, January 21, 2019, www.buzzfeednews.com/article/skarlan/heres-what-older-trans-and-nonbinary-people-want-you-to-know; Catherine Silver, "Gendered Identities in Old Age: Toward (De)gendering?," *Journal of Aging Studies* 17, no. 4 (November 2003): 379–397.

* Unless otherwise noted, all quotes that follow from the attributed individual are from the same interview(s).

INDEX

menstrual cramps, 30, 166, 179, 234, 261

menstrual cycles, 31, 38–43, 46–52, 177–182, 192, 220

menstrual flow, 25, 43, 50, 171, 178–179, 186

Menstruation and Menopause (book), 24

mental health concerns, 95, 129–151, 157–160, 224, 245–249, 265. *See also* depression

Merck Manual (book), 36

Merman, Ethel, 48

Messages from the Menopausal Universe (zine), 17

metabolic syndrome, 205

metabolism, 48, 66, 108, 158, 172, 197–198, 204–205

microbiomes, 136, 169, 173

midlife crisis, 224, 250–252

Midsommar (movie), 139

midwives, 89–90

mini-herbals, 63, 106, 126–127, 181, 279–283. *See also* herbal aids

Mirren, Helen, 214

Mishiali, Tonia, 130

mood swings, 108, 129–151, 157–158, 265, 289

Morissette, Alanis, 244

movement benefits, 60, 64–65, 73–77, 159, 173, 181, 187, 212, 224

Ms. (magazine), 34, 35

Music Man, The (musical), 73

My Big Fat Greek Wedding (movie), 215

"My Guitar Gently Weeps," 225

Nagoski, Amelia, 64–65

Nagoski, Emily, 64–65

nail care, 207–213

Naked at Our Age: Talking Out Loud About Senior Sex (book), 221

National Gay and Lesbian Task Force, 290

National Institute for Health and Care Excellence (NICE), 51, 104

National Institute on Aging, 43

National Institutes of Health, 43

"natural" menopause, 20

negative feelings, 113, 139–151, 182

Neumann, Ann, 33

neurological concerns, 66, 157, 165–170. *See also* brain

neuroplasticity, 158, 160–161

New England Journal of Medicine (magazine), 99

New York Times (newspaper), 35

Nicks, Stevie, 269

nigam, kiran, 12, 63, 66, 174–176, 203

night sweats, 6, 25, 42, 50–56, 65–70, 103–109, 113, 121–128. *See also* vasomotor issues

nonbinary identity, 6, 21, 85–86, 194, 289, 292. *See also* gender identity

nootropics, 279–280

Norsigian, Judy, 269

North American Menopause Society (NAMS), 8, 43, 50, 52, 91, 99–100, 104, 106, 115, 128

NPR, 99, 131

Nuffield Health, 246

nurse practitioners, 89–113

nutritional therapy, 12

Obama, Barack, 247

Obama, Michelle, 247, 269

O'Connor, Sinéad, 54

"Ode on a Cooling Pillow," 70

Of the Management Proper at the Cessation of the Menses (book), 25

Office of Research on Women's Health, 43

Old Town Road (song), 275

On Death and Dying (book), 71

On the End of Menstruation as the Time for the Beginning of Various Diseases (book), 25

oophorectomy, 20–21, 26, 54–55, 103, 108–110, 180

orchiectomy, 286–288

osteoporosis, 53, 103–107, 176, 265, 283, 286

Our Bodies, Ourselves (book), 6, 8, 35

Our Bodies, Ourselves: Menopause (book), 52, 97

ovarian cancer, 48, 55, 108, 186

ovaries, 20, 27, 37–55, 177–182

ovariotomy, 26

"Over the Hills and Far Away," 130

ovulation, 38–40, 47, 166, 178

pain
chronic pain, 5–6, 10, 59, 66, 71, 80, 140, 156, 165, 188, 201, 215
cramps, 30, 166, 179, 234, 261
neurology and, 165–170
reducing, 113, 165–170, 231

pandemic, 4, 9, 75, 143, 151, 156, 240, 274

panic attacks, 4–5, 65, 123, 126, 132, 151

Parker, Dorothy, 3

Parton, Dolly, 237

INDEX

INDEX

INDEX

ABOUT THE AUTHOR

Heather Corinna is an insufferable queer and nonbinary feminist activist, author, educator, artist, organizer, and innovator; a joker, an (ex-)smoker, and a midnight toker who gets their lovin' on the run. They're the founder, director, designer, and editor of the web clearinghouse and organization Scarleteen, the first comprehensive sex, sexuality, and relationships education site and resource of its kind. Heather and the team at Scarleteen have provided millions of young people accurate, inclusive information and support for over two decades. They're often tired.

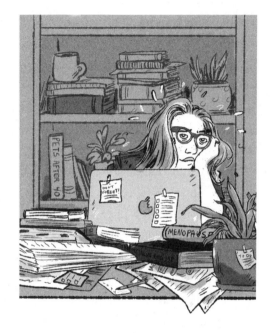

Heather's also the author of *S.E.X: The All-You-Need-To-Know Sexuality Guide to Get You Through Your Teens and Twenties* (Hachette, 2007, 2016), and, with Isabella Rotman, *Wait, What?: A Comic Book Guide to Relationships, Bodies, and Growing Up* (Oni Press/Lion Forge, 2019), for older middle readers and younger teen. They've been an early childhood educator; a sexuality, contraception, and abortion educator and counselor; a member of the editorial board for the *American Journal of Sexuality Education* and the Board of Directors for NARAL Pro-Choice Washington; a writer and contributing editor for the 2011 edition of *Our Bodies, Ourselves*; and a plaintiff for the ACLU, where they eventually got to stick it to the Bush administration, which was one of their Best Days Ever. By working themselves to a pulp, Heather has won acclaim and several awards in their field, and a lot of places and people say they're awesome. Some do not.

When not locked in a small room feverishly writing a book in a pandemic or otherwise overindulging in labor, Heather hangs out with their dog, goes outside, makes and geeks out about music, cooks, babies houseplants, and tries to enjoy the purportedly existential theater of life in Chicago.

ABOUT THE ILLUSTRATOR

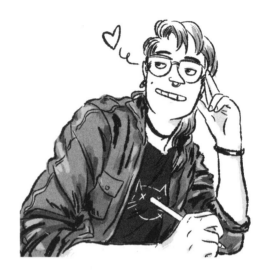

Archie Bongiovanni is a cartoonist and illustrator living in Minneapolis who has been featured in *The New Yorker*, *The Nib*, *Vice*, and *Autostraddle*. They're the co-creator of *A Quick and Easy Guide to They/Them Pronouns*, and their graphic novel, *Grease Bats*, is an ongoing monthly comic on Autostraddle.com and was released as a printed collection in 2019. Archie's newest graphic novel, *Mimosa*, is slated for publication in 2022, along with *History Comics: Stonewall*, their collaboration with A. Andrews. While their sex toy review podcast is dead (RIP), they've worked in the sex industry as a trained sexual health educator for five years through Minneapolis's favorite sex shop, The Smitten Kitten.